Advances in Neural and Behavioral Development

Volume 2

Richard N. Aslin, Editor

University of Rochester

ABLEX PUBLISHING CORPORATION
NORWOOD, NEW JERSEY

Printed in the United States of America

ISBN 0-89391-370-7

ISBN 8755-0032

Ablex Publishing Corporation
355 Chestnut Street
Norwood, New Jersey 07648

Contents

To Ellen and Bob
who provided the foundation
for my personal and professional
development

Preface to the Series

Advances in Neural and Behavioral Development is a series of volumes devoted to recent trends in neural development and the influence of neural mechanisms on the development of behavioral systems in both humans and nonhumans. The neurosciences have undergone a remarkable period of growth in the past decade as indicated by membership in professional organizations, the introduction of new journals, and the development of highly sophisticated techniques for assessing neural structure and function. Anatomical, biochemical, and electrophysiological analyses have provided a rich source of information concerning the possible causal links between brain mechanisms and behavior. A similar growth in the study of behavioral development, particularly within an evolutionary framework, has uncovered remarkable competencies in the young of many species. These behavioral analyses verify the functional significance of concomitant neural development, just as the development of underlying neural mechanisms constrains the course of behavioral development. It is to this close interaction between the behavioral and neural levels that the present series is directed.

The goal of each chapter in an *Advances* volume is to provide the author(s) with the opportunity to present empirical reviews of their own programmatic research as well as integrative summaries of others' research efforts. In addition to strictly empirical contributions, an *Advances* chapter can serve as a vehicle for addressing timely theoretical issues whose synthesis may benefit research programs in a variety of areas. Chapter length is unrestricted so that researchers can elaborate on their data, model, or theory in a way that might not be appropriate for a journal article. Book-length manuscripts will be published in a series of *Monographs on Neural and Behavioral Development*. These *Monographs* may include dissertations or other lengthy reports of research programs that exceed the page limit of a book chapter and stand alone as major contributions to the field.

All of the chapters in the first few *Advances* volumes were solicited by invitation. This enabled each volume to be organized around a particular sensory modality. However, future volumes will contain a mix of invited chapters and manuscripts submitted for editorial review. The primary determinant for inclusion will be outstanding scholarship, whether authored by a young investigator or a senior scientist. There are an enormous number of exceptionally interesting topics within the broad realm of neural and behavioral development. Thus, we can expect a series of *Advances* volumes and *Monographs* that provide up-to-date reviews for experienced scientists reading in their own particular area of research, for experienced scientists reading in research areas peripheral to their own, and for graduate students just beginning to uncover the excitement of developmental science.

I would like to express my appreciation to Ablex Publishing Corporation, including Walter Johnson, Barbara Bernstein, and Craig Van Dyck, for enabling me to bring this series into print. I would also like to thank Sandra Shea for performing numerous editorial functions, and the staffs of the Departments of Psychology at Indiana University and the University of Rochester for providing me with excellent facilities and support.

Richard N. Aslin
University of Rochester

Foreword to Volume 2

The mammalian auditory system has fascinated researchers for well over a century, due in large part to the empirical and theoretical synthesis provided by Hermann von Helmholtz. Despite the efforts of many talented researchers, however, the auditory system has not enjoyed the primary status attributed to the visual system as *the* model of sensory systems. This secondary status is in part the result of less easily recorded behavioral responses indicative of auditory function and less easily accessible neural structures. Nevertheless, the auditory system plays an extremely important role in intra- and interspecies communication as well as providing information about the location of objects in the environment. Not surprisingly, studies of the *development* of auditory function have also lagged behind analogous developmental studies of the visual system. In the past 5 years, however, there has been an intensified effort to understand the processes that influence auditory development. The purpose of this second volume of *Advances in Neural and Behavioral Development,* therefore, is to highlight these recent discoveries on the neural properties of the mammalian auditory system as well as the behavioral/perceptual correlates of these neural properites.

The first three chapters cover key features of the anatomy of the developing auditory system. Pujol and Sans provide an overview of the synaptic events that occur during the prenatal development of hair cells in both the vestibular and cochlear organs, including the processes of overproduction, competition, and specialization. Steel and Bock describe a number of defects in the developing auditory system that are caused by inherited structural anomalies, mutations, and hormonal imbalances. A strong case is made that the distinction between primary and secondary defects must be studied from a developmental perspective. Feng and Shofner present a comprehensive description of the anatomy, physiology, and ecology of the amphibian auditory system, along with the behavioral correlates of auditory development. This is a particularly fascinating species because of the metamorphosis that transforms the organism from an aquatic to a terrestrial environment, necessitating a significant alteration in the tranduction of auditory signals.

The final five chapters cover basic issues in the development of auditory structure and function. Brugge provides a detailed review of the functional development of the cat auditory nerve, emphasizing ontogenetic changes in the discharge characteristics of single neurons to variations in stimulus intensity, frequency, and phase. Buchwald and Shipley provide a detailed description of the averaged electrical potential recorded from the scalp of the cat, emphasizing the postulated neural generator sites for various components of the auditory brainstem (ABR) and midlatency wave forms. Javel, Walsh, and McGee provide an overview of the development of auditory evoked potentials in both cats and humans. Of particular interest is their attempt to normalize the ABRs in these two species, thereby providing a suitable animal model of human auditory development. Lippe, Ryals and Rubel discuss the important theoretical issue of the place principle in the coding of frequency information. Their recent work demonstrating a developmental shift in the representation of frequency along the basilar membrane has important implications for a variety of auditory functions. Finally, Kelly offers a comprehensive review of the development of sound localization abilities in a variety of species, as well as the relation between these abilities and the onset of auditory responsiveness assessed both behaviorally and neuroanatomically.

Taken together, these eight chapters provide an up-to-date overview of auditory development by the leading researchers in this growing field. Along with future volumes of the *Advances in Neural and Behavioral Development,* the reader will gain new insights through integrative reviews of current empirical research findings.

1 Synaptogenesis in the Mammalian Inner Ear*

Remy Pujol
Alain Sans
INSERM-U.254
Université de Montpellier II
Montpellier, France

INTRODUCTION

The mammalian inner ear contains two different sensory epithelia which, in adulthood, form the vestibular and the cochlear organs. Phylogenetically, the vestibular receptors first appeared in low vertebrates; complementary auditory receptors appeared when amphibians adapted to a terrestrial life. The common origin of both types of sensory organ can clearly be seen in the embryogenesis of the mammalian inner ear; both derive from the otic placodes which become the primitive otocysts on each side of the rhombencephalon. Very early in its development, the primitive otocyst differentiates into vestibular and cochlear receptors, but the very first stages of sensory cell differentiation and synaptogenesis display numerous similarities which justify a common description.

The present chapter does not intend to review the literature on vestibular and cochlear synaptogenesis but rather to stress some of the major problems related to the developmental period in the inner ear when nerve fibers and sensory cells establish and adjust their connections. The first controversial issue concerns the beginning of interactions between nerve endings and sensory cells. Do the cells, already differentiated in some aspects, attract the fibers, or do the fibers initiate cytodifferentiation after their arrival? The second issue concerns synaptogenesis itself, and here a specific description is needed for each kind of sensory organ. Nevertheless, vestibular and cochlear development exhibits parallels. In both cases, two types of sensory cells form.

*Authors are indebted to their collaborators who worked on the matter, especially D. Favre and M. Lenoir. Thanks are due to B. Etchecopar, S. Ladrech, and P. Schuman for technical participation, and to A. Bara for editorial assistance.

Correspondence to R. Pujol can be sent to INSERM, U. 254, Laboratorie de Neurobiologie de L'Audition, CHR St. Charles, 34059 Montpellier Cedex, France. Correspondence to A. Sans can be sent to INSERM, U. 254, Laboratorie de Neurophysiologie Sensorielle, USTL, Place E. Bataillon, 34060 Montpellier Cedex, France.

These sensory cells are connected by a double innervation consisting of afferents which transmit the sensory messages and of efferents which bring controlling messages from the central nervous system. Moreover, in both cases, for a highly specialized cell type, the different stages of synaptogenesis involve similar mechanisms of plasticity such as endings competing for synaptic space, temporary exuberant branching, and remodeling of synaptic specializations.

FIRST STAGES OF SENSORY CELL DIFFERENTIATION

The possible role of afferent nerve fibers in the induction of hair cell differentiation is a fundamental problem in developmental sensory neurobiology. Thornhill (1972) found that cell differentiation does not occur in the lamprey labyrinth until the cells are contacted by nerve terminals. Similarly, Sher (1971) observed nerve endings penetrating into an undifferentiated sensory epithelium in the mouse. In contrast, while observing the development of regeneration of an amphibian lateral line, Jørgensen and Flock (1976) showed that hair cells can develop and even form presynaptic bodies in the absence of innervation. This agrees with observations of *in-vitro* preparations of mouse otocysts (Van de Water, 1976) which indicate that the first step in hair cell differentiation does not depend on the presence of nerve fibers. Thus, it appears that there is a quasi-simultaneity between the growth of nerve fibers in the epithelium and the differentiation of sensory cells. As a result, it is difficult to determine which of the two events occurs first, especially since embryonic development occurs quite rapidly in most of the experimental species. It is less difficult when analyzing the slower development of the human otocyst.

We recently described the early stages of differentiation in the cochlear (Pujol & Lavigne-Rebillard, 1985) and the vestibular (Sans & Dechesne, 1985) organs in human fetuses aged 7 to 12 weeks. Both receptors follow a very similar process of differentiation, the labyrinth preceding the cochlea by 1 or 2 weeks. At embryonic week 7 (vestibule) or 9 (cochlea), the undifferentiated epithelium is characterized, in surface observations, by regular polyhedric cells with one mini-kinocilium at their center and microvilli on their edges. On transverse sections the epithelium is composed of polystratified and undifferentiated epithelial cells (Fig. 1A). There is no trace of tectorial and otoconial membranes. The apical poles of all the epithelial cells are linked by tight junctions. Desmosomelike junctions are numerous between the cells in the different layers. From the spiral and vestibular ganglion neurons, fibers can be followed up to the undifferentiated epithelium. They are packed together and pass through the basal membrane of the lower layers of the epithelial cells, with some endings even reaching the uppermost layer (Fig. 2).

In a second stage (Fig. 1B), the fibers become progressively more numerous and begin to surround the base of elongated cells in the upper layer (Fig. 3). These cells are the future hair cells, but they show an undifferentiated apical pole with microvilli and a mini-kinocilium. Numerous microvesicles of various sizes can be seen in the afferent nerve endings at this stage, some of them with dense cores.

During the next stage (Fig. 1C), hair cell cytodifferentiation becomes clear. On the top, a cuticular plate with stereocilia begins to differentiate, and at the base, presynaptic bodies can be seen surrounded by vesicles. The other epithelial cells begin to reorganize into one layer, and the thickness of the sensory epithelium decreases. From this stage on, the vestibular and the cochlear epithelium must be analyzed separately.

To summarize, these findings from human material indicate that the arrival of nerve endings in the sensory epithelia precedes hair cell differentiation. Of course, this does not necessarily mean that the fibers are needed to trigger hair cell differentiation. On the other hand, the possibility still exists that these cells, though still morphologically undifferentiated, release a biochemical signal attracting the nerve fibers to their target.

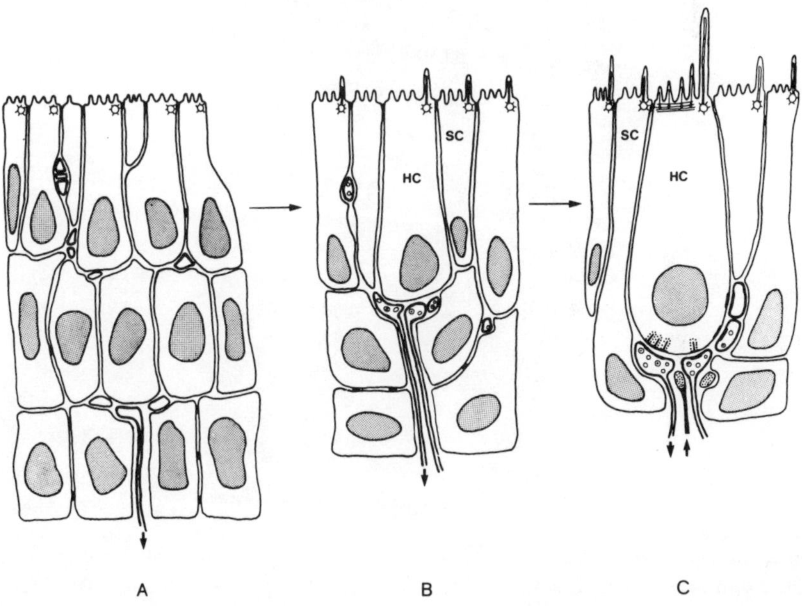

Figure 1. Schematic drawings of three early stages of the inner ear sensory epithelium innervation. A: afferent fibers (↓) enter the undifferentiated epithelium and spread out. B: afferent endings surround the base of an elongated cell. C: a differentiated primitive hair cell (HC) is contacted by afferent and efferent (↑) fibers.

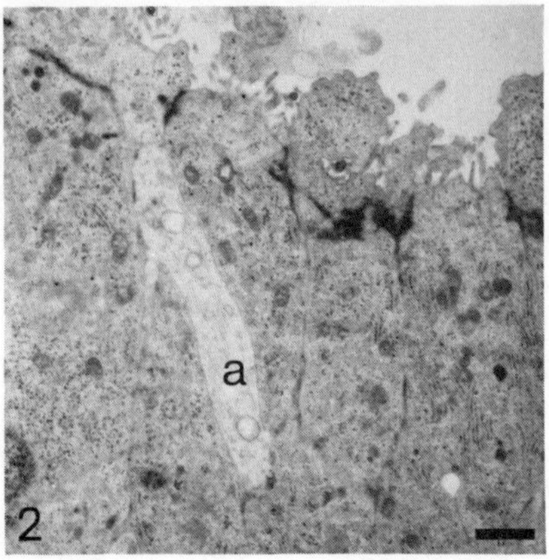

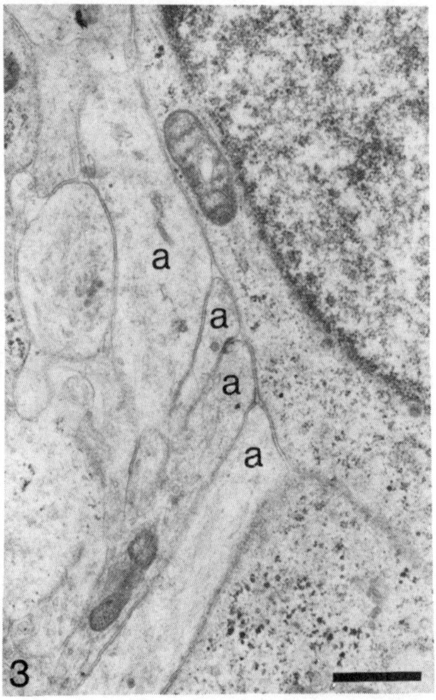

Figure 2. Afferent nerve fiber (a) reaching the apical pole of the undifferentiated epithelium in a 10-week-old human fetal cochlea (see also Fig. 1A). Scale: 2 μm.

Figure 3. The base on elongated cell is contacted by several afferent endings (a). No synaptic differentiation can be detected in a 7-week-old human fetal ampulla (see also Fig. 1B). Scale: 1 μm.

SYNAPTOGENESIS IN THE VESTIBULAR EPITHELIUM

First Stages of Afferent Synapses

The afferent synapses appear earlier in the vestibular epithelium than in the cochlea. The first sign of a synaptic contact is a slight increase in the density of the opposing membranes of the sensory cells and afferent nerves. Then an asymmetric synaptic differentiation with presynaptic bodies is observed, and the postsynaptic side is thicker than the presynaptic side. A granular material is attached to the innermost layer of membranes and the filamentous structures which exist in the synaptic cleft are progressively screened by granular electron-dense material. On the presynaptic side, microtubules reach the density-increased membranes and coexist with synaptic bodies: They are connected with the presynaptic densities (Favre, Demêmes, & Sans, 1986). At this first stage in the differentiation of vestibular afferent synapses, numerous small synaptic bodies are usually clustered in the same presynaptic structure (Fig. 4). In some species such as the cat, presynaptic bodies with round profiles are more numerous than ribbon profiles, but this is not so evident in human embryos (Fig. 4). The role of these polysynaptic bodies is not clear. At this developmental stage, it is obvious that the vestibular epithelium is not yet physiologically functional. It has been postulated by Sobkowicz, Rose, Scott, and Slapnick (1982) that the presence of a synaptic body at the cell membranes induces the formation of new synaptic bodies to stabilize the synaptic site. It is also possible to hypothesize that the synaptic bodies have a trophic effect on nerve growth, attracting the nerve fibers by chemotactism (Pujol, Carlier, & Devigne, 1979), a mechanism which implies that the early synaptic bodies are not necessarily linked to synaptic structures. This hypothesis is supported by the existence of ribbons floating in the cytoplasm of the cells (Fig. 5), and by the presence of ectopic synaptic bodies in mouse organotypic cultures when the embryonic otocyst explantation is performed on the 13th day of gestation. In the latter experiments, numerous synaptic bodies have been found attached to the membrane of well-differentiated sensory cells not contacted by the vestibular nerve (J. Raymond, personal communication, 1984). These results also suggest that the sensory cell can achieve a significant part of its differentiation on its own. This is in good agreement with a study of the terminal mitoses of rat vestibular hair cells by tritiated thymidine radioautography (Sans & Chat, 1982), showing that the differentiation into type I (HCI) and type II (HCII) cells is genetically programmed.

By the time the first afferent synapses are formed in the vestibular epithelium, the sensory cells also develop a growing hair bundle at their apex. It must be emphasized that the development of vestibular receptors shows a spatial cytodifferentiation from the center to the sides of the maculae and

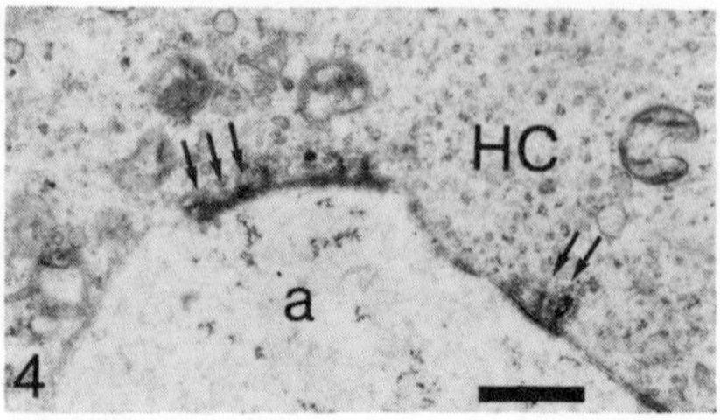

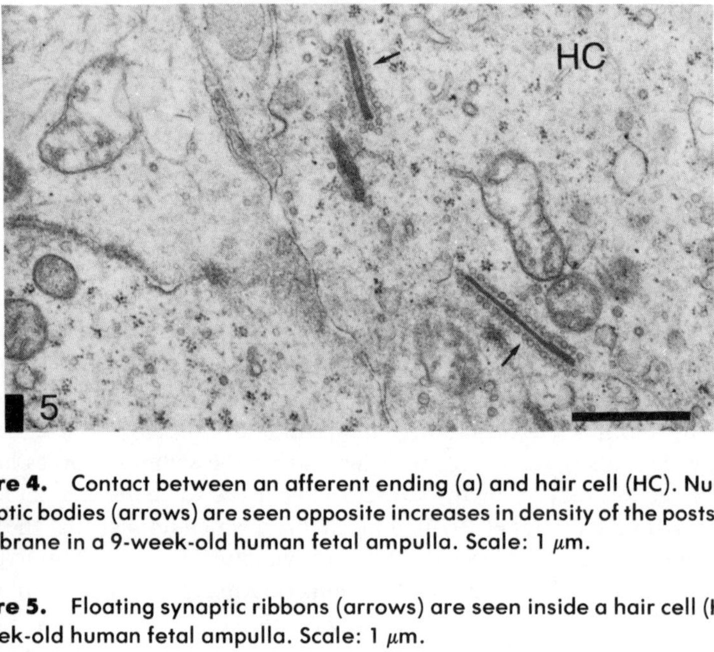

Figure 4. Contact between an afferent ending (a) and hair cell (HC). Numerous synaptic bodies (arrows) are seen opposite increases in density of the postsynaptic membrane in a 9-week-old human fetal ampulla. Scale: 1 μm.

Figure 5. Floating synaptic ribbons (arrows) are seen inside a hair cell (HC) in a 9-week-old human fetal ampulla. Scale: 1 μm.

from the top to the bottom of the cristae; the maculae start differentiating first (Sans & Chat, 1982; Mbiène, Favre, & Sans, 1984).

Arrival of Efferent Fibers

The efferent fibers are detected in the vestibular epithelium after the arrival of afferent fibers. They only appear when the first afferent synapses are well differentiated. In human embryos the first afferent synapses are observed at 8 weeks, and the first efferents are seen at 9–10 weeks. This feature indicates that the efferent system does not directly induce the formation and maturation of the afferent synapses. The efferent nerve endings establish axo-dendritic or axo-somatic contacts with afferent fiber and hair cell membranes, respectively. The early synapses show an increase in density of pre- and postsynaptic membranes, a cluster of numerous and regular micro-vesicles in the presynaptic efferent nerve endings, and a granular substance in the synaptic cleft. Nevertheless, in the future HCI the axo-somatic synapses are only transitory contacts, whereas in the HCII the efferent synapses develop a postsynaptic cistern in the soma of the hair cell during maturation. In the first stages of afferent and efferent synaptogenesis, it is impossible to distinguish between HCI and HCII in the labyrinth: All the innervated sensory cells have a type-II-like innervation.

Later Stages of HCII Synaptogenesis

During the maturation of the sensory cells, HCII preserve the main synaptic characteristics described at the end of the first stage of synaptogenesis (see Fig. 6). This also corresponds to the classic synaptic pattern of vestibular cells in lower vertebrates. Nevertheless, some structural maturation processes can be noted, such as an increase in the number of efferent terminal endings with a disappearance of growth microvesicles and a well-structured presynaptic body in each afferent synapse. With this slight ultrastructural evolution, HCII cells change in shape. They become more elongated, and their nucleus is usually deeper in the vestibular epithelium than the nucleus of the other sensory cells.

Later Stages of HCI Synaptogenesis

Spatula-shaped-growing nerve endings begin to innervate the base of some sensory cells; they eventually form the nerve chalice of HCI. This nerve ending has a growth cone with a spearheaded part which threads through supporting and hair cells (Fig. 7). From place to place, behind the growth cone, the opposing membranes show an increase in density, with granular material adhering to the inner surfaces of the two membranes. Coated vesicles which participate in the elaboration of the sensory cell membranes are also observed. In the region farthest from the growth cone, the density of the membranes further increases and becomes symmetrical, with an accumulation of granular material in the intercellular space. The number of synaptic bodies progressively decreases, while the symmetrical density of the hair cell and chalice membranes increases. During the postnatal period in the cat, the total number of synaptic bodies in HCI is reduced by 93% while the length of the specialized neuroepithelium contact increases by 300% (Favre & Sans, 1979). In a later stage, the elongated and polylamellar synaptic bodies become very rare. These features suggest that during development, the nature of the synapses and probably the synaptic transmission process change fundamentally at the HCI level. The formation of a nerve chalice around an HCI often

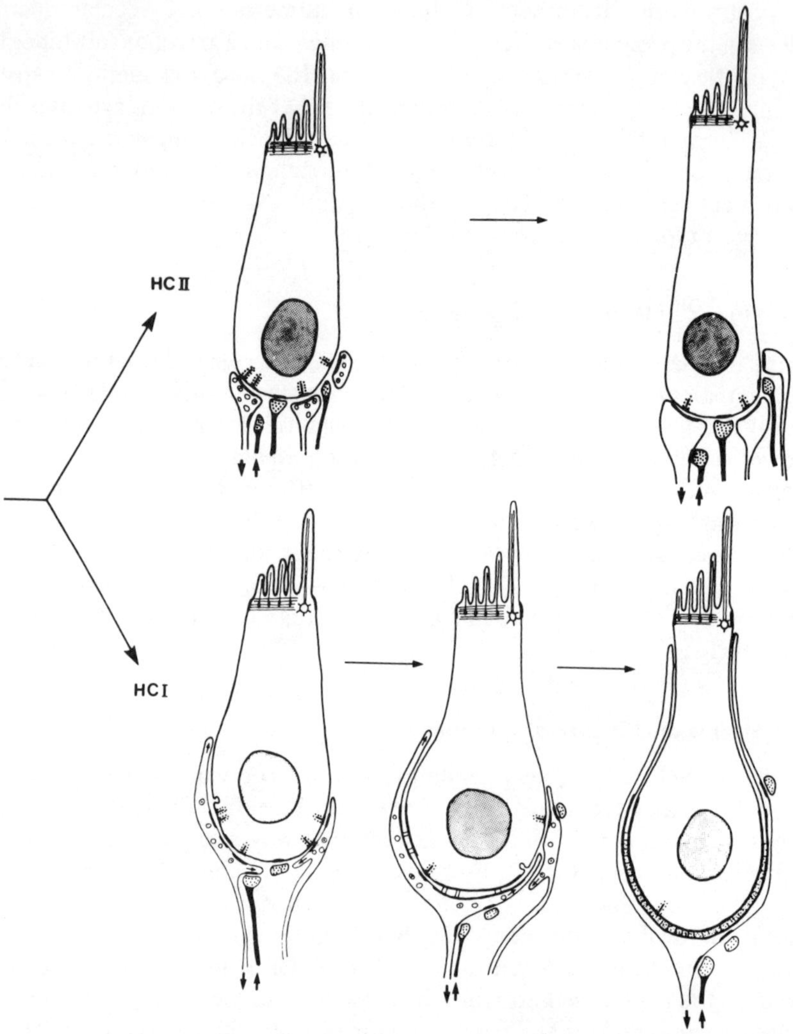

Figure 6. Evolution of vestibular hair cell synapses. The primitive HC (Fig. 1C) gives rise to an HCII and an HCI. The final stage of the HCII (upper right) does not differ significantly from the primitive HC. In contrast, HCI evolution shows a transient HCII stage (lower left), followed by the formation of a highly specialized hair cell connected only with one afferent nerve chalice (right). Symbols: ↓ = afferents; ↑ = efferents.

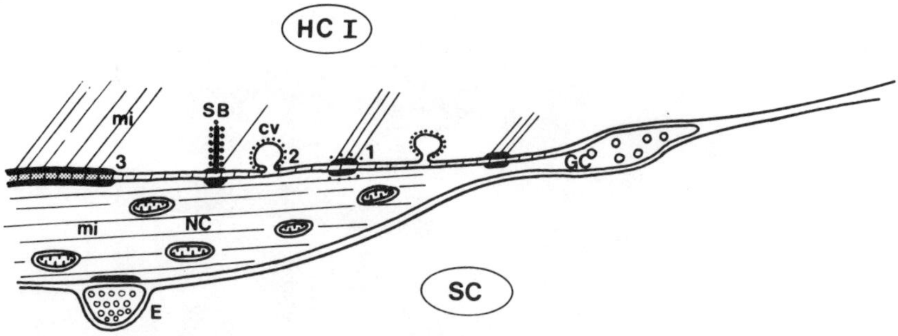

Figure 7. Different stages of formation of a nerve chalice (NC). The growth cone (GC) of an afferent separates the membranes of a hair cell (HC) and a supporting cell (SC). The different stages of synaptic differentiation are schematized and correspond successively to: (1) coated vesicles (CV) and membrane densities associated with microtubules on presynaptic side; (2) transient presynaptic bodies; (3) membrane densities on each side of the synapse and floculated material in the cleft. An efferent ending (E), previously connected with the HC synapses now with the NC. (From Favre, Dememes, & Sans, 1986, Fig. 3.)

displays competition phenomena when a multiafferentation occurs at the base of the hair cell. The growth cone of some growing nerves, which has already formed a synaptic contact with the sensory cell, detaches from the other fibers, both afferent and efferent, and finally forms the chalice (Fig. 8). During these competitive phenonema, the efferent synapses change their polarization, the axo-somatic contacts disappear, and new axo-dendritic contacts are formed between the efferent endings and the afferent nerve chalice (Favre & Sans, 1978).

In conclusion, it appears that during ontogenesis, HCI passes first through an HCII-like stage before taking on the characteristics of a highly specialized cell (Fig. 9).

SYNAPTOGENESIS IN THE COCHLEA

First Stages of Afferent Synapses

Synaptogenesis on both inner (IHC) and outer (OHC) hair cells begins very early in the mammalian cochlea. As soon as the future sensory cells connected with the radial afferents start to differentiate, membrane thickenings as well as presynaptic specializations can be observed. Thus, at least the ultrastructural features of synapses appear in the cochlea long before the onset of auditory function (see Pujol & Hilding, 1973; Pujol, 1985). Again, the

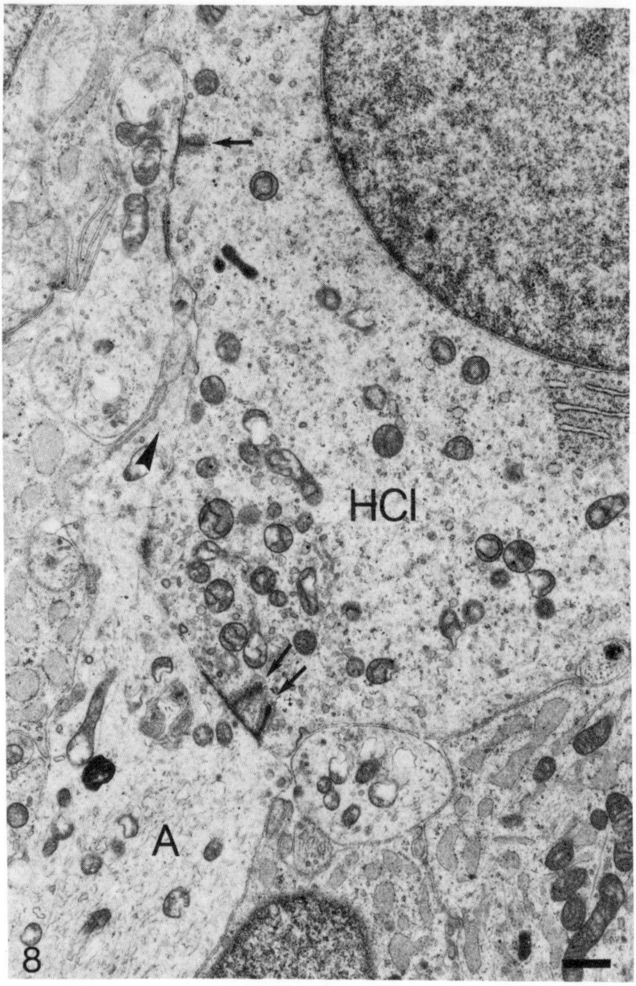

Figure 8. Chalice formation at the base of a future HCI. One afferent nerve ending (A) sends a growth cone (▲) which eventually displaces another afferent (A) from the HCI. Arrows indicate synaptic bodies. 10-week-old human fetal ampulla. Scale: 1 μm.

human cochlea, with its slow development, appears to be a good model for observing the very first stages of synaptogenesis (Pujol & Lavigne-Rebillard, 1985). The IHC mature earlier than the OHC, and in a 12-week-old fetus (i.e., at leasts 4 weeks before the onset of function) classical afferent synapses, with presynaptic bodies surrounded by vesicles, can be seen first at inner and then at outer hair cell bases. These synaptic differentiations have been observed on both types of cells even before the formation of stereocilia.

These afferent synapses follow the same developmental process for some time on both types of hair cells. The number of endings connecting the cells increases. Similarly, the number of presynaptic bodies increases temporarily on the cell side opposite the endings (Figs. 10 & 13; Pujol, Carlier, & Devigne, 1979). At this stage, afferents connected with the IHC and some of those connected with the OHC seem to belong to the same system; i.e., the radial dendrites from the type-I ganglion cells (Fig. 12). They have the same morphological characteristics and make the same type of synaptic contacts with IHC

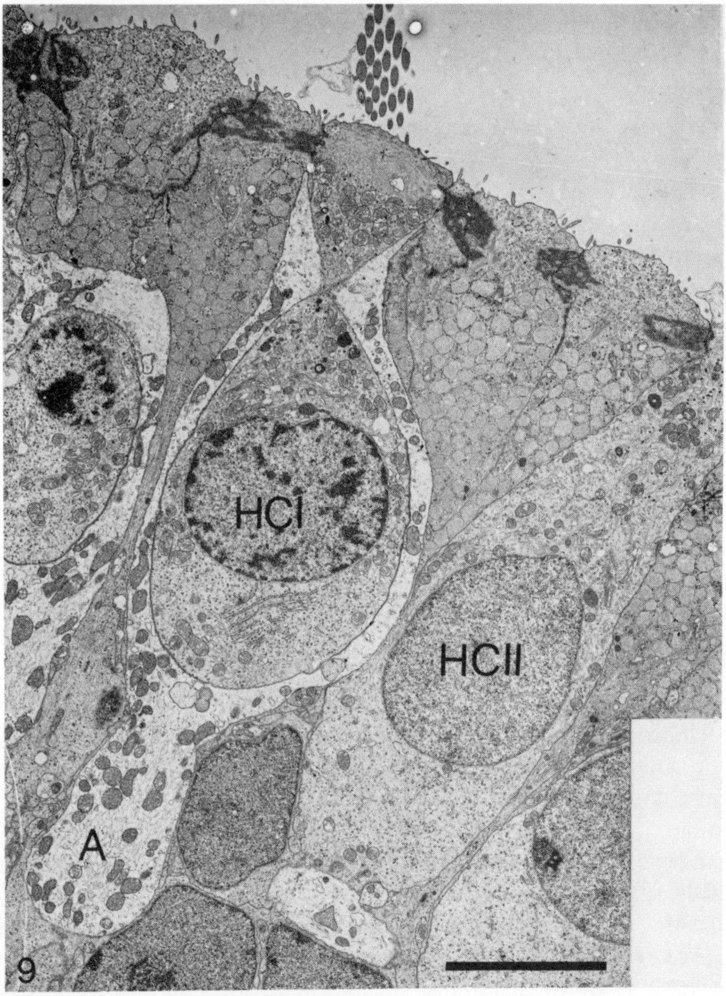

Figure 9. Final stage of HCI synaptogenesis. The afferent nerve chalice (A) is well formed. A mature HCII can be seen on the right. 20-day-old rat ampulla. Scale: 10 μm. (Courtesy of D. Demêmes, unpublished picture.)

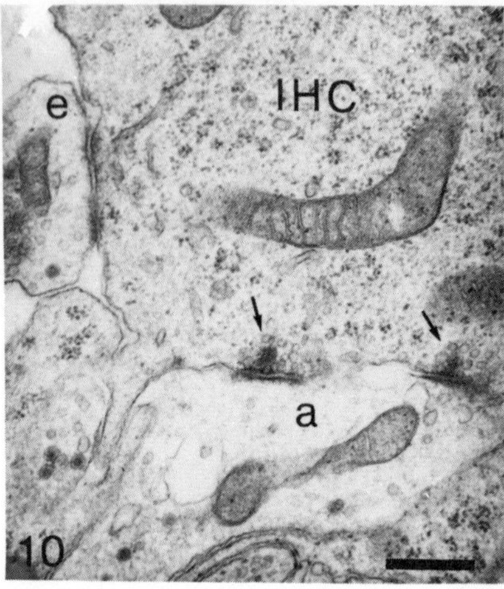

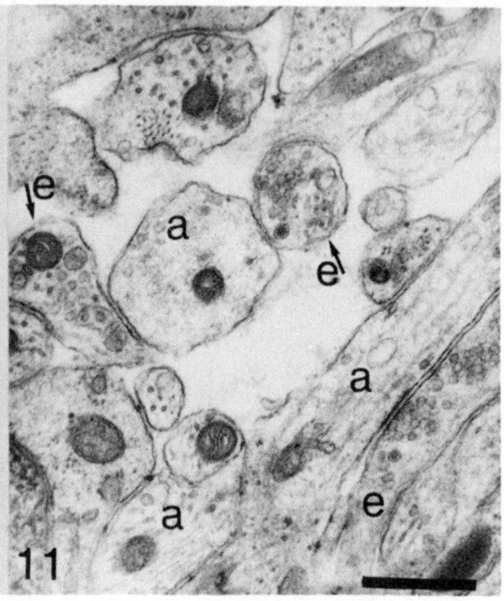

Figure 10. First afferent (a) and efferent (e) endings at the base of an inner hair cell (IHC). The afferent forms two distinct synaptic differentiations with presynaptic bodies (arrows) in the IHC. Cat fetus 10 days before birth. Scale: 5 μm. (Reproduced from Pujol, Carlier, and Devinge, 1979, by permission of the publisher.)

Figure 11. First efferent axo-dendritic synapse in the inner spiral bundle (below an IHC): a = afferents; e = efferents. 10-week-old human fetus. Scale: 5 μm.

and OHC, characterized within the sensory cell by typical presynaptic bodies (Figs. 10 & 13). In addition, they also seem to possess the same kainate receptors, or at least they react in the same way to kainic acid toxicity (Pujol, Lenoir, Robertson, Eybalin, & Johnstone, 1985).

Arrival of Efferent Fibers

Efferents can be seen at the level of the IHC at about the same time as the first specialized afferent synapses (Fig. 10) (Pujol & Lavigne-Rebillard, 1985; Shnerson, Devigne, & Pujol, 1982). Efferent endings in the plexus below the IHC contain uniformly sized clear vesicles, which contrast with irregular vesicles found in the growing afferent terminals. Since there are no data describing the neurochemistry and/or the nucleus of origin in these first efferent fibers, it is difficult to speak about a lateral or a medial system (see Warr, 1980). Nevertheless, there is good reason to suppose these endings belong to the lateral system, since they are distributed mainly, if not exclusively, below IHC, and they form numerous axo-dendritic synapses with afferents (Fig. 11). The medial system, which is essentially connected to OHC, appears to mature much later (see the section "Later-Stages of OHC Synaptogenesis").

Later Stages of IHC Synaptogenesis

As previously indicated, the first pattern of IHC innervation is not really different from what will be the adult configuration. The only noticeable differences concern an increase in the number of afferent endings connected with a single IHC (see Fig. 14). At the same time, irregular vesicles within these endings disappear almost completely, giving rise to a clear and floccu-

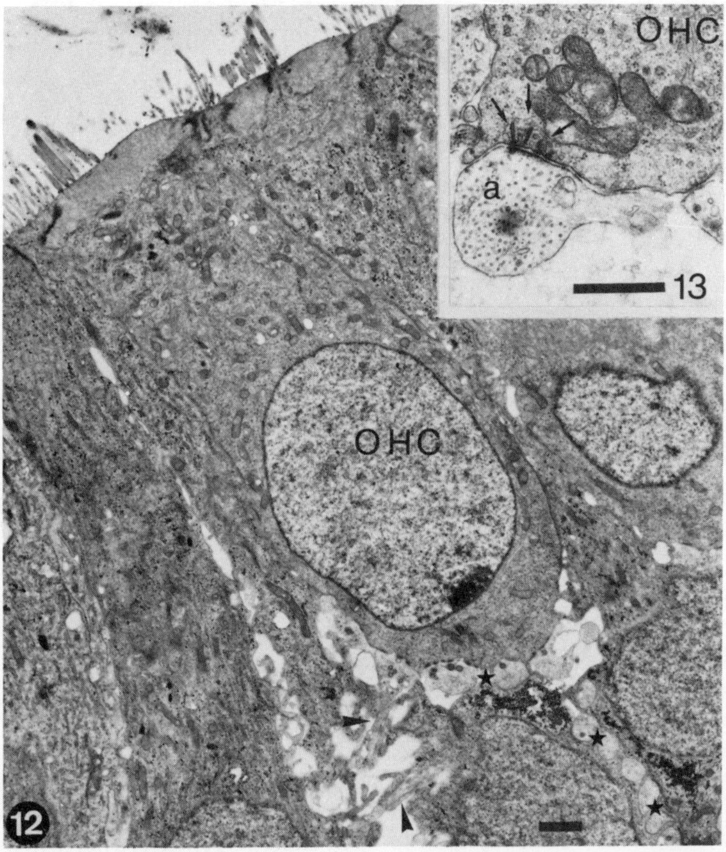

Figure 12. Immature outer hair cell (OHC) only innervated by afferent endings. Note the two kinds of afferents which reach the OHC either radially (arrowhead) or, between the Deiter's cells, spirally (stars). Cat fetus 6 days before birth. Scale: 1 μm.

Figure 13. Contact between an afferent (a) and an immature OHC. Multiple-synaptic bodies (arrows) can be seen on the cell side. The afferent has a section with clear microtubules and a growth cone. Cat fetus 6 days before birth. Scale: 5 μm.

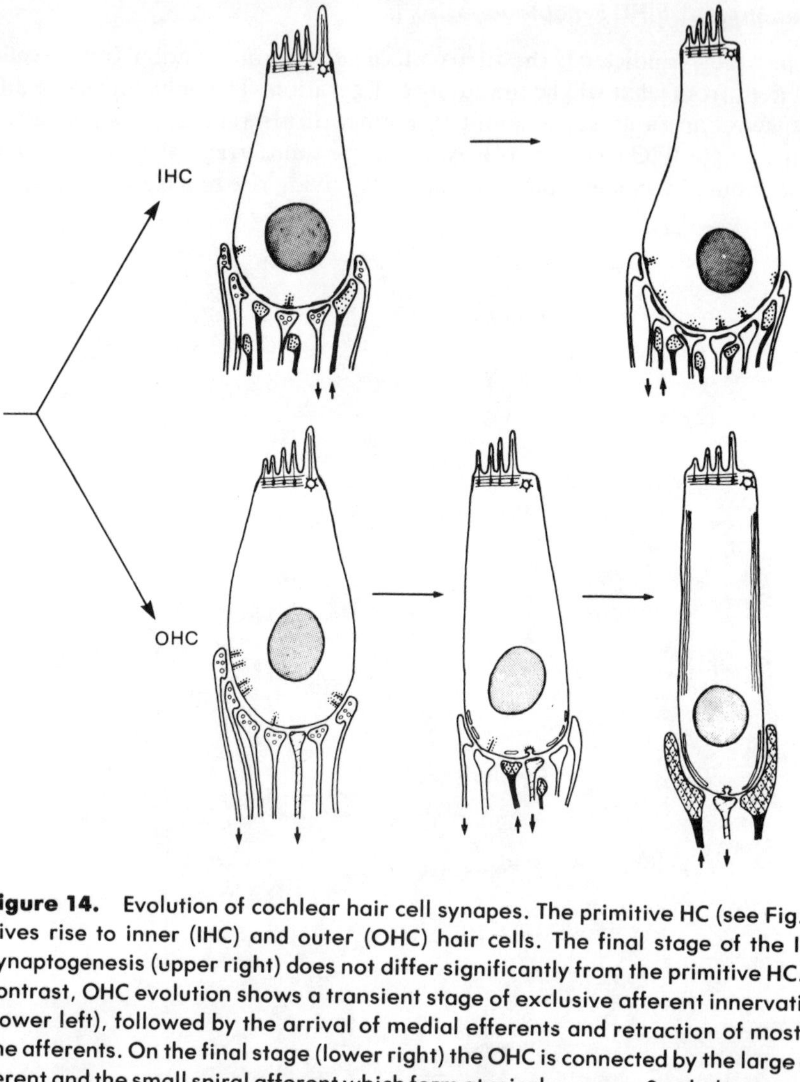

Figure 14. Evolution of cochlear hair cell synapses. The primitive HC (see Fig. 1) gives rise to inner (IHC) and outer (OHC) hair cells. The final stage of the IHC synaptogenesis (upper right) does not differ significantly from the primitive HC. In contrast, OHC evolution shows a transient stage of exclusive afferent innervation (lower left), followed by the arrival of medial efferents and retraction of most of the afferents. On the final stage (lower right) the OHC is connected by the large efferent and the small spiral afferent which form atypical synapse. Symbols: ↓ = afferents (white radial afferents; white and hatched = spiral afferents). ↑ = efferents (black with dotted endings = lateral efferents; black with dotted and hatched endings = medial efferents).

lent cytoplasmic content. Another slight evolution involves the efferent endings in the inner spiral bundle, which increase in number. Some of these endings can be seen to contact the base of IHC directly. This is merely a transient stage in some species such as the cat (Pujol, Carlier, & Devigne, 1979) or the mouse (Shnerson, Devigne, & Pujol, 1982). In other species such as the guinea pig, a few of these axo-somatic synapses can be found in adult IHC.

Later Stages of OHC Synaptogenesis

OHC synaptogenesis follows a completely different process from IHC synaptogenesis (see: Pujol, Carlier, & Devigne, 1978, 1979; Lenoir, Shnerson, & Pujol, 1980; Shnerson, Devigne, & Pujol, 1982; Pujol, 1985). Here, together with a drastic modification of the cell shape, the evolution of synapses involves the elimination of certain connections and the formation of others. The major event concerns the late arrival of fibers from the medial efferent system, which eventually form huge synapses directly with the OHC base. The successive stages of OHC synaptogenesis can be summarized. First, when the OHC is still only surrounded by afferent endings, there is a rapid and marked decrease in the number of presynaptic bodies (Pujol, Carlier, & Devigne, 1979). Second, at about the time of the onset of cochlear function, the medial efferents arrive at the OHC level; some transient axodendritic synapses can be seen. Then the efferents reach the OHC membrane and seem to push afferents away (Fig. 15). At the same time, postsynaptic cisterns are formed inside the OHC. In the final stage, most of the afferent dendrites have retracted and the OHC is surrounded by large efferent synapses showing characteristics pre- and postsynaptic specializations (Fig. 16). Opposite to the small afferents which connect the adult OHC, few, if any, presynaptic specialization can be seen. The kainic acid experiment, already mentioned (Pujol, Lenoir, Robertson, Eybalin, & Johnstone, 1985), tends to indicate that these afferents, which stay at the OHC level in adulthood, are different in nature from those which have retracted. Thus, a temporary exuberant branching of the radial afferents innervating the OHC could be hypothesized. The retraction of these afferents seems to depend only on the arrival of efferents, as demonstrated by two different sets of experiments. In hypothyroid rats (Uziel, Pujol, Legrand, & Legrand, 1982), the arrival of medial efferents at the OHC level is delayed and the hair cell is still only surrounded by numerous afferents on day 22, which corresponds to a mature stage in normal rats. Similarly, when the vestibular nerve, which carries efferents to the cochlea, is cut early in development, a supernumerous afferent innervation is also seen, around the adult OHC, which lacks its efferent innervation (Pujol & Carlier, 1982).

This description of OHC synaptogenesis deserves two more comments. First, the evolution of the synaptic pattern below the OHC reflects the evolution of the OHC itself, which, starting from a typical sensory stage, eventually at the end of maturation takes on specific properties more linked to cochlear micromechanics (see Siegel & Kim, 1982; Brownell, 1983). Second, OHC synaptogenesis may display differences depending on the level of the cochlear partition. It appears that the complete evolution schematized in Figure 14 concerns mainly the basal part of the cochlea (i.e., the portion involved in coding high or mid frequencies). In the apical part, this evolution may be incomplete, especially because fewer efferents arrive at this level. Some radial afferents may then stay, and this could account for the numerous afferent

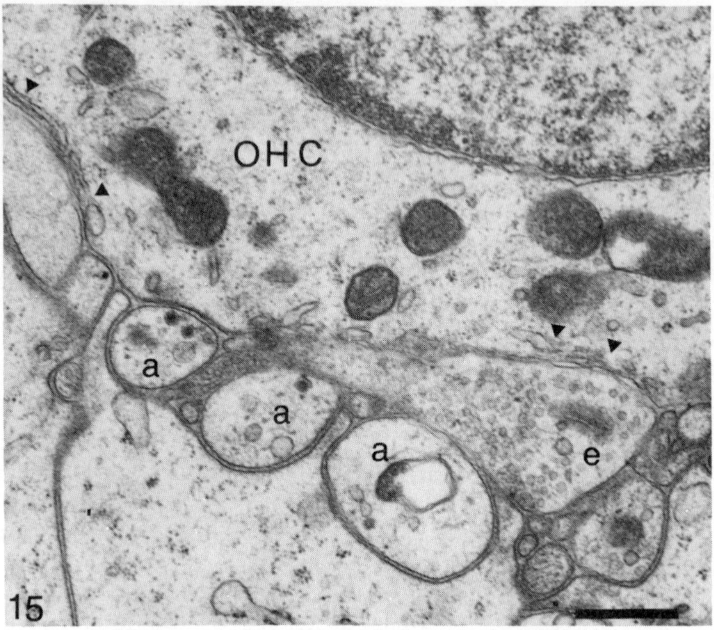

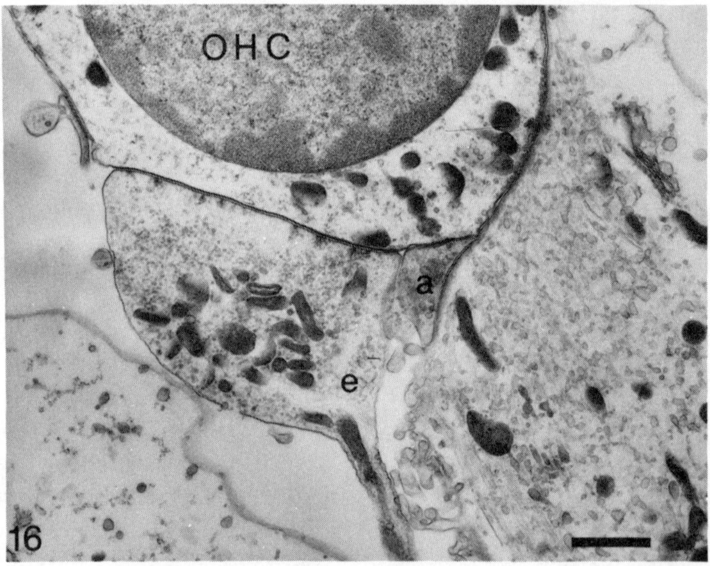

Figure 15. Arrival of the medial efferents at the OHC level. An efferent ending (e) seems to push afferents (a) away from the OHC membrane. Postsynaptic cysternae (triangles) begin to form in the OHC. 7-day-old rat. Scale: 5 μm. (Reproduced from Lenoir, Shnerson, & Pujol, 1980, by permission of the publisher.)

Figure 16. Final stage of OHC synaptogenesis. In this section the OHC is connected by a large efferent (e) ending filled with microvesicles, and a small afferent (a). One-month-old rat. Scale: 1 μm. (Courtesy of M. Lenoir, unpublished picture.)

endings found below OHC in apical turns and also for the presence of presynaptic bodies in OHC. Moreover, depending on the species, the border between a "basal" and an "apical" cochlea may vary: For example, the cat and the rat seem to have a "basal" cochlea much more extended toward the apex than the guinea pig or the chinchilla. This could explain numerous controversies found in the literature concerning the synaptic pattern of OHCs (Spoendlin, 1969; Dunn & Morest, 1975; Siegel & Brownell, 1981) and, of course, concerning their physiological properties (Russell & Sellick, 1983; Dallos, Santos-Sacchi, & Flock, 1982).

Parallel conclusions can be drawn from results in the cochlear and the vestibular organs. Both have a poorly differentiated type (IHC and HCII) and a highly differentiated type (OHC and HCI) of sensory cell. In both cases the synaptogenesis of the former follows a quite simple pattern, and that of the latter has a much more complicated development implying competitive phenomena and a remodeling of synaptic connections.

REFERENCES

Brownell, W.E. (1983). Observations on a motile response in isolated outer hair cells. In W.R. Webster & L.M. Aitkin (Eds.), *Mechanisms of hearing*(pp. 5–10). Clayton, Victoria: Monash University Press.

Dallos, P., Santos-Sacchi, J. & Flock, A. (1982). Intracellular recordings from cochlear outer hair cells. *Science, 218,* 582–584.

Dunn, R.A., & Morest, D.K. (1975). Receptor synapses without synaptic ribbons in the cochlea of the cat. *Proceeding of the National Academy of Sciences, USA, 72,* 3599–3603.

Favre, D., Demêmes, D., & Sans, A. (1986). Microtubule organization in the vestibular sensory cells during synaptogenesis. *Developmental Brain Research, 25,* 137–142.

Favre, D., & Sans, A. (1978). The development of vestibular efferent nerve endings during cat maturation: Ultrastructural study. *Brain Research, 142,* 333–337.

Favre, D., & Sans, A. (1979). Embryonic and postnatal development of afferent innervation in cat vestibular receptors. *Acta Otolaryngologica (Stockholm), 87,* 97–107.

Jørgensen, J.M., & Flock, A. (1976). Noninnervated sense organs of the lateral line: development in the regenerating tail of the salamander (*Ambystoma mexicanum*). *Journal of Neurocytology, 5,* 33–41.

Lenoir, M., Shnerson, A., & Pujol, R. (1980). Cochlear receptor development in the rat with emphasis on synaptogenesis. *Anatomy & Embryology, 160,* 253–262.

Mbiène, J.P., Favre, D., & Sans, A. (1984). The pattern of ciliary development in fetal mouse vestibular receptors. A qualitative and quantitative SEM study. *Anatomy & Embryology, 170,* 229–238.

Pujol, R. (1985). Morphology, synaptology and electrophysiology of the developing auditory periphery. *Acta Otolaryngologica (Stockholm)* (Suppl. 421), 5–9.

Pujol, R., & Carlier, E. (1982). Cochlear synaptogenesis after sectioning the efferent bundle. *Developmental Brain Research, 3,* 151–154.

Pujol, R., Carlier, E., & Devigne, C. (1978). Different patterns of cochlear innervation during the development in the kitten. *Journal of Comparative Neurology, 117,* 529–536.

Pujol, R., Carlier, E., & Devigne, C. (1979). Significance of presynaptic formations in the very early stages of cochlear synaptogenesis. *Acta Otolaryngologica (Stockholm), 89,* 317–322.

Pujol, R., & Hilding, D.A. (1973). Anatomy and physiology of the onset of auditory function. *Acta Otolaryngologica (Stockholm), 76,* 1–10.

Pujol, R., & Lavigne-Rebillard, M. (1985). Early stages of innervation and sensory cell differentiation in the human fetal organ of Corti. *Acta Otolaryngologica (Stockholm)* (Suppl. 423), 43–50.

Pujol, R., Lenoir, M., Robertson, D., Eybalin, M., & Johnstone, B.M. (1985). Kainic acid alters selectively, in the adult cochlea, auditory dendrites connected with inner hair cells. *Hearing Research, 18,* 145–151.

Russell, I.J., & Sellick, P.M. (1983). Low-frequency characteristics of intracellularly recorded receptor potentials in guinea-pig cochlear hair cells. *Journal of Physiology, 338,* 179–206.

Sans, A., & Chat, M. (1982). Analysis of temporal and spatial patterns of rat vestibular hair cells differentiation by tritiated thymidine radioautography. *Journal of Comparative Neurology, 206,* 1–8.

Sans, A., & Dechesne, C. (1985). Early development of vestibular receptors in human embryos: An electron microscopic study. *Acta Otolaryngologica (Stockholm)* (Suppl. 423), 51–58.

Sher, A.E. (1971). The embryonic and postnatal development of the inner ear of the mouse. *Acta Otolaryngologica (Stockholm)* (Suppl. 285), 1–77.

Shnerson, A., Devigne, C., & Pujol, R. (1982). Age-related changes in the C57B1/6J mouse cochlea. II. Ultrastructural findings. *Developmental Brain Research, 2,* 77–78.

Siegel, J.H., & Brownell, W.E. (1981). Presynaptic bodies in outer hair cells of the chinchilla organ of Corti. *Brain Research, 220,* 188–193.

Siegel, J.H., & Kim, D.O. (1982). Efferent neural control of cochlear mechanics? Olivocochlear bundle stimulation affects cochlear biomechanical nonlinearity. *Hearing Research, 6,* 171–182.

Sobkowicz, H.M., Rose, J.E., Scott, G.L., & Slapnick, S.M. (1982). Ribbon synapses in the developing intact and cultured organ of Corti in the mouse. *Journal of Neuroscience, 2,* 942–957.

Spoendlin, H. (1969). Innervation patterns in the organ of Corti of the cat. *Acta Otolaryngologica (Stockholm), 67,* 239–254.

Thornhill, R.A. (1972). The development of the labyrinth of the lamprey (*Lampreta fluviatilis). Proceedings of the Royal Society (London), B181,* 175–198.

Uziel, A., Pujol, R., Legrand, C., & Legrand, J. (1982). Cochlear synaptogenesis in the hypothyroid rat. *Developmental Brain Research, 7,* 295–301.

Van de Water, T.R. (1976). Effects of removal of the statoacoustic ganglion complex upon the growing otocyst. *Annals of Otology Rhinology & Laryngology, 85,* (Suppl. 33), 1–32.

Warr, W.B. (1980). Efferent components of the auditory system. *Annals of Otology Rhinology & Laryngology, 89* (Suppl. 74), 114–120.

2 Developmental Abnormalities of the Mammalian Auditory System*

Karen P. Steel
Gregory R. Bock
MRC Institute of Hearing Research
University of Nottingham
Nottingham NG7 2RD
United Kingdom

INTRODUCTION

The study of developmental abnormalities of the auditory system can facilitate our understanding of the auditory system in two main ways in addition to elucidating the process of development itself. First, the forms of pathology arising from abnormal development are often quite different from the forms of pathology that can be induced experimentally in adult animals. Developmental defects, therefore, extend the range of lesions available to the physiologist for investigating normal auditory function. Second, by studying the process of development it is possible to identify the site of the initial lesion more accurately than if only the end-point of the disease is examined. This is important, because a defect in one part of the auditory system can trigger extensive, progressive degenerative changes in other parts of the system. Knowledge about key features of the disease may form a basis for diagnosis and study of etiology of auditory abnormalities in adult humans, so as to make best use of the very limited genetic and pathological information on human developmental abnormalities.

A fundamental concept in the explanation of developmental defects is that of the critical period. A critical period is a time during development when a cell type or tissue appears to be particularly sensitive to the presence or absence of nutrients, hormones, or other factors. Different parts of the inner ear may respond to the same factor at different developmental times; for example, the critical period during which a certain minimum level of thyroxine is required in rats is 12–17 days after birth for normal synaptogenesis but 6–7 days after birth for normal tectorial membrane production (Uziel, Legrand, & Rabie, 1985). The term *critical period* is used to describe the times during which the course of gross morphogenesis or cellular differentiation may be

*We thank Professor M. P. Haggard for comments on the manuscript and Dr. Ed Rubel for some useful discussions.

qualitatively influenced by experimental manipulation as well as the times during which apparently mature cells exhibit enhanced quantitative sensitivity to damaging influences. The latter include periods of extreme sensitivity of cochlear hair cells to ototoxic drug or noise induced damage (e.g., Saunders & Bock, 1978; Henry, 1983). Since these periods extend beyond the time at which histological maturation of the inner ear is generally considered to be complete, it has been suggested that the process of functional maturation is prolonged in comparison with anatomical maturation, although definitions of maturity are constrained by the limitations of techniques currently available.

Normal development of the auditory system has been reviewed elsewhere (e.g., Rubel, 1978). The purpose of this chapter is to review briefly the main types of auditory abnormality that can be attributed to errors in the developmental process. Normal neural development is dependent upon normal sensory input, and this principle has been particularly well demonstrated in the visual system. In the present review, we intend to show how this principle applies to the auditory system by focusing upon the location of the primary defect and discussing how such defects can lead to changes in other parts of the auditory system.

OUTER AND MIDDLE EAR

A wide variety of external ear abnormalities have been described in humans (Melnick, 1980; Aase, 1980; Konigsmark & Gorlin, 1976). Many cases are of genetic origin and often involve other developmental defects and/or hearing impairment in addition to the pinna malformation. Eight of the 10 hereditary syndromes showing pinnal anomalies documented by Konigsmark and Gorlin (1976) also showed conductive hearing losses, indicative of middle ear defects. One of these syndromes was characterized by a malformation of the incudostapedial junction, while other cases showed hypoplasia of ossicles, absent ossicles, malformed ossicles, fixed stapedial footplate, or fusion of ossicles. An extensive series of middle ear abnormalities in humans, both with and without associated defects, has been described by Nadol (1980). Deformities of the outer and middle ears may also be a consequence of teratogenic agents such as thalidomide and may be associated with morphogenetic defects of the inner ear, as described in the next section (Phelps, 1974). Defects of the middle ear in humans can lead to conductive (as opposed to sensorineural) hearing loss.

In animals, pinna defects have been reported in several mouse mutants, such as the *short-ear* mutant (e.g., Green, 1981). Middle ear abnormality has also recently been found to occur spontaneously in the LP/J inbred strain of mouse (Chole & Henry, 1983). Excess bony deposits were seen on the ossicles and otic capsule, giving an appearance similar to that seen in human otosclerosis (Fig. 1). Physiological responses of LP/J mice to airborne sound stimuli showed raised thresholds, but it has not yet been shown that the raised thresholds are due to the middle ear anomaly rather than to a cochlear dysfunction.

BONY LABYRINTH

Abnormalities in which the overall structure of the labyrinth is deformed in some way are called morphogenetic abnormalities. The deformity appears to result from an interference with the normal processes of morphogenesis in early development. In some cases, normal development seems to have been halted at an immature stage, while in other cases the anomaly may be minor, with no apparent functional consequences, or major, so that the inner ear is hardly recognizable. Asymmetry between the two ears is common, and variability in extent of the deformity is also seen among mice known to be carrying the same mutation. Mouse mutants with morphogenetic inner ear defects have been reviewed by Deol (1980), and similar defects may be found in humans (e.g., Phelps, 1974; Phelps, Sheldon, & Lloyd, 1976). The range of deformities found in mice is broadly similar to the range seen in humans, and two features suggest that similar mechanisms may be responsible for the deformities in the two species: First, the lateral semicircular canal is the most commonly or most severely affected part of the labyrinth in both humans and mice (Steel & Bock, 1983; Phelps, 1974; Schuknecht, 1980; Sando,

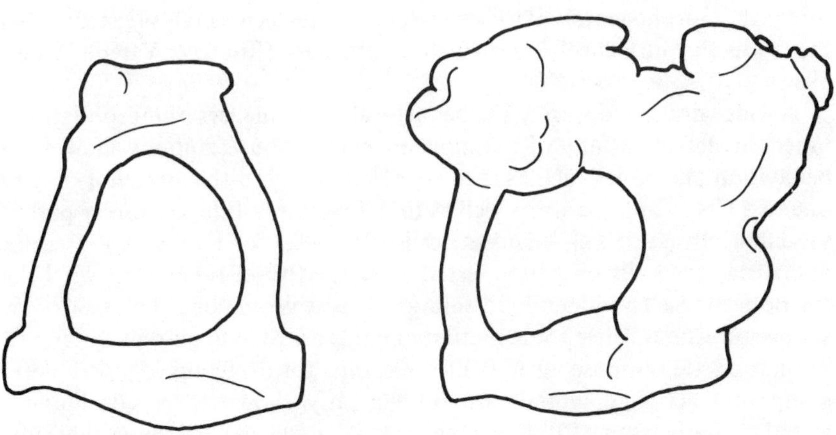

Figure 1. Diagram of a normal mouse stapes on the left, and a stapes from an LP/J mouse on the right, showing abnormal bone deposits. (Redrawn from Chole & Henry, 1983.)

1980); second, morphogenetic inner ear defects can be associated with neural tube defects in both humans and mice (Wright, Phelps, & Friedmann, 1976; Deol, 1966; Steel & Bock, 1983).

Morphogenetic defects may be caused by exposure during development to teratogenic levels of various agents such as thalidomide (Phelps, 1974), vitamin A (Morriss, 1972), or histidine (Kacser, Mya Mya, Duncker, Wright, Bulfield, McLaren, & Lyon, 1977). The critical period during which a high level of histidine can cause inner ear damage is known from experiments on maternal diet to be the second week of gestation in the mouse (gestation period is normally 20 days). Mutations may also be the cause of morphogenetic defects; for example, mutant mice with low histidase activity, leading to excess histidine levels (histidinaemia), produce offspring with morphogenetic inner ear defects (Kacser, Mya Mya, & Bulfield, 1979). The biochemical basis of the abnormality has not yet been described in any other case of hereditary inner ear deformity.

There is some evidence that morphogenetic defects may be mediated by abnormal inductive influences of the neural tube. Observations of correlations between morphogenetic defects of the inner ear and abnormal structural development of the neural tube in several different groups of animals suggest that the neural tube can induce normal development of the inner ear (Deol, 1966; Kacser et al., 1979). Support for such an inductive effect comes from experiments in which the developing labyrinth (otocyst) is removed from normal foetal mice at 9.5 to 10 days of gestation and incubated in culture. These cultured otocysts will only continue to develop normally if part of the neural tube, the rhombencephalon, is also cultured in the same dish. When a filter is placed between the otocyst and rhombencephalon in the culture dish, morphogenesis of the otocyst continues as normal, suggesting that the "inductive influence" is a diffusible substance (Ruben & Van de Water, 1983).

A wide variation occurs in the behavioral consequences of morphogenetic inner ear defects. Many of the morphogenetic mouse mutants show gross behavioral anomalies such as shaking or circling, but this behavior may be due to a CNS abnormality as well as to deformities of the vestibular part of the labyrinth (see Steel, Niaussat, & Bock, 1982, for references). Hearing ability has generally only been tested using the Preyer reflex (ear twitch) or startle response to sudden loud sounds. This is not a good indicator of response threshold, since some mutant animals are able to give an apparently normal startle response when their thresholds for detection of eighth nerve compound action potentials are subsequently shown to be considerably raised in comparison with control animals. Nonetheless, morphogenetic mutants in which only the vestibular labyrinth is affected usually show normal startle responses, and in those in which the cochlea is also malformed, startle responses vary considerably (Steel et al., 1982).

ORGAN OF CORTI

Abnormal maturation of the hair cells and supporting cells of the organ of Corti has been demonstrated in cases of hereditary deafness of the neuroepithelial type (Steel & Bock, 1983). To show that the abnormality is a defect in the late stages of cellular differentiation, it is necessary to use transmission electron microscopy. Previous studies using light microscopy suggested that the hair cells developed normally and then began to degenerate at some point after normal histological maturation was complete. This group of mutants was therefore called the degenerative group (Grüneberg, 1956). However, each of the mutants of this type that has since been examined with transmission electron microscopy has been shown to display clear signs of abnormal hair cell maturation, and so it has been suggested that the term *neuroepithelial* would be a more appropriate name for the group (Steel & Bock, 1983). Degeneration of hair cells usually does follow the abnormal development, but "degenerative" seems to be a misleading description since it may be taken to imply normal development.

Two patterns of developmental anomaly have been reported in neuroepithelial mutants. The first of these patterns has been described in the *deafness, shaker-1,* and *Ames waltzer* mouse mutants (Bock & Steel, 1983; Shnerson, Lenoir, Van de Water, & Pujol, 1983; Kikuchi & Hilding, 1965; Osako & Hilding, 1971; Pujol, Shnerson, Lenoir, & Deol, 1983). The abnormality in these animals is characterized by retarded regression of the finger-like processes of Deiters' cells (supporting cells beneath the hair cells) between the rows of outer hair cells (OHCs) and retarded formation of the tunnel and Nuel fluid-filled areas (that is, the fluid areas between the pillar cells and around the OHCs, within the organ of Corti), plus failure of the OHCs to mature to the long thin shape normally seen in the adult organ of Corti. OHCs remain short and rounded and often show early degenerative signs such as vacuole formation (Fig. 2). The appearance of stereocilia may be relatively normal in some parts of the cochlea even though, at least in the *deafness* mutant, no OHCs show a normal appearance below the reticular lamina. This observation suggests that even scanning electron microscopy may be of limited use in revealing developmental organ of Corti defects (Bock & Steel, 1983). Inner hair cell (IHC) anomalies are not so clearly defined and consist mainly of early degenerative signs within the hair cell rather than a change in size or shape compared with normal inner hair cells. Innervation of hair cells is also abnormal and is described later.

The second pattern of developmental anomaly of the organ of Corti has been uniquely described in the *Bronx waltzer* mutant mouse. As for *shaker-1, deafness,* and *Ames waltzer,* the *Bronx waltzer* is best classified as a neuroepithelial mutant, because the primary defect occurs in the neuroepithelial tissues. In contrast to the mutants described in the previous paragraph, the

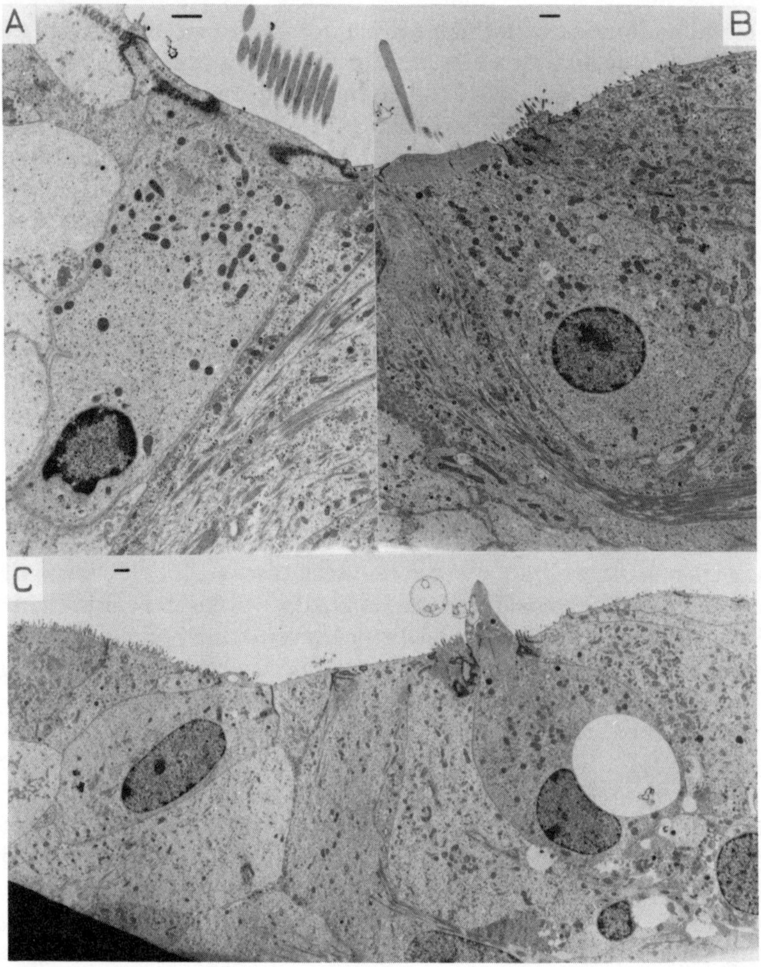

Figure 2. Ultrathin sections of the organ of Corti of a *deafness* (dn/dn) mouse mutant aged 20 days. Scale bar represents 1 μm. (A) An outer hair cell. Stereocilia have a normal appearance, but the cell body is abnormally short and there is no sign of formation of the Nuel fluid areas around the sides of the hair cell. These fluid spaces develop at 6–10 days after birth in normal mice. (B) An inner hair cell of reasonably normal appearance. (C) Organ of Corti, showing a degenerating inner hair cell, with a large vacuole and fused stereocilia, on the right. The tunnel and Nuel spaces have failed to open, and no outer hair cells can be recognized in this region.

Bronx waltzer inner ear has largely normal OHCs, and the developmental defect occurs in the IHCs and pillar cells (Deol & Gluecksohn-Waelsch, 1979; Deol, 1981; Lenoir & Pujol, 1984; Keithley & Feldman, 1983; Fig. 3). Very few IHCs develop, and estimates of the number of normal IHCs present vary from about 5–25% of the number in normal mice. In addition to these, some abnormally small IHCs may be found. The deficit of IHCs is a developmental anomaly, because the abnormality or absence of these cells may be detected at birth (Deol & Gluecksohn-Waelsch, 1979; Lenoir & Pujol, 1984), and there are few signs of any degenerative changes with age (Lenoir & Pujol, 1984; Keithley & Feldman, 1983). The pillar cells also show a developmental abnormality, especially the inner pillar cells, which may be malformed or missing. OHCs have normal innervation, while IHC synapse formation is abnormal even in those cells with an otherwise reasonably normal appearance (Lenoir & Pujol, 1984).

Many of the neuroepithelial mutants show overt behavioral peculiarities such as waltzing or circling, as suggested by their names. Hearing ability in many of them has only been assessed using the startle response, which, as previously noted, is a rather poor indicator of hearing. Those which have been studied physiologically fall into two categories: Some have a limited period during early adulthood when some response can be obtained, while others show no signs of response at any time during development (Steel et al., 1982). In *Bronx waltzer,* cochlear potentials can be recorded in adult animals, but the responses are abnormal at all stages (Bock, Yates, & Deol, 1982).

TECTORIAL MEMBRANE

The most striking example of abnormal development of the tectorial membrane is seen when an animal is made hypothyroid during the period of formation of the membrane. The tectorial membrane (TM) is an acellular, gel-like matrix composed largely of protein (Steel, 1980, 1983), which has a distinct shape and structure, and lies over the sensory hair cells in the cochlea. Ultrastructurally, it consists of two types of fibril: type A and type B, the latter often appearing as amorphous material. These fibrils appear to be produced by the underlying epithelial ridge cells during development. During this period, the epithelial cells (with the exception of the future hair cells) appear to be metabolically very active and have long microvilli on their apical surfaces showing close connections with the fibrillar TM material (Hinojosa, 1977). During normal development, the microvilli become shorter and less closely linked to the TM, while some of the greater epithelial ridge cells begin to degenerate and retract, allowing the inner spiral sulcus fluid-filled area to form.

When the animal is made hypothyroid by administration of an antithyroid drug such as propyl-thiouracil during the period of secretion of the TM mate-

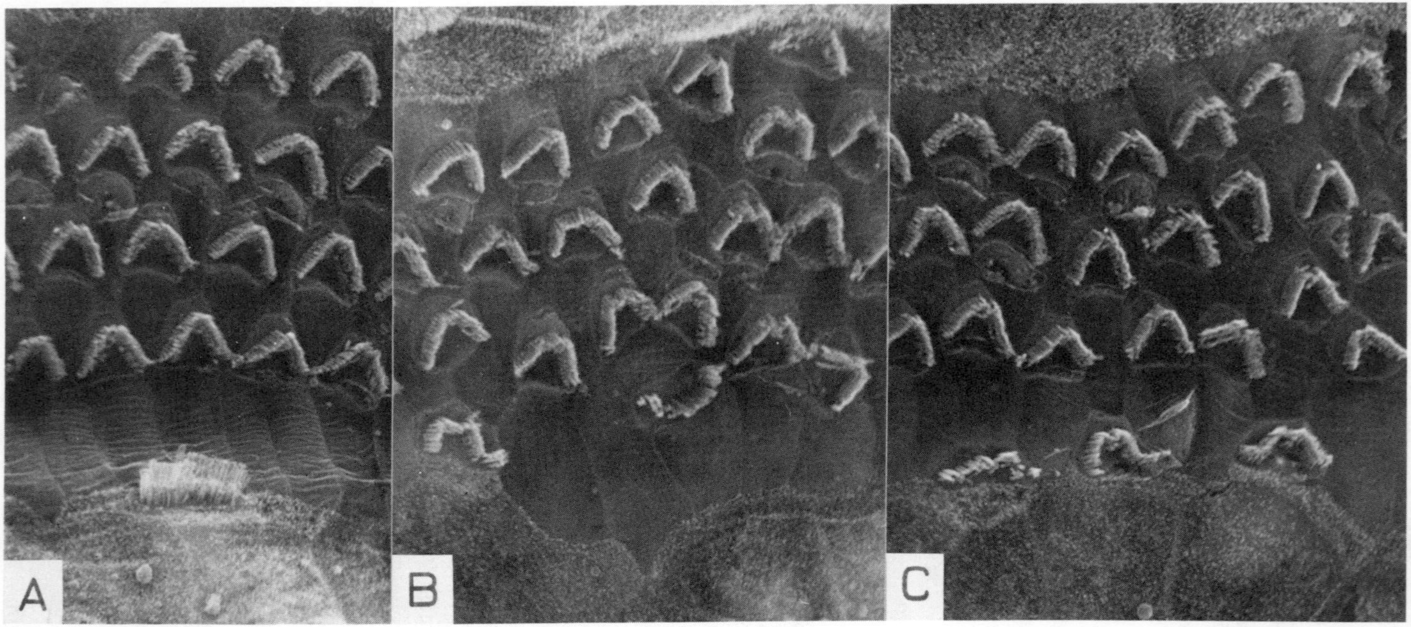

Figure 3. Three scanning electron micrographs taken from different regions of a *Bronx waltzer* (bv/bv) mouse mutant aged 8 months. (A) Only a few inner hair cells are present in bv/bv mice. Four rows of outer hair cells are often seen. (B) and (C) Outer hair cells are irregularly arranged in some regions of the cochlea, although most of them are present. Some of the hair cells which lie in the position of inner hair cells look like displaced outer hair cells.

rial, the process of secretion seems to be prolonged (Deol, 1973, 1976; Uziel, Gabrion, Ohresser, & Legrand, 1981; Steel, 1979). In particular, the epithelial cells filling the future inner spiral sulcus continue to secrete TM material for a much longer period than normal, which results in a large bulge of TM over this region. These cells eventually retract much later than they do in normal animals, but the abnormal bulge in the middle part of the TM remains. The distorted shape of the TM persists and is found in old animals, even when the period of experimentally induced hypothyroidism was limited to the critical period of development during which the TM was being secreted. Observations on these hypothyroid animals suggest that (a) regression of the epithelial cells to form the inner spiral sulcus is thyroxine-dependent, and (b) that the overall shape of the tectorial membrane is set in some unknown way at about the time that its secretion is normally completed. If the TM material is abnormal in size or shape at this point in development, then the abnormality is preserved, and this feature is illustrated in Figure 4. Hypothyroidism results in a delay in maturation of the middle ear and external ear canal and a delayed onset of cochlear potentials in the rat (Uziel, Rabie, & Marot, 1980). Cochlear potentials with raised thresholds can be recorded in adult mice made hypothyroid throughout development (Steel, 1979).

TM abnormalities may also be found in adult animals following degenerative changes in other parts of the cochlear duct. Some of these changes would probably be expected. For example, in cases in which OHCs and their stereocilia are degenerating, the TM often loses its close connections to the underlying organ of Corti and floats freely in the scala media, attached only by its connection to the limbus. More dramatic changes may be found in cochleo-saccular degeneration, where the TM may retract into the inner spiral sulcus following the progressive collapse of Reissner's membrane. Pederson, Mair, and Elverland (1980) observed in the deaf white cat that the TM collapsed onto the surface of the organ of Corti, with formation of deep indentations over stereocilia and microvilli, before Reissner's membrane had collapsed sufficiently to "push" the TM down in this region. They suggested that these changes, along with the appearance of calcium-containing spheres, may be a consequence of changes in endolymph. It seems most likely that most of the TM changes described in pathological adult cochleas are secondary to earlier changes in other parts of the cochlear duct and so represent degenerative changes rather than abnormalities of tectorial membrane development per se.

COCHLEAR INNERVATION

At the IHC base, both afferent and efferent nerve endings may be found at first during development, but the efferent endings progressively retract and

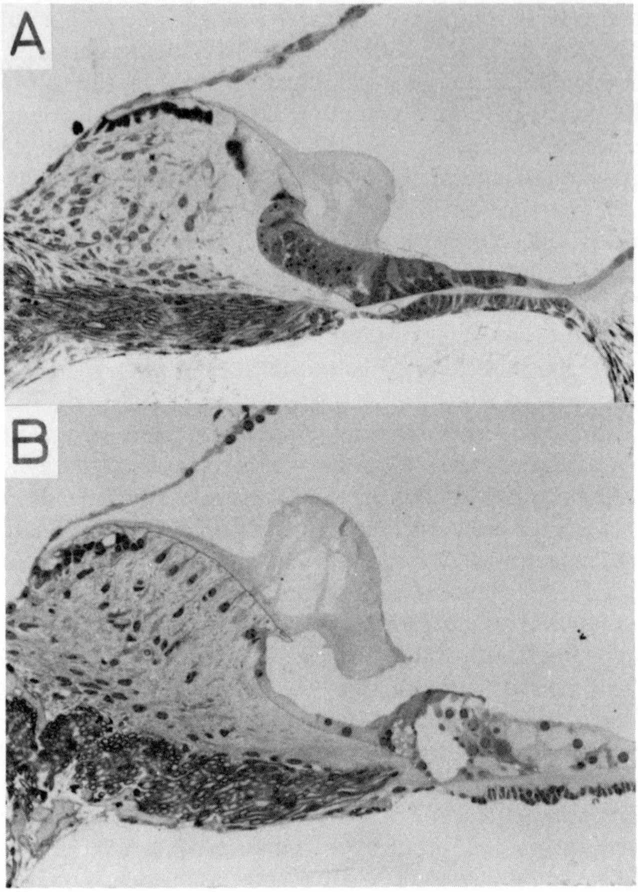

Figure 4. The tectorial membrane in mice treated with 6-n-propyl-2-thiouracil to induce hypothyroidism throughout their development. (A) 12 days after birth: Kolliker's organ has not yet retracted to form the inner spiral sulcus, and its abnormally long persistence appears to be associated with a prolonged period of secretion of the tectorial membrane material. This leads to an abnormal bulge in the tectorial membrane directly above Kolliker's organ. (B) 25 weeks old: The distorted shape of the tectorial membrane has been preserved, although the cells of Kolliker's organ have now retracted.

form synapses directly onto the afferent dendrites just below the hair cell (Lenoir, Shnerson, & Pujol, 1980; Pujol, Carlier, & Lenoir, 1980). The base of the OHC forms many synapses with afferent nerve endings during early development, but these later retract and are replaced by the large efferent nerve endings which are characteristic of adults. In an elegant experiment,

Pujol and Carlier (1982) prevented the arrival of the efferent endings by cutting the efferent bundle early in development. Efferents subsequently failed to arrive at the base of the OHCs, and the afferent nerve endings remained in place. OHC synapses with the persistent afferent nerve endings were not normal, however, because the hair cell developed postsynaptic cisterns.

Failure of efferent nerve endings to reach OHCs at the normal time or in the normal quantity has also been reported in rats made hypothyroid during the normal period of development (Uziel, Pujol, Legrand, & Legrand, 1983). In this case, the neurons may be physically hampered in their outgrowth toward OHCs by the retardation in the opening of tunnel and Nuel fluid spaces and the presence of amorphous material around the hair cells. IHC innervation is relatively normal in the hypothyroid rats.

Late arrival of efferents at the OHCs has also been reported in the *shaker-1* mouse mutant (Kikuchi & Hilding, 1965; Shnerson et al., 1983). It is interesting to note that this mutant, like the hypothyroid rats, showed a delayed opening of the Nuel and tunnel fluid areas. OHC afferent innervation is normal in 3-day-old mutants, but thereafter both afferent and efferent nerve endings progressively degenerate along with the hair cells. An abundance of efferent nerve endings appear on IHCs while IHC afferents degenerate. In the *deafness* mutant mouse, afferent and efferent synapses are present on IHCs at birth, although the afferent nerve endings are swollen; by 7 days old both types of nerve ending are degenerating (Pujol, Shnerson, Lenoir, & Deol, 1983). Innervation of OHCs in *deafness* mice shows retarded development (Pujol et al., 1983), and very few nerve endings remain in a recognizable condition by 15 days of age (Bock & Steel, 1983). In the *Bronx waltzer* mutant mouse, OHC innervation is nearly normal, while IHCs, where present, show distinctly abnormal synapses (Lenoir & Pujol, 1984).

Several reports have indicated early spiral ganglion cell degenerative changes or developmental anomalies in animals with hereditary deafness (i.e., animals with raised thresholds for behavioral or physiological responses to sound). In the *Bronx waltzer* mutant, the spiral ganglion cell population is about 50% that of normal mice and contains a larger proportion of type-II cells (those which innervate OHCs) than normal (Keithley & Feldman, 1983; Lenoir & Pujol, 1984). The reduction in cell numbers is apparent at birth, so it is most likely a developmental anomaly rather than the result of retrograde degeneration. In the *shaker-1* and *deafness* mouse mutants, spiral ganglion abnormalities parallel those of the organ of Corti, consisting of retarded maturation coupled with early onset of degeneration (Pujol et al., 1983; Shnerson et al., 1983). Certain deaf white cats show very early signs of spiral ganglion degeneration (Pujol, Rebillard, & Rebillard, 1977; Rebillard, Pujol, & Rebillard, 1981), although others do not, showing only retrograde degeneration (Elverland & Mair, 1980).

STRIA VASCULARIS

Abnormal strial development is frequently seen in animals with cochleo-saccular, or Scheibe type, degeneration of the inner ear. During the course of development of such animals, one of the earliest histological anomalies seen is atrophy of the stria, associated with a poor vascular supply (Mair & Elverland, 1977; Sugiura & Hilding, 1970; Johnsson, Hawkins, Muraski, & Preston, 1973; Hilding, 1973). The strial defect may be considered to be the primary abnormality in cochleo-saccular degeneration (Steel & Bock, 1983; Steel et al., 1983), since Reissner's membrane collapses and damage to the organ of Corti usually occurs after the strial abnormality becomes evident. An example of strial abnormality is shown in Figure 5.

A clue to the possible cause of the strial defect is provided by the fact that cochleo-saccular degeneration is generally associated with white spotting of the coat, caused by lack of recognizable melanocytes in the white areas. The spotting extends to internal organs which would normally be pigmented (Deol, 1971), including the stria vascularis. In mice carrying a spotting mutation, Deol (1970) reported that pigmentation of the stria was closely correlated with its condition: Unpigmented regions of the stria appeared thin with a reduced vascularity, while the few pigmented regions of the stria to be found had a normal histological appearance. The intermediate cells of the stria are similar to melanocytes (Hilding & Ginzberg, 1977), so a melanocyte defect might be associated with an intermediate cell defect, in turn leading to strial dysfunction and atrophy.

There are two observations supporting the suggestion that strial dysfunction might occur in animals with cochleo-saccular degeneration. Firstly, the scala media fluid volume is not maintained at its normal level, as shown by the usual collapse of Reissner's membrane, eventually obliterating scala media, or occasionally by dilation of scala media. Second, Suga and Hattler (1970) failed to record an endocochlear potential in a small number of animals with cochleo-saccular degeneration (2 deaf white cats and 3 deaf Dalmatian dogs). However, both of these observations have a number of alternative explanations, and so the evidence for strial dysfunction in cochleo-saccular degeneration can only be regarded as circumstantial at the moment.

Various physiological and behavioral tests have been used to assess hearing in animals with cochleo-saccular defects (e.g., Rebillard, Rebillard, & Pujol, 1981; Suga & Hattler, 1970; Flottorp & Foss, 1979). In general, there appears to be some variability in the expression of the defect, with some animals showing normal hearing, some unilateral impairment, and some bilateral impairment. All affected ears show either raised thresholds or no sign of responses to sound stimuli.

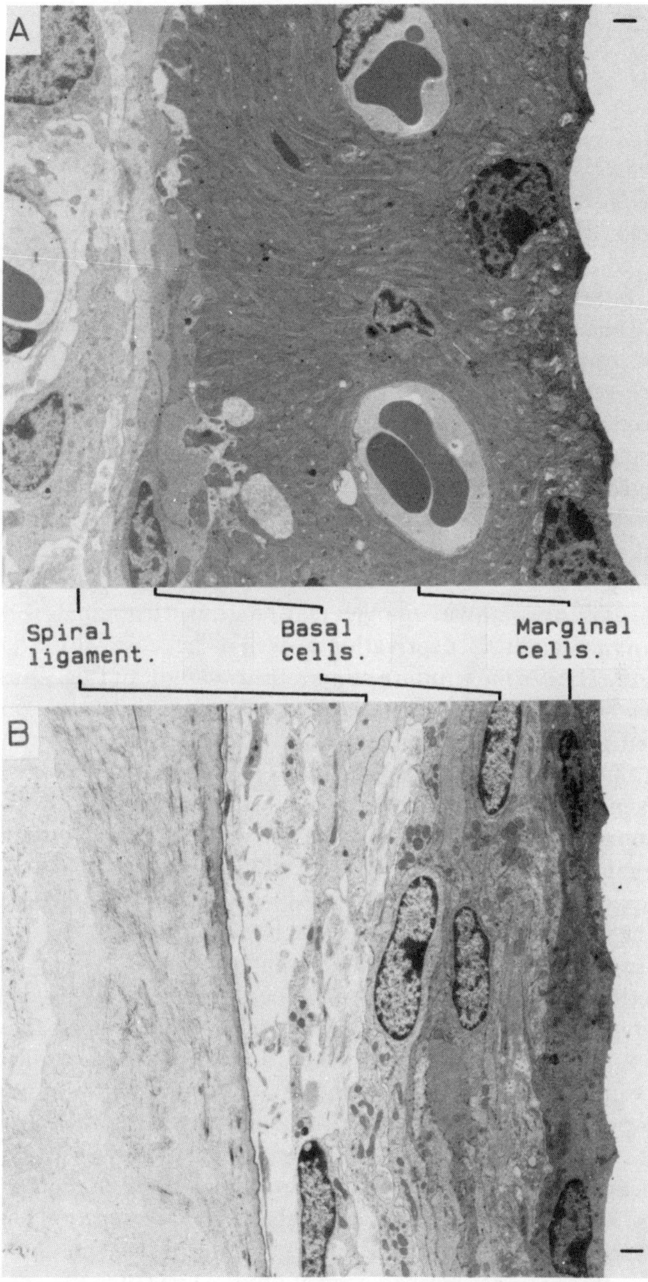

Figure 5. (A) The normal mouse stria vascularis. (B)Stria vascularis of the *viable dominant spotting* (W^v/W^v) mouse mutant, an example of cochleo-saccular degeneration, showing an abnormally thin marginal cell layer. Scale bar represents 1 μm.

CENTRAL AUDITORY PATHWAYS

The normal maturation of central auditory pathways is dependent upon normal sensory input during development. When the sound levels reaching the inner ear are attenuated by experimental interference or when the cochlea is destroyed, a range of anatomical anomalies in brainstem auditory nuclei are observed (e.g. Webster & Webster, 1977, 1979; Trune, 1983; Coleman, Blatchley, & Williams, 1982; Kitzes, Nordeen, & Arnaud, 1983). The specific qualitative changes in brainstem auditory nuclei following auditory deprivation are only found when the deprivation occurs sufficiently early in development (e.g., Webster, 1983), although the central auditory pathways may be subject to transneuronal degeneration following damage to the cochlea of adult animals. Physiological changes may also occur as a result of experimental auditory deprivation during development: For example, responses to high-intensity sounds have been reported to be larger in deprived animals compared with controls (Henry & Saleh, 1973; Saunders, Bock, James, & Chen, 1972).

Central auditory pathway changes may be studied in animals with genetically determined auditory deprivation as well as in those with experimental deprivation. The *deafness* mouse mutant is an example of this. *Deafness* mutants show no signs of stimulus-related cochlear activity at any time during the normal period of development (Steel & Bock, 1980), and there are no gross histological CNS abnormalities (Steel & Bock, 1984). However, evoked responses measured in the inferior colliculus in response to direct electrical stimulation of the contralateral cochlear nerve are considerably larger in the *deafness* mutants than in control mice (Steel & Bock, 1984). The larger evoked response is most likely due to an increased rate of discharge of single units in the inferior colliculus (Horner & Bock, 1984b).

More specific genetically determined central auditory system defects have been described in several other animals. The most extensively studied of these is the *quivering* mouse mutant. In *quivering* mice, cochlear anatomy and function appear to be normal, while there are minor anomalies in single unit responses in the cochlear nucleus and major abnormalities in inferior colliculus responses (Bock, Frank, Steel, & Deol, 1983; Horner & Bock, 1984a, 1985). The combination of normal response thresholds of the cochlea and elevated thresholds in the inferior colliculus of *quivering* mutants suggests that this mouse has a central deafness. Central auditory dysfunction has been described in several other animals, although in none of these has it been clearly shown that there is a deafness of central origin. The Gunn rat, which develops neonatal hyperbilirubinemia, shows normal cochlear anatomy and function, but surface responses show an abnormal waveform and amplitude of waves II to IV, suggesting functional damage in the brainstem auditory pathways (Uziel, Marot, & Pujol, 1983). Surface responses to clicks in the *quaking* mutant mouse show an increased latency of the first four far-field potentials compared with normal mice (Shah & Salamy, 1980). However, there was apparently no difference in threshold between the abnormal animals and controls in the latter two examples. Extensive degeneration of the central auditory pathways has been described in hereditary epilepsy in *Peromyscus* mice (Ross, 1962), and morphological defects have been demonstrated in the cochlear nucleus of the *reeler* mouse mutant (Martin, 1981a, b), but it is not known whether the central defects in these two animals were a consequence of a peripheral cochlear abnormality. Finally, various anatomical abnormalities have been observed in brainstem auditory nuclei of albino animals (Conlee, Parks, Romero, & Creel, 1984); the brainstem evoked potentials to monaural stimuli recorded from ipsi- and contralateral electrodes suggest that there may be asymmetries in central auditory function in both albino cats (Creel, Conlee, & Parks, 1983) and humans (Creel, Garber, King, & Witkop, 1980).

Experimental interference with brain development can affect the auditory pathways. For example, rats treated with p-chlorophenylalanine and phenylalanine during the critical period of development show reduced myelin deposition and increased latencies of brainstem evoked potentials in comparison with that of control rats (Shah, Bhargava, Johnson, & McKean, 1978).

CONCLUSION

Although this review has focused upon the location of the primary (or at least the earliest detectable) abnormality, defects in any part of the auditory system might be expected to lead to changes in other parts of the auditory system. The secondary changes may be developmental or degenerative in character.

Some examples of developmental changes which seem likely to be secondary in origin were described in the previous section, where central auditory pathway development appears to be dependent upon normal peripheral function. However, secondary anomalies are not restricted to the effects of ascending afferents; for example, the failure of efferent nerve endings to reach OHCs in animals showing retarded development of the organ of Corti may be a direct consequence of the hair cell anomaly.

Secondary degenerative changes are also commonly found. For instance, early stria vascularis defects as found in cochleo-saccular degeneration lead eventually to collapse of Reissner's membrane and damage to the organ of Corti. Hair cell abnormalities often lead to retrograde degeneration of the afferent nerve endings and spiral ganglion cells (e.g., Steel & Bock, 1984), while transneuronal degeneration may extend to second or higher order neurons in the auditory system (e.g., Kitzes et al., 1983).

We have seen that a simple developmental defect may lead to a complex combination of pathological features in the mature auditory system. The array of secondary changes may obscure the original site of the lesion, and so if an understanding of the primary defect is sought, it will usually be necessary to study the course of development. A better understanding of which defects are primary and which are secondary in the range of pathologies which exist in humans might indicate ways in which the abnormal course of development might be modified by clinical intervention. Since developmental studies of particular diseases are virtually impossible in humans, such studies on animals with auditory system defects can be extremely valuable for our understanding of abnormal developmental processes.

REFERENCES

Aase, J.M. (1980). Microtia-clinical observations. In: R.J. Gorlin (Ed.) *Morphogenesis and malformation of the ear* (pp. 289–297). New York: Liss.

Bock, G.R., Frank, M.P., Steel, K.P., & Deol, M.S. (1983). The quivering mutant mouse: Hereditary deafness of central origin. *Acta Otolaryngologica, 96,* 371–377.

Bock, G.R., & Steel, K.P. (1983). Inner ear pathology in the deafness mutant mouse. *Acta Otolaryngologica, 96,* 39–47.

Bock, G.R., Yates, G.K., & Deol, M.S. (1982). Cochlear potentials in the Bronx waltzer mutant mouse. *Neuroscience Letters, 34,* 19–25.

Chole, R.A., & Henry, K.R. (1983). Otosclerotic lesions in the inbred LP/J mouse. *Science, 221,* 881–882.

Coleman, J., Blatchley, B.J., & Williams, J.E. (1982). Development of the dorsal and ventral cochlear nuclei in rat and effects of acoustic deprivation. *Developmental Brain Research, 4,* 119–123.

Conlee, J.W., Parks, T.N., Romero, C., & Creel, D.J. (1984). Auditory brainstem anomalies in albino cats: II. Neuronal atrophy in the superior olive. *Journal of Comparative Neurology, 225,* 141–148.

Creel, D., Conlee, J.W., & Parks, T.N. (1983). Auditory brainstem anomalies in albino cats: I. Evoked potential studies. *Brain Research, 260,* 1–9.

Creel, D., Garber, S.R., King, R.A., & Witkop, C.J. (1980). Auditory brainstem anomalies in human albinos. *Science, 209,* 1253–1255.

Deol, M.S. (1966). Influence of the neural tube on the differentiation of the inner ear in the mammalian embryo. *Nature, 209,* 219–220.

Deol, M.S. (1970). The origin of the acoustic ganglion and effects of the gene dominant spotting (W^v) in the mouse. *Journal of Embryology and Experimental Morphology, 23,* 773–784.

Deol, M.S. (1971). Spotting genes and internal pigmentation patterns in the mouse. *Journal of Embryology and Experimental Morphology, 26,* 123–133.

Deol, M.S. (1973). An experimental approach to the understanding and treatment of hereditary syndromes with congenital deafness and hypothyroidism. *Journal of Medical Genetics, 10,* 235–242.

Deol, M.S. (1976). The role of thyroxine in the differentiation of the organ of Corti. *Acta Otolaryngologica, 81,* 429–435.

Deol, M.S. (1980). Genetic malformations of the inner ear in the mouse and in man. In R.J. Gorlin (Ed.), *Morphogenesis and malformation of the ear* (pp. 243–261).

Deol, M.S. (1981). The inner ear in Bronx waltzer mice. *Acta Otolaryngologica, 92,* 331–336.

Deol, M.S., & Gluecksohn-Waelsch, S. (1979). The role of inner hair cells in hearing. *Nature, 278,* 250–252.

Elverland, H.H., & Mair, I.W.S. (1980). Hereditary deafness in the cat. An electron microscopic study of the spiral ganglion. *Acta Otolaryngologica, 90,* 360–369.

Flottorp, G., & Foss, I. (1979). Development of hearing in hereditarily deaf white mink (Hedlund) and normal mink (standard) and the subsequent deterioration of the auditory response in Hedlund mink. *Acta Otolaryngologica, 87,* 16–27.

Grcen, M.C. (1981). *Genetic variants and strains of the laboratory mouse.* Stuttgart, W. Germany: Gustav Fischer.

Grüneberg, H. (1956). Hereditary lesions of the labyrinth in the mouse. *British Medical Bulletin, 12,* 153–157.

Henry, K.R. (1983). Abnormal auditory development resulting from exposure to ototoxic chemicals, noise, and auditory restriction. In R. Romand (Ed.), *Development of auditory and vestibular systems.* New York: Academic Press.

Henry, K.R., & Saleh, M. (1973). Recruitment deafness: Functional effect of priming-induced audiogenic seizures in mice. *Journal of Comparative and Physiological Psychology, 84,* 430–435.

Hilding, D.A. (1973). Vascular abnormalities in animal inherited deafness. In A.J.D. de Lorenzo (Ed.), *Vascular disorders and hearing defects.* Baltimore, MD: University Park Press.

Hilding, D.A., & Ginzberg, R.D. (1977). Pigmentation of the stria vascularis: The contribution of neural crest melanocytes. *Acta Otolaryngologica, 84,* 24–37.

Hinojosa, R. (1977). A note on development of Corti's organ. *Acta Otolaryngologica, 84,* 238–251.

Horner, K.C., & Bock, G. R. (1984a), Single unit responses in the cochlear nucleus of the deaf *quivering* mouse. *Hearing Research, 13,* 63–72.

Horner, K.C., & Bock, G.R. (1984b). Inferior colliculus single unit responses to peripheral electrical stimulation in normal and congenitally deaf mice. *Developmental Brain Research, 15,* 33–43.

Horner, K.C., & Bock, G.R. (1985). Combined electrophysiological and autoradiographic delimitation of retrocochlear dysfunction in a mouse mutant. *Brain Research, 331,* 217–223.

Johnsson, L.G., Hawkins, J.E., Muraski, A.A., & Preston, R.E. (1973). Vascular anatomy and pathology of the cochlea in Dalmatian dogs. In A.J.D. de Lorenzo (Ed.), *Vascular disorders and hearing defects.* Baltimore, MD: University Park Press.

Kacser, H., Mya Mya, K., & Bulfield, G. (1979). Endogenous teratogenesis in maternal histidinaemia. In F.A. Hommes (Ed.), *Models for the study of inborn errors of metabolism* Amsterdam, The Netherlands: Elsevier.

Kacser, H., Mya Mya, K., Duncker, M., Wright, A.F., Bulfield, G., McLaren, A., & Lyon, M.F. (1977). Maternal histidine metabolism and its effect on foetal development in the mouse. *Nature, 265,* 262–266.

Keithley, E.M., & Feldman, M.L. (1983). The spiral ganglion and hair cells of Bronx waltzer mice. *Hearing Research, 12,* 381–391.

Kikuchi, K., & Hilding, D.A. (1965). The defective organ of Corti in shaker-1 mice. *Acta Otolaryngologica, 60,* 287–303.

Kitzes, L.M., Nordeen, K.W., Arnaud, A., & Semple, M.N. (1983). Structural and functional consequences of neonatal cochlear ablation. In W.R. Webster & L.M. Aitkin (Eds.), *Mechanisms of hearing.* (pp. 120–122). Melbourne, Australia: Monash University Press.

Konigsmark, B.W., & Gorlin, R.J. (1976). *Genetic and metabolic deafness.* Philadelphia: Saunders.

Lenoir, M., & Pujol, R. (1984). Age-related structural investigation of the *Bronx waltzer* mutant mouse cochlea: Scanning and transmission electron microscopy. *Hearing Research, 13,* 123–134.

Lenoir, M., Shnerson, A., & Pujol, R. (1980). Cochlear receptor development in the rat with emphasis on synaptogenesis. *Anatomy and Embryology, 160,* 253–262.

Mair, I.W.S., & Elverland, H.H. (1977). Hereditary deafness in the cat. An electron microscopic study of the stria vascularis and Reissner's membrane. *Archives of Otorhinolaryngology, 217,* 199–217.

Martin, M.R. (1981a). Acetylcholinesterase-positive fibers and cell bodies in the cochlear nuclei of normal and reeler mutant mice. *Journal of Comparative Neurology, 197,* 153–167.

Martin, M.R. (1981b). Morphology of the cochlear nucleus of the normal and reeler mutant mouse. *Journal of Comparative Neurology, 197,* 141–152.

Melnick, M. (1980). The etiology of external ear malformations and its relation to abnormalities of the middle ear, inner ear, and other organ systems. In R.J. Gorlin (Ed.), *Morphogenesis and malformation of the ear* (pp. 303–331). New York: Liss.

Morriss, G.M. (1972). Morphogenesis of the malformations induced in rat embryos by maternal hypervitaminosis A. *Journal of Anatomy, 113,* 241–250.

Nadol, J.B. (1980). Pathoembryology of the middle ear. In R.J. Gorlin (Ed.), *Morphogenesis and malformation of the ear* (pp. 181–209). New York: Liss.

Osako, S., & Hilding, D.A. (1971). Electron microscopic studies of capillary permeability in normal and Ames waltzer deaf mice. *Acta Otolaryngologica, 71,* 365–376.

Pedersen, E.K., Mair, I.W.S., & Elverland, H.H. (1980). Hereditary deafness in the cat: An electron-microscopic study of the tectorial membrane. *Archives of Otorhinolaryngology, 229,* 55–68.

Phelps, P.D. (1974). Congenital lesions of the inner ear, demonstrated by tomography. *Archives of Otolaryngology, 100,* 11–18.

Phelps, P.D., Sheldon, P.W.E., & Lloyd, G.A.S. (1976). Hearing in patients with congenital deformity of the inner ear. *Clinical Otolaryngology, 1,* 31–38.

Pujol, R., & Carlier, E. (1982). Cochlear synaptogenesis after sectioning the efferent bundle. *Developmental Brain Research, 3,* 151–154.

Pujol, R., Carlier, E., & Lenoir, M. (1980). Ontogenetic approach to inner and outer hair cell function. *Hearing Research, 2,* 423–430.

Pujol, R., Rebillard, M., & Rebillard, G. (1977). Primary neural disorders in the deaf white çat cochlea. *Acta Otolaryngologica, 83,* 59–64.

Pujol, R., Shnerson, A., Lenoir, M., & Deol, M.S. (1983). Early degeneration of sensory and ganglion cells in the inner ear of mice with uncomplicated genetic deafness (dn): Preliminary observations. *Hearing Research, 12,* 578–63.

Rebillard, M., Pujol, R., & Rebillard, G. (1981). Variability of the hereditary deafness in the white cat. II. Histology. *Hearing Research, 5,* 189–200.

Rebillard, M., Rebillard, G., & Pujol, R. (1981). Variability of the hereditary deafness in the white cat. I. Physiology. *Hearing Research, 5,* 179–187.

Ross, M.D. (1962). Auditory pathways of the epileptic waltzing mouse: I. A comparison of the acoustic pathways of the normal mouse with those of the totally deaf epileptic waltzer. *Journal of Comparative Neurology, 119,* 317–339.

Rubel, E.W. (1978). Ontogeny of structure and function in the vertebrates auditory system. In M. Jacobson (Ed.), *Handbook of sensory physiology* (Vol. 9) (pp. 135–237). Berlin: Springer-Verlag.

Ruben, R.J., & Van de Water, T.R. (1983). Recent advances in the developmental biology of the inner ear. In S.E. Gerber & G. T. Mencher (Eds.), *Development of auditory Behaviour* (pp. 3–35). New York: Grune & Stratton.

Sando, I. (1980). Discussion of inner ear anomalies—Reply to Dr. Schuknecht. In R.J. Gorlin (Ed.), *Morphogenesis and malformation of the ear* (pp. 73–82). New York: Liss.

Saunders, J.C., & Bock, G.R. (1978). Influences of early auditory trauma on auditory development. In G. Gottlieb (Ed.), *Studies on the development of behavior and the nervous system* (Vol. 4, pp. 249–287). New York: Academic Press.

Saunders, J.C., Bock, G.R., James, R., & Chen, C.S. (1972). Effects of priming for audiogenic seizure on auditory evoked responses in the cochlear nucleus and inferior colliculus of BALB/c mice. *Experimental Neurology, 37,* 388–394.

Schuknecht, H.F. (1980). Dysmorphogenesis of the inner ear. In R.J. Gorlin (Ed.), *Morphogenesis and malformation of the ear* (pp. 47–71). New York: Liss.

Shah, S.N., Bhargava, V.K., Johnson, R.C., & McKean, C.M. (1978). Latency changes in brain stem auditory evoked potentials associated with impaired brain myelination. *Experimental Neurology, 58,* 111–118.

Shah, S.N., & Salamy, A. (1980). Auditory-evoked far-field potentials in myelin deficient mutant quaking mice. *Neuroscience, 5,* 2321–2323.

Shnerson, A., Lenoir, M., Van de Water, T.R., & Pujol, R. (1983). The pattern of sensorineural degeneration in the cochlea of the deaf shaker-1 mouse: Ultrastructural observations. *Developmental Brain Research, 9,* 305–315.

Steel, K.P. (1979). An animal model for congenital deafness with hypothyroidism. Unpublished data.

Steel, K.P. (1980). The proteins of normal and abnormal tectorial membranes. *Acta Otolaryngologica, 89,* 27–32.

Steel, K.P. (1983). Review. The tectorial membrane of mammals. *Hearing Research, 9,* 327–359.

Steel, K.P., & Bock, G.R. (1980). The nature of inherited deafness in deafness mice. *Nature, 288,* 159–161.

Steel, K.P., & Bock, G.R. (1983). Hereditary inner ear abnormalities in animals. Relationships with human abnormalities. *Archives of Otolaryngology, 109,* 22–29.

Steel, K.P., & Bock, G.R. (1984). Electrically evoked responses in animals with progressive spiral ganglion degeneration. *Hearing Research, 15,* 59–67.

Steel, K.P., Niaussat, M.M., & Bock, G.R. (1983). The genetics of hearing. In J.F. Willott (Ed.), *The auditory psychobiology of the mouse* (pp. 341–394). Springfield, IL: Charles C. Thomas.

Suga, F., & Hattler, K.W. (1970). Physiological and histopathological correlates of hereditary deafness in animals. *Laryngoscope, 80,* 81–104.

Sugiura, A., & Hilding, D.A. (1970), Stria vascularis of deaf Hedlund mink. *Acta Otolaryngologica, 69,* 160–171.

Trune, D.R. (1983). Influence of neonatal cochlear removal on the development of mouse cochlear nucleus: III. Its efferent projections to inferior colliculus. *Developmental Brain Research, 9,* 1–12.

Uziel, A., Gabrion, J., Ohresser, M., & Legrand, C. (1981). Effects of hypothyroidism on the structural development of the organ of Corti. *Acta Otolaryngologica, 92,* 469–480.

Uziel, A., Legrand, C., & Rabie, A. (1985). Corrective effects of thyroxine on cochlear abnormalities induced by congenital hypothyroidism in the rat. I. Morphological study. *Developmental Brain Research, 19* 111–122.

Uziel, A., Marot, M., & Pujol, R. (1983). The Gunn rat: an experimental model for central deafness. *Acta Otolaryngologica, 95,* 651–656.

Uziel, A., Pujol, R., Legrand, C., & Legrand, J. (1983). Cochlear synaptogenesis in the hypothyroid rat. *Developmental Brain Research, 7,* 295–301.

Uziel, A., Rabie, A., & Marot, M. (1980). The effect of hypothyroidism on the onset of cochlear potentials in developing rats. *Brain Research, 182,* 172–175.

Webster, D.B. (1983). Late onset of auditory deprivation does not affect brainstem auditory neuron soma size. *Hearing Research, 12,* 145–147.
Webster, D.B., & Webster, M. (1977). Neonatal sound deprivation affects brain stem auditory nuclei. *Archives of Otolaryngology, 103,* 392–396.
Webster, D.B., & Webster, M. (1979). Effects of neonatal conductive hearing loss on brain stem auditory nuclei. *Annals of Otology, Rhinology and Laryngology, 88,* 684–688.
Wright, J.L.W., Phelps, P.D., & Friedmann, I. (1976). Temporal bone studies in anancephaly. *Journal of Laryngology and Otology, 90,* 919–927.

3 Development of the Anuran Auditory System*

Albert S. Feng
William P. Shofner
Department of Physiology and Biophysics
University of Illinois
524 Burrill Hall
407 S. Goodwin Avenue
Urbana, IL 61801

INTRODUCTION

Anurans (frogs and toads) typically exist in two different forms during their life cycle after hatching from the egg, first as aquatic larvae or tadpoles and then following metamorphosis as terrestrial organisms. As the ecology of the anuran changes during metamorphosis, there are parallel changes in the morphology, physiology, and biochemistry of the anuran's organ systems (see Gilbert & Frieden, 1981, for reviews) which allow the animal to live successfully in these respective environments.

One important aspect of an animal's ecology is the acoustic environment. Sound consists of a far-field pressure wave and a near-field particle displacement wave. In air, the far field generally predominates while the near field is negligible. On the other hand, both the far and near fields are strongly present underwater. The sound detecting systems change during development from the lateral line and auditory system in tadpoles which detect the near and far fields of underwater sound, respectively, to an auditory system in terrestrial adults which is specialized for the detection of airborne pressure waves. The detection of airborne sound presents an additional problem to anurans exiting from water to land due to the impedance mismatch between the air and fluid-filled inner ear. This problem, however, is solved by the development of a middle ear apparatus during metamorphosis. As the body size (and age) of postmetamorphic anurans continues to increase, there are concurrent changes in the size of the auditory structures resulting in changes

---

* Research in the authors' laboratory is supported by grants from the National Science Foundation and the Research Board of the University of Illinois. We thank Pat Due for her typing and Gerhard Neuweiler for his helpful comments on an earlier draft of this article.

Current address for W. Shofner: Department of Biomedical Engineering, The Johns Hopkins University School of Medicine, 720 Rutland Avenue, Baltimore, MD 21205.

in auditory function. This chapter describes our present understanding of the morphological and physiological development of the anuran auditory system as well as the development of acoustically guided behavior in anurans through their aquatic and terrestrial life. The development of the lateral line system has been previously reviewed (M.R. Wright, 1951; Russell, 1976) and will not be discussed here.

Larvae of various anuran species develop at varying paces, and their life spans in larval form range from 1–3 months to 1–2 years depending in part on the geographical location and climate of the breeding area. Thus, when discussing the development of larval anurans, it is often useful to follow the course of development by presenting stage numbers based on the external morphology of the tadpole, and several investigators have described a variety of staging schemes. Shumway (1940) presents a staging scheme from fertilization through the embryonic period (prior to limb bud formation), while Taylor and Kollros (1946) describe a scheme for the metamorphic period from limb bud formation through metamorphosis. Complete staging schemes encompassing the entire larval period from fertilization through metamorphosis have been described by Witschi (1956) and Gosner (1960). A comparison of the staging schemes along with those of other authors can be found in Just, Kraus-Just, and Chech (1981). In the following sections, the stage number of tadpoles will follow the scheme of Witschi (Fig. 1).

ONTOGENY OF ACOUSTICALLY GUIDED BEHAVIOR

Phylogenetically, anurans represent the first terrestrial vertebrates to produce and use vocalizations as part of their behavioral repertoire. In many species, vocal communication plays an important role in behaviors ranging from territorial defense to reproduction, and calls are classifiable according to the particular behaviors that they subserve. For example, adult male anurans produce a species-specific mating call which is used to attract conspecific females during the mating season, and this call serves as a mechanism in maintaining reproductive isolation from other sympatric anuran species. Mating call discrimination is primarily based on the animal's ability to detect the differences in the spectral and temporal patterns of the calls (Capranica, 1965, 1966; Gerhardt, 1974, 1981; Straughan, 1975). Other calls can play a role in male–male interactions. Territorial calls, for instance, are used by a dominant male in the defense of high-quality oviposition sites, while release calls are given by a male when clasped by another male. Unreceptive females also can produce a release call when clasped by a male. Warning calls are produced by anurans during escape behaviors. These calls vary from one another in their spectral and temporal characteristics. Tadpoles are not known to produce sonic signals, but they appear to be equipped with an acoustic apparatus

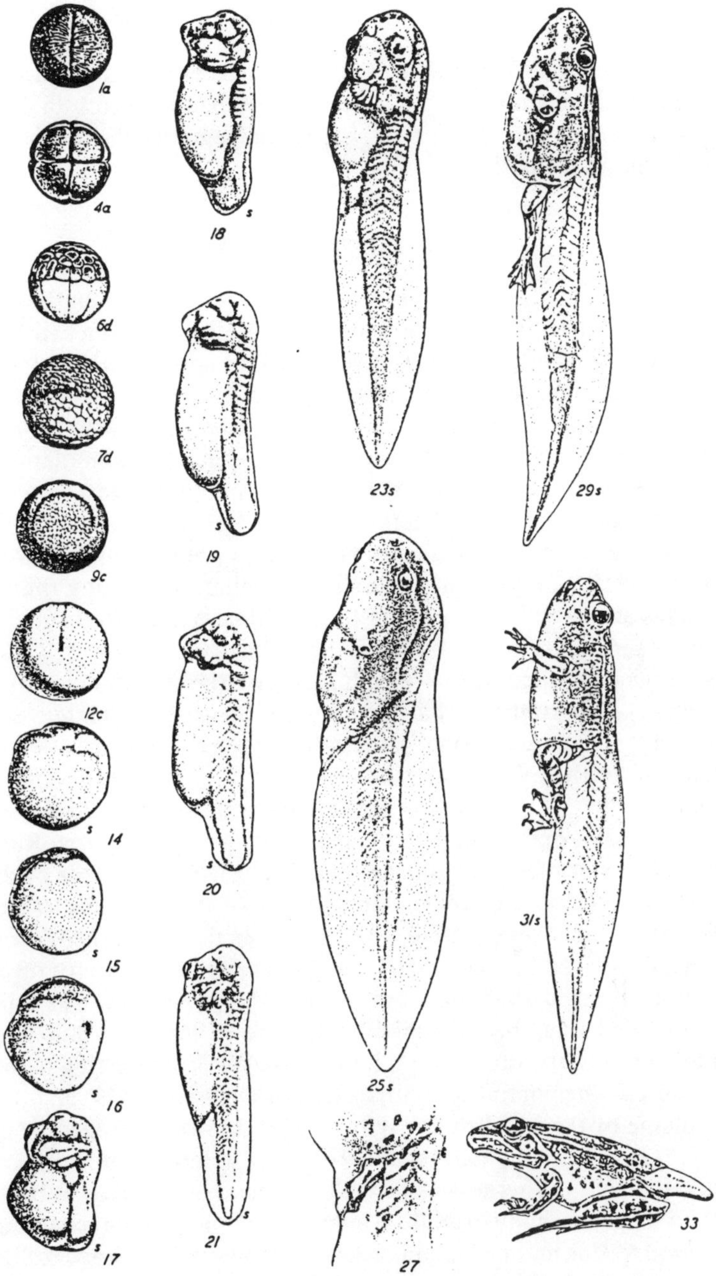

Figure 1. Schematic diagrams showing body (or hindleg) morphologies at various embryonic stages (1–33) of anuran development: a: frontal view; c: caudal view; d: dorsal view; s: lateral view; v: ventral view. (Modified from Witschi, 1956, by permission of the publisher.)

for sound detection. We shall first examine the potential for underwater acoustic communication in tadpoles, which will be followed by a discussion on how apparent age may affect acoustically guided behavior in post-metamorphic anurans.

Underwater Acoustic Communication in Tadpoles

Before examining the behaviors in tadpoles which may be acoustically guided, we first must ask whether the tadpole auditory system can detect underwater acoustic pressure waves. A review of the adult's underwater hearing capacity may help us to understand such potential in tadpoles. While the auditory system of adult bullfrogs (*Rana catesbeiana*) is adapted for detecting airborne sounds, it is also sensitive to underwater acoustic stimulation (Lombard, Fay, & Werner, 1981), and the effective stimulus appears to be pressure rather than particle velocity (Hetherington & Lombard, 1982). Recordings made from both whole animal and partial head preparations show that the amplitude of the microphonic potential is similar, suggesting that the air-filled lungs and mouth cavity are not involved in pressure transduction. On the other hand, when the air-filled middle ear cavity is filled with water, there is a significant reduction in the amplitude of the microphonic response. These observations indicate that pulsations of the air-filled middle ear cavity may directly stimulate the inner ear (Hetherington & Lombard, 1982). Thus, the function of the middle ear cavity of adult anurans in the water may be analogous to that of the gas-filled swim bladder in fish (van Bergeijk, 1967). A similar type of operation may be present in anuran tadpoles. Ranid tadpoles possess a bronchial columella (Fig. 5) at their later stages of development which connects the bronchial membrane of the bronchus to the round window of the inner ear (Witschi, 1949, 1955), analogous to the Weberian ossicles in fish (see van Bergeijk, 1967, and Fay & Popper, 1980, for reviews). It is therefore thought that the lungs in the tadpole may serve as a pressure transducer and that the bronchial columellae in turn transmit vibrations from the lungs to the inner ear (Witschi, 1949). It is interesting to note that the measured lung volume in bullfrog tadpoles (stages 28–29) and the measured volume of the middle ear cavity in adult bullfrogs ranged from 0.14–0.42 cm^3 (van Bergeijk, 1957) and 0.2–0.4 cm^3 (Hetherington & Lombard, 1982), respectively. Therefore, one might expect that the lungs of the tadpole and the middle ear cavity in adults would have similar resonance frequencies. In addition to this middle ear apparatus, tadpoles in later stages of development also possess hair cells and neural connections, which will be discussed in more detail in later sections. Thus, it appears that morphologically, tadpoles have the potential for detecting an underwater acoustic pressure wave, but conclusive evidence for such capacity is not available.

At the present time, little is known about the behavior of anuran tadpoles in response to underwater sound. Spaeti (1978) played pure tones between 1000–2000 Hz of unknown sound pressure levels to *Rana temporaria* tadpoles. Tadpoles in later stages of development (stages 26–27) possessing completely formed bronchial columellae showed wriggling and swimming movements in response to tones. However, it is unclear whether the tadpoles were responding to near-field particle displacements or to the far-field pressure wave.

One potential use of underwater sound by tadpoles is in aggregation behaviors. Katz, Potel, and Wasserug (1981) have shown that in the dark, aggregates of *Xenopus laevis* tadpoles still show parallel orientation with respect to their nearest neighbors. The lateral line system was presumed to be involved in this behavior. In addition, anuran tadpoles have also been shown to prefer to aggregate with sibling tadpoles over nonsiblings (Waldman & Adler, 1979; Waldman, 1981; Blaustein & O'Hara, 1982). However, neither Katz et al. (1981) nor Blaustein and O'Hara (1982) found any evidence that tadpoles produce sounds. They therefore concluded that auditory cues are not important in these aggregation behaviors but rather chemical cues appear to be more essential for kin recognition. In the following section we shall review how sound progressively influences the life of terrestrial anurans.

Ontogeny of Airborn Acoustic Communication

The behavioral responses of newly metamorphosed anurans is poorly understood. Bullfrogs (*Rana catesbeiana*), for example, do not begin to produce a mating call until they are one year past metamorphosis (Dickerson, 1969), which shall be considered as the age when they become capable of mating. While newly metamorphosed bullfrogs have been heard to give an alarm call (Wright, 1914), the spectral structure of this juvenile call is unknown. As bullfrogs grow older, their body size continues to increase and their mating call changes accordingly. Unfortunately, the exact age–body-size relationship has not been established for this species, and generally the body size is used to depict the developmental stage of an individual. In this chapter, adult bullfrogs will be those which are 2–3 years past metamorphosis and beyond. The ontogeny of various anuran species typically follows a species-specific time course.

The mating success of reproductively mature male anurans appears to be related to age for at least some species. For example, in *Rana catesbeiana* (Howard, 1978, 1979), *Rana sylvatica* (Howard, 1980), *Rana clamitans* (Wells, 1977), *Physalaemus postulosus* (Ryan, 1980), *Bufo quercicus* (Wilbur, Rubenstein, & Fairchild, 1978), *Bufo woodhousei fowleri* (Fairchild, 1981), and *Bufo americanus* (Gatz, 1981), the larger and older males are more successful in mating than are smaller, younger males (Fig. 2). However, the reproductive success of males in other species does not appear to be

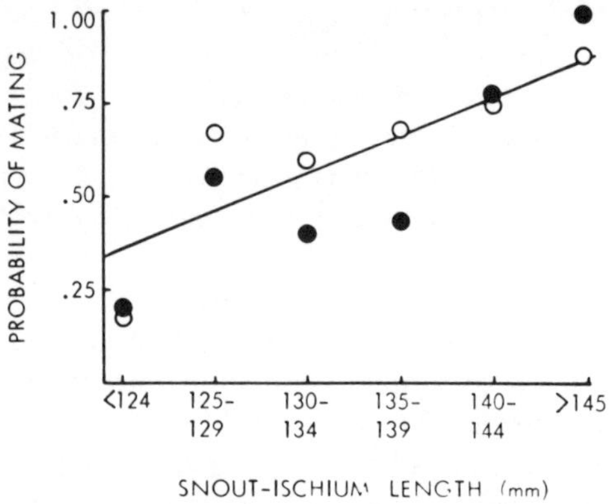

Figure 2. Regression analysis of the probability of mating success in males versus male size. Closed circles = males in 1975; open circles = males in 1976. Regression equation is $Y = 0.02X - 2.64$; $R^2 = .72$; $p = .0005$; $SE = 0.14$. (Reproduced from Howard, 1978, by permission of the publisher.)

related to age or size, i.e., *Bufo woodhousei* (Sullivan, 1981, 1983b), *Bufo cognatus* (Sullivan, 1983a), *Bufo americanus* (Wilber et al., 1978; Kruse, 1981), *Bufo terrestris* (Wilbur et al., 1978), *Hyla cinerea* (Gerhardt, 1982) and *Hyla versicolor* (Fellers, 1979). For *Bufo americanus,* it is unclear why Gatz (1981) found a positive correlation with size (age) and mating success, while Kruse (1981) and Wilber et al. (1978) found no correlation. Perhaps this discrepancy is related to differences in the ecology of different geographic regions. In several species the greater mating success of larger males is primarily because they are stronger and can more readily displace smaller males in amplexus (Davies & Halliday, 1979) or they defend superior quality of territory or resource (Howard, 1978).

In the rest of anurans studied thus far, however, the greater success of larger, older males in mating appears to be related to characteristics of their mating calls. For example, larger males often call for longer periods of time than do smaller males (Gatz, 1981) and produce calls with lower pulse rates and longer call durations (Fairchild, 1981). In addition, larger males produce mating calls having lower dominant frequency components (Capranica, 1965, 1966; Oldham & Gerhardt, 1975; Ryan, 1980; Fairchild, 1981), in part due to their more massive vocal cords (Martin, 1971). Of these studies, the most conclusive evidence showing that females indeed select larger males on the basis of the quality of the male's call has come from the Ryan's (1980) study of *Physalaemus postulosus.*

In bullfrogs, behavioral significance of the lower-frequency components in the mating calls of larger, older males has been elegantly demonstrated (Capranica, 1965, 1966, 1968). The mating call of a large adult male bullfrog

(> 150 mm) has a bimodal spectral energy distribution with low and high frequency peaks centered around 200–300 Hz and 1400–1500 Hz, respectively, as shown in Figure 3C. When the bullfrog mating call is presented to a group of adult male bullfrogs, it evokes a high level of mating calls from the males (Capranica 1965, 1966). Using synthetic mating calls, Capranica (1965, 1966) has demonstrated that the spectral features of the mating call are most essential for the evoked vocal response in males. Both low and high frequency peaks must be present in the call, and the low frequency peak of energy must be below 500 Hz. In addition, the acoustic energy in the intermediate frequency range of 500–900 Hz must be small. This last factor is interesting, since the addition of a frequency component of 500 Hz to the synthetic call can partially or totally suppress the evoked vocal response, depending on the relative amplitude of the 500 Hz component to the low-frequency peak. Smaller, younger males (89–102mm) produce a bimodal mating call with a low frequency peak around 500–700 Hz (Figure 3D) rather than at 200–300 Hz as in the older adults (152–178 mm). Thus the call of the younger frogs is unattractive to the larger adults.

The evoked vocal response of male bullfrogs has some interesting parallels with the physiological properties of their auditory periphery. Primary auditory fibers of adult bullfrogs can be grouped into 3 populations: low-frequency sensitive fibers having best excitatory frequencies (BEFs) around 200–300 Hz, intermediate-frequency sensitive fibers with BEFs of 500–900 Hz, and high-frequency sensitive fibers with BEFs of 1000–1700 Hz (Feng, Narins, & Capranica, 1975; see also Fig. 11). The low-frequency population is thus maximally excited by the low-frequency energy of the species mating call and the high frequency population by the high frequency energy of the call. Thus for eliciting vocal responses in male bullfrogs, both low- and high-frequency populations of primary auditory fibers must be excited simultaneously, mimicking an AND operation in electronic circuitry (Frishkopf, Capranica, & Goldstein, 1968). Furthermore, excitation of low frequency fibers as needed for a successful AND operation requires that there should be minimal energy at intermediate frequencies around 500–900 Hz. These tones, which represent the dominant low frequency energy of juvenile's mating calls, are known to suppress responses of adult's low frequency fibers, mediating the phenomenon of two-tone suppression (see Fig. 13).

It is also interesting to note that the dominant spectral energies of the adult mating call match the frequency ranges of the low- and intermediate-frequency populations of auditory fibers in the younger bullfrog (Shofner & Feng, 1981; see the following sections). Not only does this match exist, but ecologically, juvenile and younger adult bullfrogs apparently are present during at least part of the adult mating season (A.J. Wright, 1914; Willis, Moyle, & Baskett, 1956; Dickerson, 1969; Howard, 1978). Typical behavior for the newly metamorphosed frogs is to hide themselves during the day and

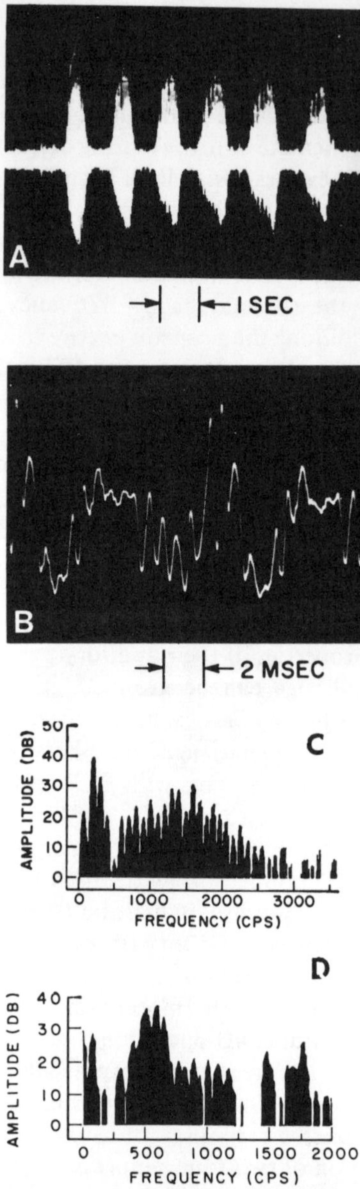

Figure 3. Field-recorded bullfrog mating call. (A) A mating call, composed of 6 similar croaks in its entirety. (B) Representative expansion of the croak waveform showing the waveshape in a single fundamental period. Note that the pulsatile waveform has a periodicity of approximately 10/s. (C) Spectrographic section taken through the middle of a croak. The harmonic structure of the spectrum reflects the quasiperiodic nature of the croak waveform. (D) Spectrographic section representative of the croak in the calls made by the smaller male bullfrog. (Modified from Capranica, 1966, by permission of the publisher.)

to venture out at night (Dickerson, 1969), the time when males are calling for a sustained period (Howard, 1978). Since adult bullfrogs are known to prey on smaller frogs (Dickerson, 1969), one might speculate that when juveniles come out of hiding, the adult mating call may guide their ventures of identifying the presence and locations of the potential adult male predators. That is, assuming that the peripheral mechanisms of call recognition are the same in juveniles as in adults, the adult mating call will be unattractive to juveniles. This is because the high frequency peak of the adult's mating call is closely matched to the range of best suppression frequencies in juveniles (Shofner & Feng, 1981; see Fig. 13) and hence will suppress the responses of low frequency fibers through the mechanism of two-tone suppression. However, there is no report of behavioral observation which supports this hypothesis.

DEVELOPMENT OF THE AUDITORY SYSTEM

The auditory system of anurans undergoes changes throughout their life. There is a continuous change in the morphology and function of the auditory apparatus starting from early embryos to tadpoles and into adulthood. The most dramatic changes occur during metamorphosis when the waterborne acoustic detection system is transformed into an airborne pressure sensing system. The details of these developmental changes will be discussed in the following sections.

Peripheral Auditory System

The peripheral auditory system of postmetamorphic anurans (see Capranica, 1976, for review) is divided into an external ear, middle ear, and inner ear (Fig. 4). The external ear consists of the tympanic membrane and the surrounding cartilaginous ring (tympanic annulus). The middle ear is comprised of an air-filled cavity containing three fused middle ear bones: plectrum, columella, and operculum. The distal end of the plectrum attaches to the tympanic membrane, and the proximal end of the plectrum, which is called the extracolumella, is fused to the distal end of the columella. The proximal end of the columella is fused via the columellar footplate to the operculum, which is connected to the oval window of the inner ear.

The fluid-filled inner ear is suspended within the bony otic capsule by loose connective tissue. The sensory epithelia of the auditory receptor organs are bathed in endolymphatic fluid, which is separated from the perilymphatic fluid by the membrane of the perilymphatic sac. Vibrations set up in the perilymph by the movement of the oval window are transmitted to the endolymph through the contact membranes.

Unlike higher vertebrates, anurans possess two distinct auditory organs,

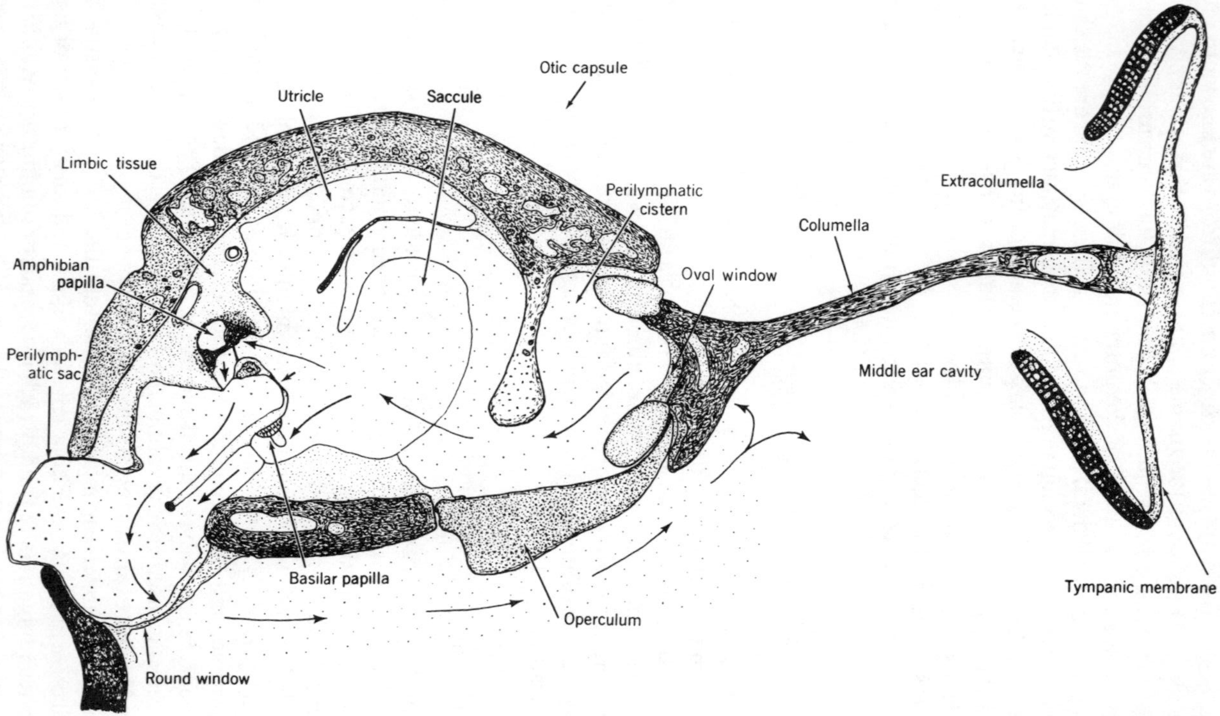

Figure 4. A schematic representation of the ear and labyrinth of *Rana pipiens,* in frontal section. The large arrows indicate the paths of fluid flow for an inward thrust of the columella. (Modified from Wever, 1973, by permission of the publisher.)

namely, the amphibian and basilar papillae (Geisler, van Bergeijk, & Frishkopf, 1965; Wever, 1973). The amphibian papilla gives rise to low- and intermediate-frequency selective auditory fibers (Feng et al., 1975; Lewis, Baird, Leverenz, & Koyama, 1982; Lewis, Leverenz, & Koyama, 1982) and is tonotopically organized (Lewis, Baird, Leverenz, & Koyama, 1982; Lewis, Leverenz, & Koyama, 1982). Recent anatomical (Shofner & Feng, 1983; Lewis, 1984) and physiological data (Hillery & Narins, 1984) indicate that the basis of such tonotopy partly lies in the presence of a traveling wave attributed to the graded change of tectorial membrane mass or volume along the length of this organ. The basilar papilla is innervated by high-frequency selective auditory fibers (Feng, et al., 1975; Lewis, Baird, Leverenz, & Koyama, 1982) and acts as a tuned resonant structure (Capranica & Moffat, 1977). Auditory nerve fibers are found exclusively in the posterior ramus of the eighth nerve (Boord, Grochow, & Frishkopf, 1971) and project to the dorsal medullary nucleus (Gregory, 1972; Matesz, 1979; Lewis, Leverenz, & Koyama, 1980; Fuzessery & Feng, 1981).

Anatomical Development. The anuran auditory periphery begins to differentiate in the late neurula (stage 16) and early tailbud stages (stage 17) when the ectodermal otic placode invaginates to form the otic vesicle (Witschi, 1949). At this stage (stage 17), the otic vesicle is attached to the ectoderm and lies ventral to the brain (Streeter, 1921). During the differentiation of the otic vesicle, the vesicle becomes detached from the ectoderm and migrates to a location dorsal to the hindbrain when it is fully differentiated into the membranous labyrinth (Streeter, 1921). It is worth noting that the position of the membranous labyrinth appears to be determined by the surrounding environment of the otic vesicle. When the primitive otic vesicle is removed and rotated about its normal axes, it still differentiates into a normal membranous labyrinth with normal relations to the brain and surrounding structures (Streeter, 1907).

The medial wall of the otic vesicle gives rise to neuroblasts which will aggregate and differentiate into the eighth nerve ganglion (Witschi, 1949). From stage 20, when the anuran larva hatches, to stage 23, when the operculum fold is apparent, fibers from the eighth nerve ganglion project into the medulla forming the ventral (vestibular) root of the eighth nerve (Larsell, 1934). Around this time (stages 23–25), the amphibian papilla begins to differentiate off the medial wall of the primitive saccule, although dorsal auditory root fibers of the eighth nerve have not formed at this time. When the hindlimb buds begin to form (stage 25), the dorsal root of the eighth nerve begins to develop as a few fibers connect the medulla with the amphibian papilla (Larsell, 1934). Near this stage of development, tadpoles have been shown to be sensitive to sound (Weiss, Stuart, & Strother, 1973, see later discussion).

As the hindlimb buds grow, the amphibian papilla epithelium begins to evaginate and the tectorial membrane begins to appear. About stage 26, the tectorial membrane of the amphibian papilla thickens and the basilar papilla begins to differentiate off the ventrocaudal wall of the saccule (Larsell, 1934). Interestingly, the sensory epithelium of the amphibian papilla develops from two separate patches of epithelium, which correspond to the rostral triangular patch and the caudal S-segment of epithelium, while the basilar papilla sensory epithelium develops from a single patch (Li and Lewis, 1974).

At the time when the hindlimb buds first form (stage 25), the bronchial columellae begin to differentiate (Witschi, 1949). Embryologically, the bronchial columellae differentiate from the pulmonary (7th) pharyngeal pouch (Witschi, 1955). A bronchial columella is a solid rod made up of mesodermal fibers which passes through the dorsal aorta and connects the bronchus to the round window. As previously mentioned, it is thought that the lungs function as pressure detectors and that the bronchial columellae transmit vibrations from the lungs to the iner ear (Witschi, 1949). The presence of the bronchial columella in larval anurans appears to be limited to Ranids (Witschi, 1955). However, larval *Xenopus* possess bronchial diverticula which also connect the bronchus to the round window, although the diverticula appear to be more primitive than the bronchial columellae (Witschi, 1950). The bronchial columellae are fully developed between the time the hindlimbs differentiate (stage 26) until the time the forelimbs are fully developed (stage 31). During the climatic period of metamorphosis (stages 32–32), the bronchial columellae degenerate while the tympanic middle ear apparatus develops (Witschi, 1949).

The development of the middle ear and middle ear cavity (Fig. 5) begins after the larva hatches (stage 21), and these structures originate from the dorsal recess of the first pharyngeal pouch (Witschi, 1949). This dorsal recess forms the rudimentary tympanic organ (Figure 5A), and it remains a rudimentary organ until the metamorphic period. Around stage 30 when the forelimbs begin to emerge, the tympanic annulus and tympanic membrane begin to differentiate from a mesenchymal disc. Since this disc is attached to the quadrate bone, which is located under the nose in tadpoles, it is carried caudally during metamorphosis (stages 31–32) as the mouth of the tadpole widens (Figure 5B). During this time, the tympanic annulus and tympanic membrane differentiate from the rudimentary mesenchymal disc while the middle ear cavity and Eustachian tube develop from an endodermal rudiment. The columella and plectrum differentiate from mesenchymal masses, and in Ranids, the middle ear bones are completely developed at the end of metamorphosis (Witschi, 1949). However, in the Egyptian toad (*Bufo regularis* Reuss), the middle ear is not completely developed until the toad is half grown, or about one year after metamorphosis (Sedra & Michael, 1959). Thus, there may be a period during postmetamorphic growth when the mid-

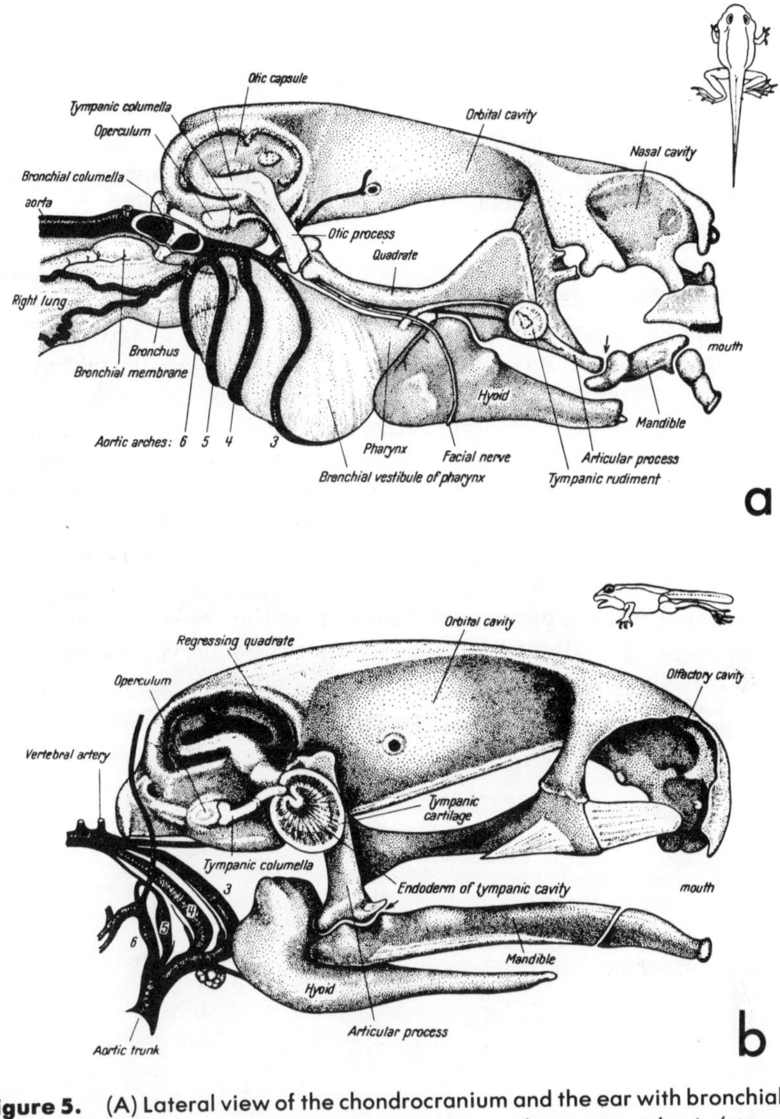

Figure 5. (A) Lateral view of the chondrocranium and the ear with bronchial and tympanic accessory organs of *Rana clamitans* in early metamorphosis (stage 31). Part of the wall of the right dorsal aorta is cut away to show the bronchial columella and its attachment to the round window. The tympanic columella ends in a mesenchymatic cord that follows the course of the facial nerve. (B) *Rana clamitans* during metamorphosis (stage 32); chondrocranium and early ossifications; articular process of the quadrate and tympanic organ are on their way to the final positions; the endodermal tympanic cavity and the ring cartilage (tympanic annulus) are differentiating and have attained a considerable size. The plectrum, distal segment of the columella, lies in a notch of the cartilage and projects toward a fold in the wall of the tympanic cavity. The bronchial columella has disappeared. (Modified from Witschi, 1949, by permission of the publisher.)

dle ear may be inefficient in transmitting sounds to the inner ear, resulting in a relative insensitivity to airborne sounds (Capranica, 1976). It would be interesting to study the changes in mechanical sensitivity of the middle ear (to both airborne and waterborne sounds) in various anuran species prior to, during, and following the metamorphosis, a period when radical changes of structures occur.

While the middle ear may be completely developed in Ranids by the end of metamorphosis, considerable growth may still occur during postmetamorphic development. For example, in the bullfrog, there can be as much as a 10-fold increase in the diameter of the tympanic membrane between newly metamorphosed and large adult frogs as shown in Figure 6 (Shofner & Feng, 1981). This implies that the middle ear bones attaching to this membrane accordingly grow in size and mass. Hence the middle ear transfer function will likely change continuously with postmetamorphic age.

Not only does the middle ear continue to grow during postmetamorphic development, the auditory organs also continue to grow as body size increases. The postmetamorphic development of the amphibian and basilar papillae in the bullfrog has been recently studied (Shofner & Feng, 1984). In the basilar papilla (Fig. 7), lumen volume, tectorial membrane volume (or mass), and contact membrane area increase dramatically with postmetamorphic

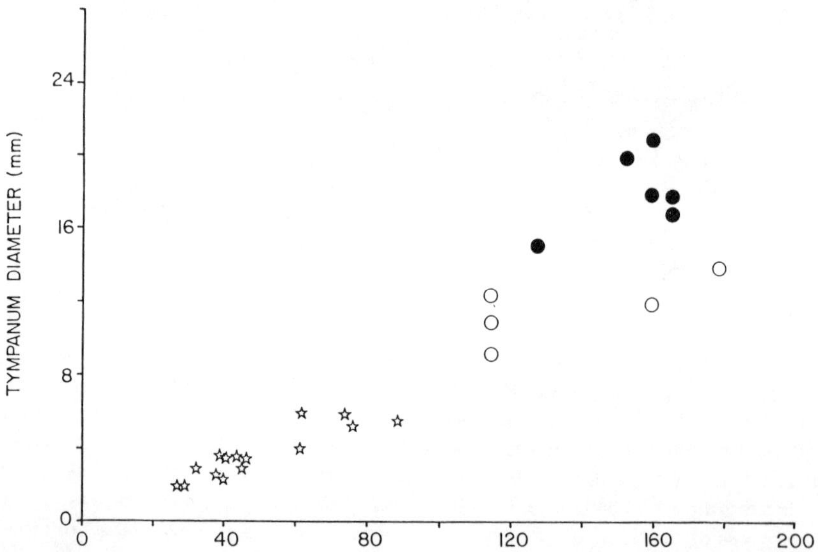

Figure 6. The diameter of the tympanum as a function of body size for the bullfrog. Measurements were taken using a caliper. Females (o); males (•); sex not determined (*). (Reproduced from Shofner & Feng, 1981, by permission of the publisher.)

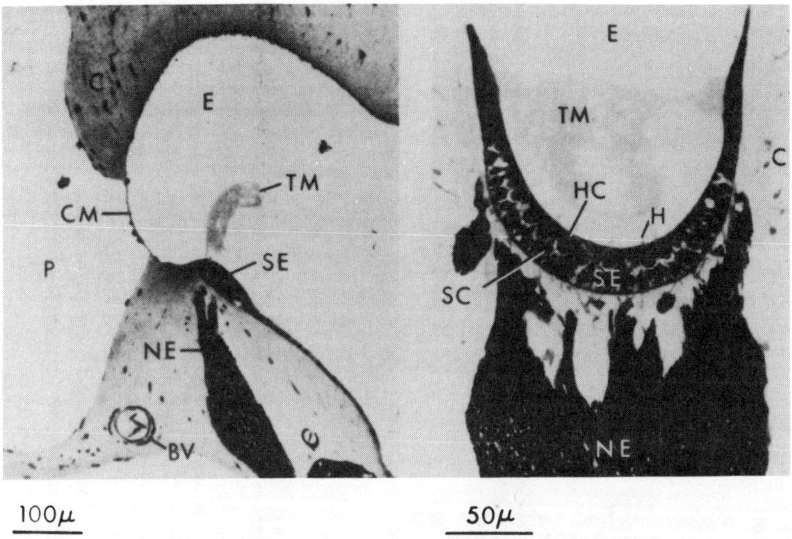

Figure 7. Photomicrograph sections through the basilar papilla, taken in orthogonal planes. (A) Longitudinal section showing the tubular shape of the papilla as it begins to open into the saccule (to the right of figure (not seen here). The tectorial membrane overlying the sensory crest extends halfway across the lumen. Myelinated nerve fibers approach the papilla from below. Small blood vessels are found in the cartilaginous wall. (B) Cross-section of the papilla through its sensory epithelium. The roof of the papilla is not shown. The sensory crest consists of hair cells and supporting cells. Several hair bundles are evident. The tectorial membrane extends from the lower half of the tube and is attached to the wall of the papilla. BV, blood vessel: C, cartilage: CM, contact membrane: E, endolymph: H, sensory hair bundle: HC, hair cell: NE, nonmyelinated nerves: P, perilymph: SC, supporting cell: SE, sensory epithelium: TM, tectorial membrane. (Reproduced from Frishkopf et al., 1968, by permission of the publisher, © 1968 IEEE.)

growth (Fig. 9). There are also slight increases in the size of the sensory epithelium and the number of hair cells. In the amphibian papilla (Fig. 8), there are local increases in the mass of the tectorial membrane along the length of the organ (Fig. 10). Furthermore, the height of one type (type D) of hair cell's stereociliary bundles of the predominant hair cell type increases by 50–75% in the caudal regions of the papilla, but not in the rostral regions. There is a gradual, albeit slight, increase in the length of the organ and in the number of hair cells as body size increases. The growth of the sensory epithelia occurs primarily at the outer edges of the organs. It is only along the organ's outer margins that "immature" hair cells are observed (Shofner & Feng, 1984). This growth pattern is identical to that of larval anurans (Li & Lewis, 1974), suggesting that hair cell growth is a continuous process throughout an anuran's

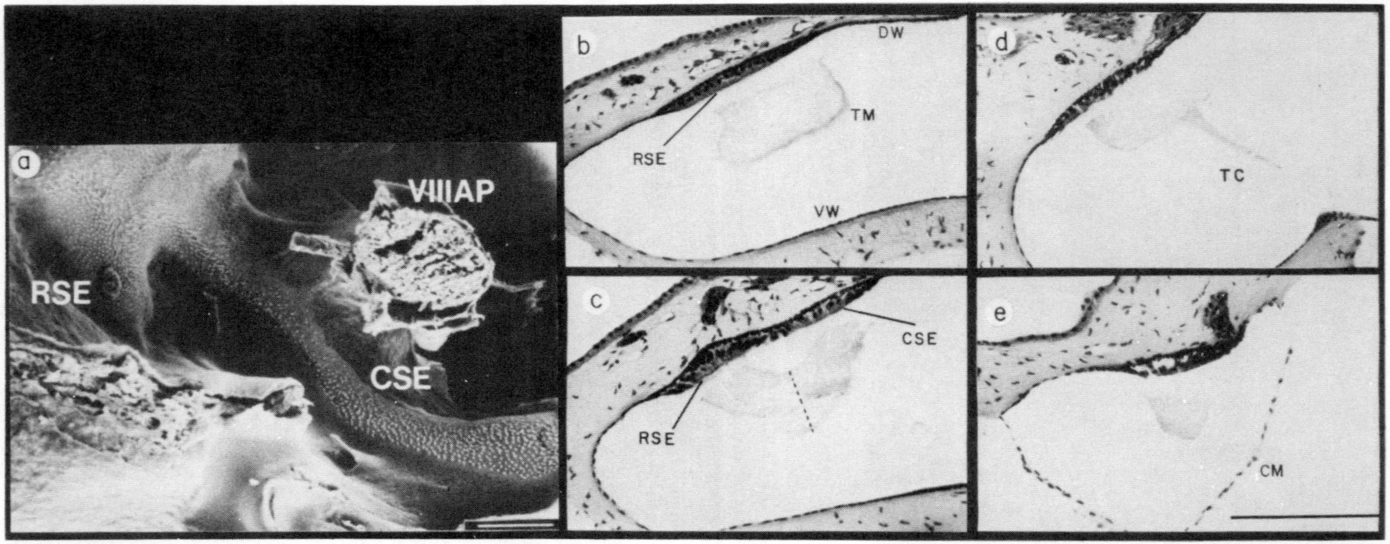

Figure 8. (A) Scanning electron micrograph of the bullfrog amphibian papilla. The tectorial membrane has been excised to observe the sensory epithelium. RSE, rostral triangular patch of sensory epithelium; CSE, caudal *S*-segment of sensory epithelium; VIIIAP, branch of eighth cranial nerve which innervates the sensory epithelium. Calibration mark: 100 μm. (B–E) Frontal sections of the amphibian papilla along its rostro-caudal length starting with the more rostral frontal section (B), to the bimodal region (C), where two separate patches of organs, RSE and CSE, are observed, to more caudal section in D where the tectorial membrane (TM) makes contact with the dorsal limbic wall forming a tectorial curtain (TC), and lastly to the caudal most section of the organ where contact membrane (CM) can be seen. Calibration mark for these sections = 250 μm. (Modified from Shofner & Feng, 1983, by permission of the publisher.)

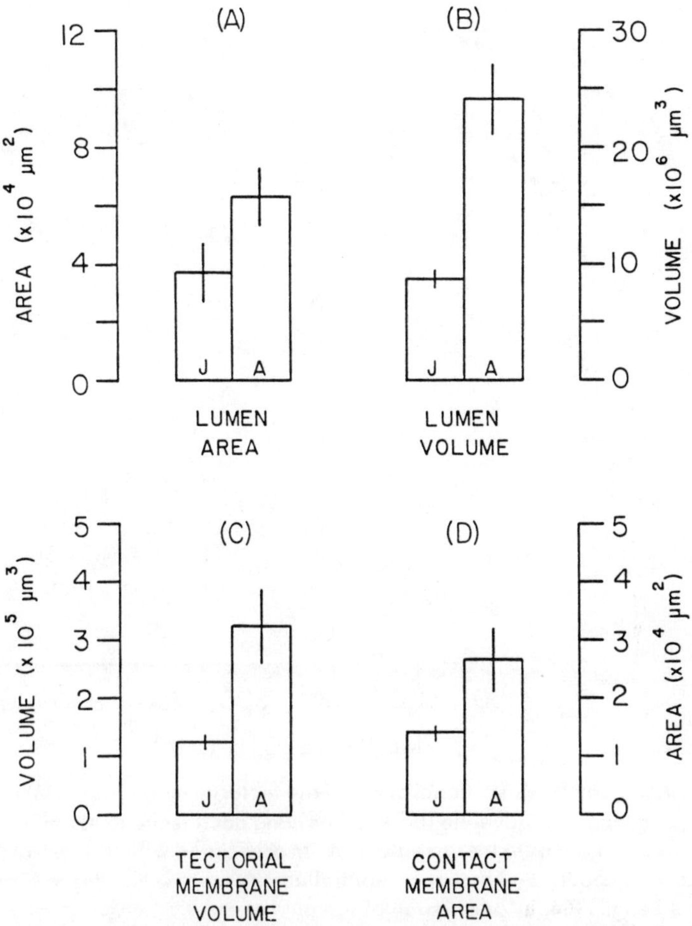

Figure 9. Histograms of the mean lumen area (A), the mean lumen volume (B), mean tectorial membrane volume (C), and mean contact membrane area (D) for juvenile (J) and adult (A) basilar papillae. Vertical lines show standard deviations. (Reproduced from Shofner & Feng, 1984, by permission of the publisher.)

life. Comparative data have also shown that among different anuran species the size of auditory organs and the number of sensory cells are proportional to the adult body size (Alfs, 1978; Alfs & Schneider, 1973).

This discussion reveals that anatomical changes in the auditory periphery occur prior to and during growth after metamorphosis. These changes undoubtedly will alter the mechanical characteristics of the middle ear and micromechanics of the inner ear organs and hence the physiological properties of the auditory system.

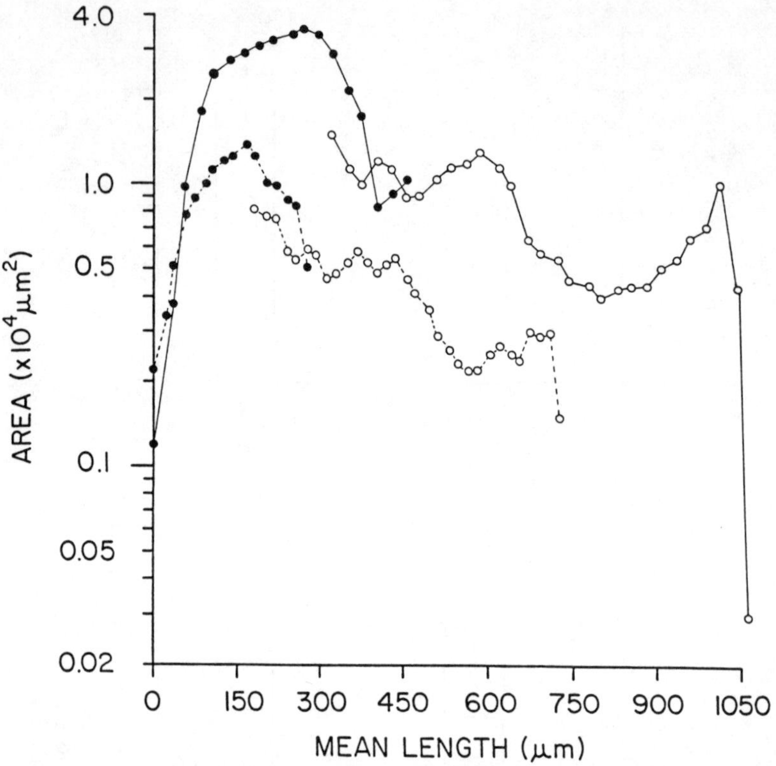

Figure 10. Mean cross-sectional areas of the tectorial membrane (TM) as a function of mean length for juvenile (broken line) and adult (solid line) amphibian papillae. Filled and open circles are values of TM associated with the rostral triangular patch and caudal *S*-segment of epithelium, respectively. (Reproduced from Shofner & Feng, 1984, by permission of the publisher.)

Physiological Development. The development of auditory sensitivity in larval anurans is poorly understood. Weiss et al. (1973) recorded microphonic potentials from the inner ear of bullfrog tadpoles having no limb growth (i.e., before stage 25) in response to pure tones of varying frequencies and intensities. Comparison of their results with those from adult bullfrogs (Strother, 1959) show that the tadpoles are typically 20–40 dB less sensitive than adults. Unfortunately, the tadpoles in the study were not submerged underwater and were presented with airborne stimulation rather than with waterborne sounds. As already described, the auditory periphery of the Ranid tadpole appears to be specialized for the detection of waterborne sounds. Since the tadpole does not possess a tympanic middle ear as impedance transformer for airborne sounds and since sectioning the columella in adults can result in a 40-dB loss in sensitivity (Strother, 1959), one might expect tadpoles to be less sensitive than adults to airborne stimulation. Thus, it is unclear whether the relative insensitivity of the bullfrog tadpole to sound reflects an immature inner ear and/or the absence of an impedance transformer for airborne sounds. From this discussion, it is clear that more conclusive experiments are needed in order to elucidate the tadpole's ability to hear underwater sound.

The large increase in the size of the tympanic membrane and middle ear bones in the bullfrog during postmetamorphic development presumably increases the masses of these structures resulting in an attenuation of high frequency vibrations. While the transfer function of the middle ear has not been studied during postmetamorphic development in any anuran species, comparative studies indicate that in a closed acoustic system, the middle ear acts as a low pass filter with an upper cutoff frequency that is correlated with species size (Saunders & Johnstone, 1972; Moffat & Capranica, 1978; also see Chung, Pettigrew, & Anson, 1981; Pinder & Palmer, 1983, for free-field studies). The upper cutoff frequency is higher in smaller species which have less massive middle ear structures. One would therefore expect that in the growing postmetamorphic anuran, a similar situation may be found.

In addition to likely changes in the mechanics of the middle ear of growing frogs, recent neurophysiological studies have suggested that the tuning properties of the organs in the inner ear as reflected by the tuning of auditory nerve fibers (Shofner & Feng, 1981; Wilczynski, Zakon, & Brenowitz, 1983) also change during postmetamorphic growth. Auditory nerve fibers in anurans possess V-shaped tuning curves (Fig. 11) which are characterized by the best excitatory frequency (BEF), i.e., the frequency to which a fiber has its lowest threshold of excitation. In most anurans the BEFs of auditory fibers fall into three groups or populations (Capranica, 1976). The distributions of these populations appear to be related to the size (age) of the anuran. In bullfrogs, for example, there is a gradual downward shift in the distributions of BEFs during postmetamorphic development (Fig. 12), particularly for intermediate- and high-frequency populations (Shofner & Feng, 1981). A similar correlation occurs in the spring peeper (*Hyla crucifer*) where the distribution of the high-frequency population of auditory fibers is centered around lower frequencies in larger females than in small females (Wilczynski et al., 1983). Low-frequency fibers generally exhibit two-tone suppression (Fig. 13), namely, responses to the unit's BEF can be suppressed by the simultaneous presence of a higher frequency tone. For these fibers, the best suppression frequencies (BSFs) are also shifted downward with age as shown in Figure 13 (Shofner & Feng, 1981).

What may be the contributing factors to the downward shifts in BEFs and BSFs with age? The increases in size and mass of the middle ear with postmetamorphic age presumably decrease the upper cutoff frequency of the auditory periphery (see earlier discussion) which can explain the decrease in

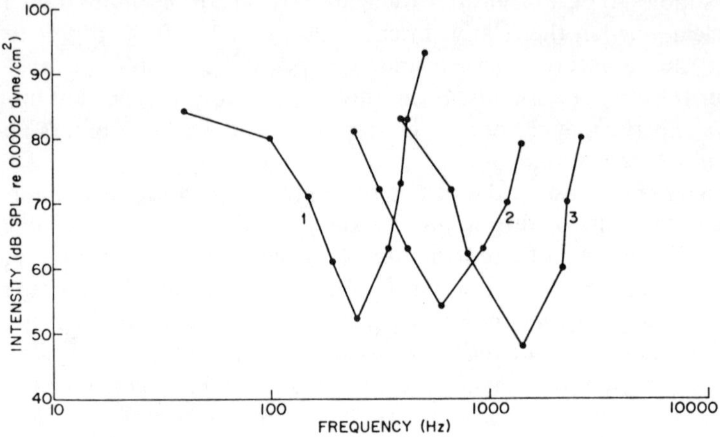

Figure 11. Representative excitatory tuning curves for the three populations of auditory nerve fibers in the bullfrog. The low-frequency sensitive fiber (unit 1) has a best excitatory frequency of 250 Hz, the mid-frequency sensitive fiber (unit 2) has a best excitatory frequency of 600 Hz, and the high-frequency sensitive fiber (unit 3) has a best excitatory frequency of 1400 Hz. The response of unit 1 to a tone at its best excitatory frequency could be totally suppressed by the simultaneous addition of a second (inhibitory) tone around 700 Hz, when presented at an intensity 10 dB greater than the excitatory tone. The responses of units 2 and 3 to excitatory tones could not be suppressed by the addition of a second tone, regardless of its frequency or level (for relative intensities of up to 30 dB above the level of the excitatory tone). (Reproduced from Feng et al., 1975, by permission of the publisher.)

the upper limit of hearing. However, these changes alone cannot account for the developmental shifts in the more refined tuning properites of individual auditory fibers. The changes in the morphologies and physical characteristics of various tissues within the inner ear conceivably are more influential in changing the tuning characteristics of the two organs. The increases in the organ volume, the size and mass of the tectorial membrane, the height and stiffness of hair cells, and the number of hair cells per unit organ area all contribute to lowering the frequency selectivities of the two organs with development (see Shofner & Feng, 1984, for a more detailed discussion).

In addition to the changes in the frequency selectivities of fibers from the two auditory papillae, the sensitivities of these fibers also vary with age (Shofner & Feng, 1981). In newly metamorphosed bullfrogs, a relatively large percentage of fibers from each organ have poor excitation thresholds (i.e., exceeding 100 dB SPL). Whereas in large adults, almost all fibers have thresholds below 90–100 dB SPL. The anatomical attributes of this shift in response sensitivity remain to be studied and may involve both mechanical factors of the middle ear and neuronal factors from the inner ear such as the height of stereocilia and the innervation density of maturing hair cells.

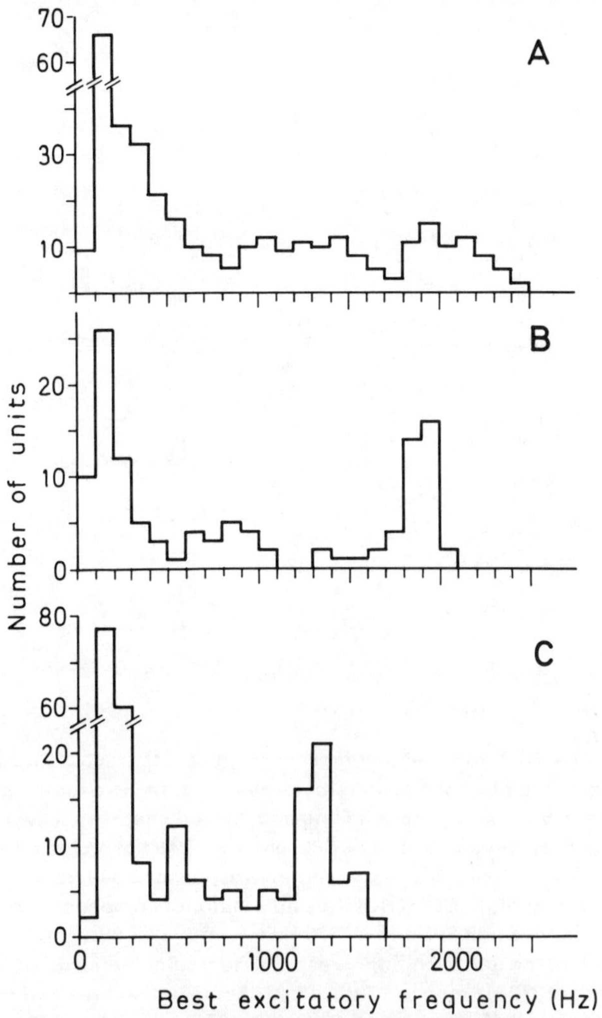

Figure 12. Histograms of the distributions of best excitatory frequencies of primary auditory nerve fibers in the bullfrog during postmetamorphic development. Bin width-100 Hz. (A) BEF distribution of 346 fibers in newly metamorphosed bullfrogs (27–46 mm snout-vent length). Low-frequency selective fibers with BEFs ranging from 100 to 800 Hz; intermediate-frequency selective fibers with BEFs ranging from 1000–1700 Hz; high-frequency selective fibers with BEFs ranging from 1800–2500 Hz. (B) BEF distribution of 117 fibers from intermediate-sized (62–67 mm) frogs. Low-frequency selective fibers ranging from 100–500 Hz; intermediate-frequency fibers ranging from 600–1100 Hz; high-frequency selective fibers ranging from 1300–2100 Hz. Note that the high-frequency population is centered around 1800–2000 Hz, with no fibers having BEFs above 2050 Hz. (C) BEF distribution of 242 auditory fibers from large adult bullfrogs (152–178 mm). Low-frequency selective fibers with BEFs ranging from 100–400 Hz; intermediate-frequency fibers with BEFs ranging from 500–900 Hz; high-frequency selective fibers with BEFs ranging from 1000–1700 Hz. Note that the high-frequency population is centered around 1200–1400 Hz, with no fibers having BEFs above 1700 Hz. (Modified from Shofner & Feng, 1981, by permission of the publisher.)

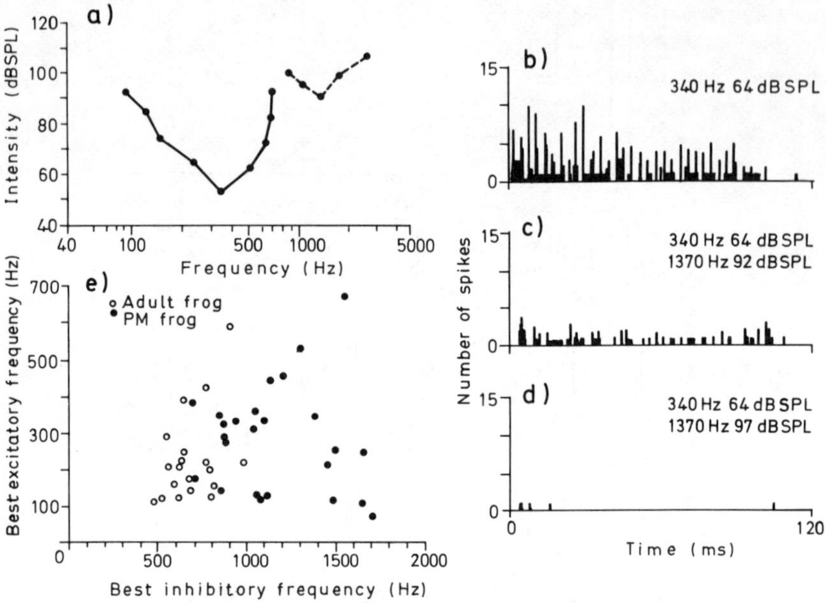

Figure 13. (A–D) Two-tone suppressive response characteristics from a low-frequency selective fiber of a postmetamorphic frog. (A) Excitatory and inhibitory tuning curves are shown by the solid line and dashed line, respectively. BEF = 340 Hz at an excitatory threshold of 54 dB SPL. BSF = 1370 Hz at an inhibitory threshold of 92-dB SPL. (B) PSTH of the unit's excitatory response to 340 Hz tone at 64 dB SPL (10 dB above threshold). (C) PSTH of the unit's inhibitory response to a combination of a 340 Hz tone at 64 dB SPL and a 1370 Hz tone at 92 dB SPL (threshold of inhibition). (D) PSTH of the unit's inhibitory response to a combination of a 340-Hz tone at 64 dB SPL and a 1370-Hz tone at 97-dB SPL (5 dB above the threshold of inhibition). All PSTHs shown are for 20 presentations of a 100-ms tone burst. Bin width = 0.5 ms. (E) Scatter diagram of the distributions of best suppression frequencies (BSFs) for adults (o) and froglets (•). BSFs ranged from 485 to 990 Hz in adults and 700 and 1700 Hz in froglets. N = 19 for adults, N = 25 for froglets. PSTH is abbreviation for post-stimulus time histogram. (Mofified from Shofner & Feng, 1981, by permission of the publisher.)

Central Auditory System

The central auditory pathways of anurans are similar to those of other vertebrates, and the auditory nuclei and the major projections (Fig. 14) have been fairly well described (Northcutt, 1980; Wilczynski & Capranica, 1984). Primary afferent fibers of the eighth nerve terminate exclusively in the ipsilateral dorsal medullary nucleus (DMN). The axons of DMN neurons send bilateral projections to the superior olivary nuclei (SON) with a more dominant projection to the contralateral SON. The SON neurons project predominantly to its ipsilateral torus semicircularis. The DMN also has axons which project directly to the contralateral torus. The torus is comprised of five nuclei: subependymal, commissural, principal, magnocellular, and laminar nuclei. The laminar, magnocellular, and principal nuclei are auditory centers (Potter, 1965). Golgi analysis has revealed that a variety of cell types are found in the torus, and each of these nuclei have neurons with distinct characteristics (Feng, 1983). The major projection from the torus is to the ipsilateral posterocentral or central nucleus of the thalamus. The axons of the posterocentral nucleus project via the lateral forebrain bundle and terminate in the ipsilateral striatum.

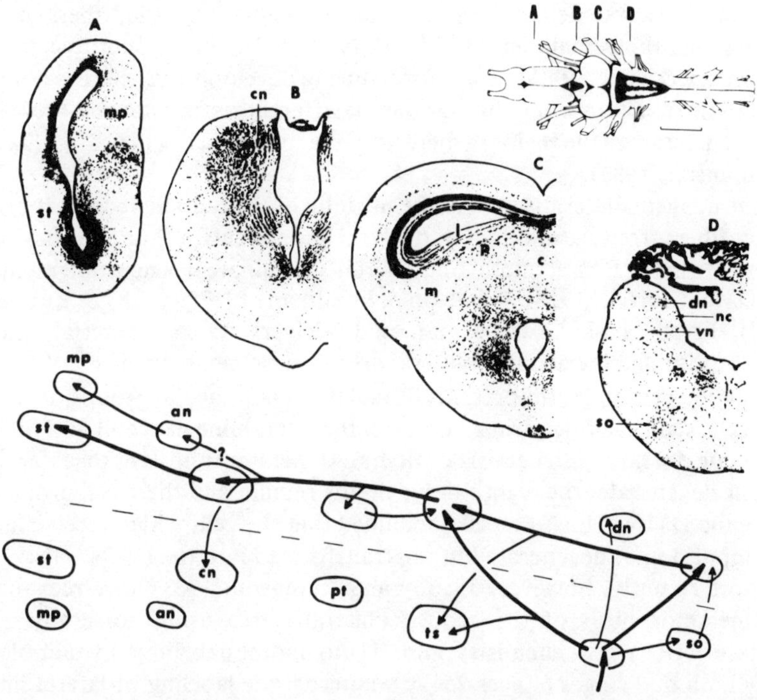

Figure 14. Photomicrographs of transverse sections through the brain of the bullfrog, *Rana catesbeiana* illustrating major auditory centers and their interconnections. The levels of the various sections are indicated in the dorsal view of the brain. Bar scale equals 10 mm. Abbreviations: an-anterior thalamic nucleus; c-commissural toral nucleus; cn-central thalamic nucleus; dn-dorsal octavus nucleus (dorsal medullary nucleus); l-laminar toral nucleus; m-magnocellular toral nucleus; mp-medial pallium; nc-caudal octavus nucleus; p-principal toral nucleus; pt-pretectum; so-superior olive; st-striatum; ts-torus semicircularis; vn-ventral octavus nucleus. (Reproduced from Northcutt, 1980, by permission of the publisher.)

Anatomical Development. Ontogenetically, anatomical changes of the caudal auditory brainstem have been noted. The changes in the morphology of the termination sites of lateral line and auditory nerve afferent fibers which occur at metamorphosis represent one of the most interesting problems in developmental neurobiology. These changes will be described in the following section; however, little else is known about the development of other nuclei in the anuran central auditory system.

During development, there is a change in the locations of the sites of termination of basilar and amphibian papillae afferent fibers. In tadpoles (stage 26) the basilar papilla fibers project to the dorsolateral DMN, while amphibian papilla fibers terminate in the ventrolateral DMN, as shown in Figure 15 (Jacoby & Rubinson, 1983). However, in adults, basilar papilla fibers terminate in the dorsomedial DMN, while amphibian papilla fibers project throughout the remainder of the DMN (Fig. 16) in a tonotopic fashion (Fuzessery & Feng, 1981). Therefore, during development, there is a medial shift in the position where basilar papilla afferents terminate and there is an overall increase in the regions where amphibian papilla fibers project (Jacoby & Rubinson, 1983).

The acousticolateralis area in the medulla of the tadpole receives both afferent fibers from the auditory and lateral line systems. While auditory fibers terminate in the DMN, lateral line afferents terminate in a neuropil medial to the DMN (Larsell, 1934; Rubinson & Friedman, 1977; Jacoby & Rubinson, 1983). From Nissl, Golgi, Cajal, and Weigert stained material, Larsell (1934) examined the acousticolateral area during metamorphosis. While the lateral line system is still present, dorsolateral and medial groups of medullary cells send their dendrites into both the lateral line neuropil and into the incoming dorsal eighth nerve root fibers. At metamorphosis as the lateral line organs degenerate, the eighth nerve inputs remain and these cell groups become the DMN. Thus, Larsell concluded that the cells which receive lateral line input do not degenerate but are transformed into the DMN cells.

More recently, however, Jacoby and Rubinson (1983) have reexamined the metamorphosis of the acousticolateralis area using horseradish peroxidase (HRP) histochemistry and ^{3}H-thymidine labeling. In tadpoles of early limb bud stages (stages 25–26), anterograde labeling of lateral line fibers fill the acousticolateralis neuropil medial to the DMN, while HRP labeling of the posterior ramus (i.e., the auditory branch) of the eighth nerve shows afferent projections to the entire DMN but no projections into the lateral line neuropil. Retrograde filling of DMN neurons (through HRP injections into the contralateral DMN and superior olive) and lateral line neurons (through injection into the contralateral tegmentum) show that dendritic fields of DMN neurons are confined to the DMN and that those of lateral line neurons are confined to the lateral line neuropil. No cells with dendritic fields in the lateral line neuropil have somata within the DMN. Furthermore,

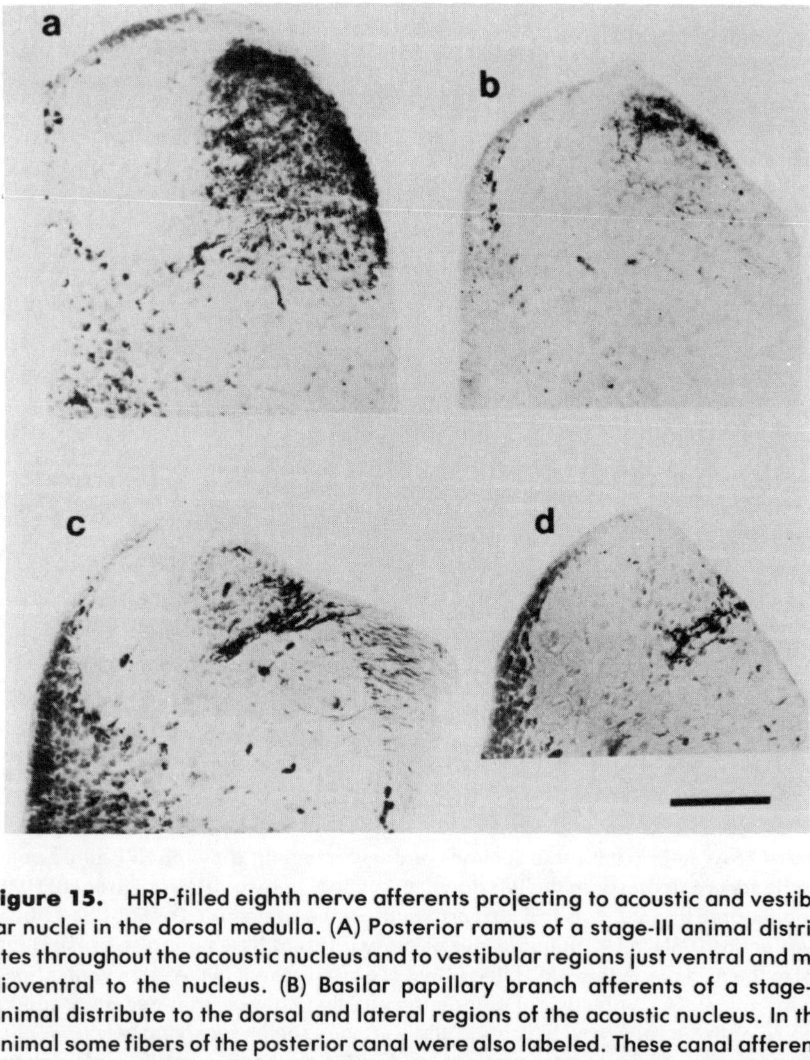

Figure 15. HRP-filled eighth nerve afferents projecting to acoustic and vestibular nuclei in the dorsal medulla. (A) Posterior ramus of a stage-III animal distributes throughout the acoustic nucleus and to vestibular regions just ventral and medioventral to the nucleus. (B) Basilar papillary branch afferents of a stage-III animal distribute to the dorsal and lateral regions of the acoustic nucleus. In this animal some fibers of the posterior canal were also labeled. These canal afferents distribute to regions ventral and medioventral to the nucleus. (C) Amphibian papillary branch afferents of a stage-II animal at the level of entrance of eighth nerve distribute within the extreme ventral and lateral regions of the acoustic nucleus. (D) The same amphibian papillary branch fill, 140 μm caudal to C. Caudal to their entrance these afferents are confined to the ventral one third of the nucleus. Scale bar = 100 μm. (Reproduced from Jacoby & Rubinson, 1983, by permission of the publisher.)

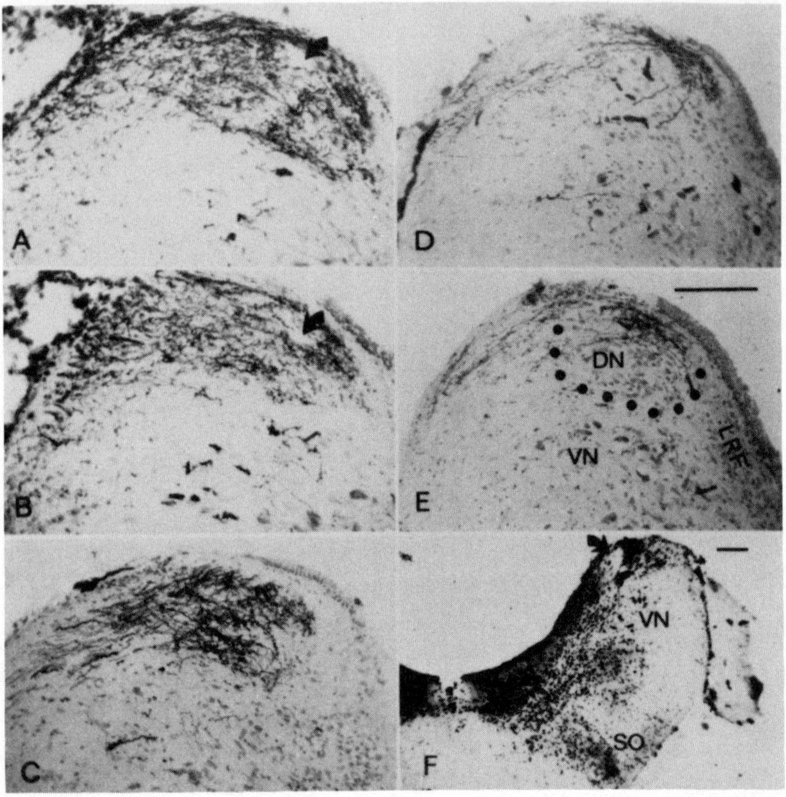

Figure 16. A–E. Transverse sections of dorsal medulla showing HRP-filled auditory fibers projecting onto the left dorsal medullary nucleus (DMN). Extent of DMN as delineated by solid dots in E is approximately the same in A–D. HRP-filled fibers cover entire DMN in (A,B): numerous primary afferent fibers are also present lateral to the nucleus. A few HRP-filled fibers are also present in the more ventral vestibular nuclei. (A) Projection of amphibian papilla (AP) fibers immediately caudal to the eighth nerve. Arrow indicates lightly stained region receiving basilar papilla (BP) afferents. (B) Same preparations as A; AP fiber projections at midpoint between the eighth and ninth nerves. (C) More lightly stained AP preparation showing a suggestion of dorsal and ventral divisions of the terminal field. (D) BP fiber projections immediately caudal to the eighth nerve. (E) Same preparations as D. BP fiber projections at midpoint between the eighth and ninth nerves. DN, dorsal medullary nucleus; LRF, lateral reticular formation; VN, ventral (magnocellular) nucleus. Bar is 250 μm. (Reproduced from Fuzessery & Feng, 1981, by permission of the publisher.)

^{3}H-thymidine labeling shows that newly generated auditory cells occupy the DMN within several hours of their formation throughout the period when lateral line neuropil concurrently grows and regenerates. These results suggest that lateral line and auditory neurons in the medulla are morphologically independent throughout early development (Jacoby & Rubinson, 1983). Thus, transformation of function, from a displacement sensitive system into a pressure sensitive system, seems to involve two separate processes. How these processes are regulated and how they interact remain to be studied.

Phylogenetically, the superior olive is a nucleus which first appears in anurans, and the ontogeny of the olive has been examined by Larsell (1934). The superior olive begins to develop around stage 25, when a group of cells first appear. By stage 26, there is an increase in the number of olivary cells with their dendrites directed toward the periphery. As development progresses, most cells will eventually possess small dendritic fields limited to within the olive itself, while other cells will develop having ventrolateral or dorsolateral processes that extend outside of the nucleus.

Physiological development. The functional development of the central auditory system is an area that has yet to be examined in anurans. The adult central auditory system has been studied extensively, especially regarding the neural mechanisms of recognition and localization of species-specific mating calls. Neurons in the DMN possess V-shaped excitiatory tuning curves, much like the primary afferent fibers (Feng & Capranica, 1976; Fuzessery & Feng, 1983). However, some DMN neurons only respond to the transient onset of an acoustic stimulus instead of sustained responses like primary afferents. Furthermore, about half of DMN neurons are sensitive to binaural stimuli (Feng & Capranica, 1976). Most of the binaural neurons are excited by ipsilateral stimulation, while contralateral stimulation either produces excitation (E–E) or inhibition of ipsilateral response (E–I). The E–I neurons are sensitive to interaural disparities of time of arrival and intensity, two acoustic cues which are essential for sound localization in space. Frogs have been shown to have the ability to accurately locate a sound source in the horizontal plane (Feng, Gerhardt, & Capranica, 1976; Rheinlaender, Gerhardt, Yager, & Capranica, 1979) as well as in the vertical plane (Gerhardt & Rheinlaender, 1982), and that azimuthal sound localization involves binaural processing, because blocking the sound input to one ear renders the organism incapable of locating a sound source (Feng et al., 1976).

The superior olivary nucleus represents the next stage of auditory processing. While most neurons possess V-shaped tuning curves (Feng & Capranica, 1978; Zakon & Capranica, 1981), a small group of SON neurons possess complex excitatory and/or inhibitory tuning curves resembling the neurons in the torus semicircularis (Fuzessery & Feng, 1983). One probable reason for having complex response curves is that the SON receives prominent descending projection from the principal and laminaris nuclei of the torus semicircularis (Feng, in press; Rubinson, personal communication). A larger percentage of SON neurons are binaural neurons, and they are excited predominantly by contralateral stimulation in contrast to binaural DMN neurons (Feng & Capranica, 1978). Most binaural neurons in the SON are E–I neurons which are excited by the contralateral ear and inhibited by the ipsilateral ear, and all of these E–I cells have best excitatory frequencies from one ear which match the best inhibitory frequencies from the other ear. These E–I cells are also sensitive to minute interaural time and intensity differences. A smaller proportion of binaural neurons in SON are of the E–E type, and they generally possess matching best excitatory frequencies from the two ears.

Zakon and Capranica (1981) recently demonstrated that when one of the auditory nerves is severed in adult bullfrogs, the severed nerve steadily regenerates and, furthermore, the binaural connectivity is eventually fully restored within 3–6 months. Immediately following the initial surgery, all SON neurons are found to be monaurally excited by the intact ear. After sufficient recovery, however, many SON neurons are again binaural with approximately the same proportion of E–E and E–I cells as in control animals. Moreover, the best frequencies (excitatory or inhibitory) are matched again from the two ears, suggesting that systematic reorganization of connectivity at the level of DMN and SON occurs after the injury. Such reorganization takes place in a step by step fashion by first regaining normal innervation density by the sixth week postoperation, followed by narrowing of tuning curves associated with the operated ear by the eighth week, and finally achieve matching of best frequencies for the two ears by the twelfth week (Zakon, 1983). The corresponding anatomical changes and the mechanism(s) by which a binaural frequency match is achieved by the nervous system during regeneration and/or ontogeny have yet to be determined. It is uncertain whether the primary factor(s) which influences the axonal growth and synaptic formation during regeneration is genetic, electrical, chemical, or mechanical. This system offers an excellent opportunity to gain further insights into this fundamental issue of regeneration (as well as development), since the time course of regeneration is relatively slow (hence there are ample opportunities to manipulate the system) and anuran's neurons regenerate readily following axotomy. Behaviorally, it is not known if operated animals would lose and eventually regain the ability to locate a sound source. Such observations along with the behavioral time course would certainly enrich our knowledge of structural and functional relationships during development. Bullfrogs, however, would not be the ideal species for this particular behavioral observation, since their sound localization ability has never been demonstrated.

Torus semicircularis occupies a strategic position along the auditory pathway, and it plays a critical role for recognition and localization of complex sound. Many torus neurons have complex excitatory and inhibitory tuning curves (Walkowiak, 1980; Fuzessery & Feng, 1982). Some torus neurons are temporally tuned with respect to the duration of BEF tones (Narins & Capranica, 1980), repetition rate (Walkowiak, 1980), and the rate of amplitude modulation (Rose & Capranica, 1983). The optimal temporal tuning corresponds well to the temporal characteristics of the mating calls. A small number of neurons in the torus and thalamus require specific tone combinations to excite them (Fuzessery & Feng, 1982, 1983). The required frequencies of the combination tones closely match the dominant spectral energies found in the species-specific calls. Since there are downward shifts in the distributions of the three populations of auditory fibers during postmetamorphic growth, will there be a corresponding change in the specificity of the combination tones for maximal excitation of the central auditory neurons? Or, for that matter, will there be a concurrent change in the evoked vocal response? These and other questions raised earlier are just a few of the many interesting developmental questions which await the attention of neurobiologists.

CONCLUSIONS

During their life cycle, anurans typically exist in two forms and live in two separate ecological niches, namely, as tadpoles in aquatic environments and as adults in terrestrial environments. This chapter has described our present understanding of the morphological, physiological, and behavioral development of the anuran auditory system. It should be apparent from this discussion that our present knowledge in most areas is limited, while other areas have not even begun to be studied.

The developmental approach to the study of the auditory system may be a useful tool for gaining some insights into the neural mechanisms underlying the encoding of biologically significant sounds. Anurans offer the potential for making correlations among morphology, physiology, behavior, and ecology. Thus, in future years, the neural and behavioral development of the anuran auditory system will likely be an exciting area of research in comparative neurobiology.

REFERENCES

Alfs, B. (1978). Electroneumikroskopische Utersuchungen zur Ultrastruktus der Sinnesendstellen im labyrinth des Laubfreoches *Hyla arborea savingnyi* (Andouin) *Zoologischer. Anzeiger Jena, 200,* 145–172.

Alfs, B. and Schneider H. (1973). Vergleichend-anatomische Untersuchungen am labyrinth zentraleuro paischer Froschlurch-Arten. *Zeitschrift fuer Morphologie der Tiere, 76,* 129–143.

Blaustein, A.R., & O'Hara, R.K. (1982). Kin recognition cues in *Rana cascadae* tadpoles. *Behavioral Neural Biology, 36,* 77–87.

Boord, R.L., Grochow, L.B., & Frishkopf, L.S. (1971). Organization of the posterior ramus and ganglion of the VIIIth cranial nerve of the bullfrog *Rana catesbeiana. MIT Research Laboratory of Electronics Quarterly Progress Report, 99,* 180–192.

Capranica, R.R. (1965). The evoked vocal response of the bullfrog: A study of communication by sound. *MIT Research Monograph* No. 33.

Capranica, R.R. (1966). Vocal response of the bullfrog to natural synthetic mating calls. *Journal of the Acoustical Society of America, 40,* 1131–1139.

Capranica, R.R. (1968). The vocal repertoire of the bullfrog (*Rana catesbeiana*). *Behaviour, 31,* 302–325.

Capranica, R.R. (1976). Morphology and physiology of the auditory system. In R. Llinas & W. Precht (Eds.), *Frog Neurobiology* (pp. 551–575). Berlin: Springer-Verlag.

Capranica, R.R., & Moffat, A.J.M. (1977). Place mechanism underlying frequency analysis in the toad's inner ear. *Journal of Acoustical Society of America,* 62 (Suppl.): S36.

Chung, S.H., Pettigrew, A.G. and Anson, M. (1981). Hearing in the frog: dynamics of the middle ear. *Proceedings of the Royal Society of London, 212,* 459–485.

Davies, N.B., & Halliday, T.R. (1979), Competitive mate searching in male common toads, *Bufo bufo. Animal Behavior, 27,* 1253–1267.

Dickerson, M.C. (1969). *The frog book, North American toads and frogs.* New York: Dover.

Fairchild, L. (1981). Mate selection and behavioral thermoregulation in Fowler's toads. *Science, 212,* 950–951.

Fay, R.R., & Popper, A.N. (1980). Structure and function in teleost auditory structures. In A.N. Popper & R.R. Fay (Eds.), *Comparative studies of hearing in vertebrates.* New York: Springer-Verlag.

Fellers, G.M. (1979). Mate selection in the gray treefrog, *Hyla versicolor. Copeia,* 286–290.

Feng, A.S. (1983). Morphology of neurons in the torus semicircularis of the northern leopard frog, *Rana pipiens pipiens. Journal of Morphology,* 175, 253–269.

Feng, A.S., & Capranica, R.R. (1976). Sound localization in anurans. I. Evidence for binaural interaction in the dorsal medullary nucleus of bullfrogs (*Rana catesbeiana*). *Journal of Neurophysiology, 39,* 871–881.

Feng, A.S., & Capranica, R.R. (1978). Sound localization in anurans. II. Binaural interactions in superior olivary nucleus of the green treefrog (*Hyla cinerea*). *Journal of Neurophysiology, 41,* 43–54.

Feng, A.S., Narins, P.M., Capranica, R.R. (1975). Three populations of primary auditory fibers in the bullfrog (*Rana catesbeiana*): Their peripheral origins and frequency sensitivities. *Journal of Comparative Physiology, 100,* 221–229.

Feng, A.S., Gerhardt, H.C., & Capranica, R.R. (1976). Sound localization behavior of the green treefrog (*Hyla cinerea*) and the barking treefrog (*H. gratiosa*). *Journal of Comparative Physiology, 107,* 241–252.

Frishkopf, L.S., Capranica, R.R., & Goldstein, M.H., Jr. (1968). Neural coding in the bullfrog's auditory system — A teleological approach. *Proceedings of the Institute of Electrical and Electronics Engineers, 56,* 969–980.

Fuzessery, Z.M., & Feng, A.S. (1981). Frequency representation in the dorsal medullary nucleus of the leopard frog, *Rana pipiens. Journal of Comparative Physiology, 143,* 339–347.

Fuzessery, Z.M., & Feng, A.S. (1982). Frequency selectivity in the anuran auditory midbrain: Single unit responses to single and multiple tone stimulation. *Journal of Comparative Physiology, 146,* 471–484.

Fuzessery, Z.M., & Feng, A.S. (1983). Mating call selectivity in the thalamus and midbrain of the leopard frog (*Rana p. pipiens*): Single and multiunit analysis. *Journal of Comparative Physiology, 150,* 333–344.

Gatz, A.J., Jr. (1981). Non-random mating by size in American toads, *Bufo americanus. Animal Behavior, 29,* 1004–1012.

Geisler, C.D., van Bergeijk, W.A., & Frishkopf, L.S. (1964). The inner ear of the bullfrog. *Journal of Morphology, 114,* 43–58.

Gerhardt, H.C. (1974). The significance of some spectral features in mating call recognition in the green treefrog (*Hyla cinerea*). *Journal of Experimental Biology, 61,* 229–241.

Gerhardt, H.C. (1981). Mating call recognition in the barking treefrog (*Hyla gratiosa*): Responses to synthetic calls and comparisons with the green treefrog (*Hyla cinerea*). *Journal of Comparative Physiology, 144,* 17–25.

Gerhardt, H.C. (1982). Sound pattern recognition in some North American treefrogs (Anura: Hylidae): Implications for mate choice. *American Zoologists, 22,* 581–595.

Gerhardt, H.C., & Rheinlaender, J. (1982). Localization of an elevated sound source by the green treefrog. *Science, 217,* 663–664.

Gilbert, L.I., & Frieden, E. (Eds.). (1981). *Metamorphosis. A Problem in Developmental Biology* (2nd ed.). New York: Plenum Press.

Gosner, K.L. (1960). A simplified table for staging anuran embryos and larvae with notes on identification. *Herpetologica, 16,* 183–190.

Gregory, K.M. (1972). Central projections of the eighth nerve in frogs. *Brain, Behavior and Evolution, 5,* 70–88.

Hetherington, T.E., & Lombard, R.E. (1982). Biophysics of underwater hearing in anuran amphibians. *Journal of Experimental Biology, 98,* 49–66.

Hillery, C.M., & Narins, P.M. (1984). Neurophysiological evidence for a travelling wave in the amphibian inner ear. *Science, 225,* 1037–1039.

Howard, R.D. (1978). The evolution of mating strategies in bullfrogs, *Rana catesbeiana. Evolution, 32,* 850–871.

Howard, R.D. (1979). Estimating reproductive success in natural populations. *American Naturalist, 114,* 221–231.

Howard, R.D. (1980). Mating behaviour and mating success in woodfrogs, *Rana sylvatica. Animal Behavior, 28,* 705–716.

Jacoby, J., & Rubinson, K. (1983). The acoustic and lateral line nuclei are distinct in the premetamorphic frog, *Rana catesbeiana. Journal of Comparative Neurology, 216,* 152–161.

Just, J.J., Kraus-Just, J., & Chech, D.A. (1981). Survey of chordate metamorphosis. In L.I. Gilbert & E. Freiden (Eds.), *Metamorphosis. A problem in developmental biology.* New York: Plenum Press.

Katz, L.C., Potel, M.J., & Wassersug, R.J. (1981). Structure and mechanisms of schooling in tadpoles of the clawed frog, *Xenpous laevis. Animal Behavior, 29,* 20–33.

Kruse, K.C. (1981). Mating success, fertilization potential, and male body size in the American toad (*Bufo americanus*). *Herpetologica, 37,* 228–233.

Larsell, O. (1934). The differentiation of the peripheral and central acoustic apparatus in the frog. *Journal of Comparative Neurology, 60,* 473–527.

Lewis, E.R. (1984). On the frog amphibian papilla. *Scanning Electron Microscopy, 4,* 1899–1913.

Lewis, E.R., Baird, R.A., Leverenz, E.L., Koyama, H. (1982). Inner ear: Dye injection reveals peripheral origins of specific sensitivities. *Science, 215,* 1641–1643.

Lewis, E.R., Levernez, E.L., & Koyama, H. (1980). Mapping functionally identified auditory afferents from their peripheral origins to their central terminations. *Brain Research, 197,* 223–229.

Lewis, E.R., Leverenz, E.L., & Koyama, H. (1982). The tonotopic organization of the bullfrog amphibian papilla, an auditory organ lacking a basilar membrane. *Journal of Comparative Physiology, 145,* 437–445.

Li, C.W., & Lewis, E.R. (1974). Morphogenesis of auditory receptor epithelia in the bullfrog. *Scanning Electron Microscopy, 3,* 791–798.

Lombard, R.E., Fay, R.R., & Werner, Y. (1981). Underwater hearing in the frog, *Rana catesbeiana. Journal of Experimental Biology, 91,* 57–71.

Martin, W.F. (1971). Mechanics of sound production in toads of the genus *Bufo*: Passive elements. *Journal of Experimental Zoology, 176,* 273–294.

Matesz, C. (1979). Central projections of the VIIIth cranial nerve in the frog. *Neuroscience, 4,* 2061–2071.

Moffat, A.J.M., & Capranica, R.R. (1978). Middle ear sensitivity in anurans and reptiles measured by light scattering spectroscopy. *Journal of Comparative Physiology, 127,* 97–107.

Narins, P.M., & Capranica, R.R. (1978). Communicative significance of the two-note call of the treefrog *Eleutherodactylus coqui. Journal of Comparative Physiology, 127,* 1–9.

Narins, P.M., & Capranica, R.R. (1980). Neural adaptations for processing the two-note call of the Puerto Rican treefrog, *Eleutherodactylus coqui. Brain, Behavior and Evolution, 17,* 48–66.

Northcutt, R.G. (1980). Central auditory pathways in anamniotic vertebrates. In A.N. Popper & R.R. Fay (Eds.), *Comparative studies of hearing in vertebrates.* New York: Springer-Verlag.

Oldham, R.S., & Gerhardt, H.C. (1975). Behavioral isolating mechanisms of the treefrogs *Hyla cincerea* and *H. gratiosa. Copeia 1975,* 223–231.

Pinder, A.C., & Palmer, A.R. (1983). Mechanical properties of the frog ear: Vibration measurements under free and closed field acoustic conditions. *Proceedings of the Royal Society of London B 219,* 371–396.

Potter, H.D. (1965). Mesencephalic auditory region of the bullfrog. *Journal of Neurophysiology, 28,* 1133–1154.

Rheinlaender, J., Gerhardt, H.C., Yager, D.D., & Capranica, R.R. (1979). Accuracy of phonotaxis by the green treefrog (*Hyla cinerea*). *Journal of Comparative Physiology, 133,* 247–255.

Rose, G., & Capranica, R.R. (1983). Temporal selectivity in the central auditory system of the leopard frog. *Science, 219,* 1087–1089.

Rubinson, K., & Friedman, B. (1977). Vagal afferent projections in *Rana pipiens, Rana catesbeiana,* and *Xenopus mulleri. Brain, Behavior, and Evolution, 14,* 368–380.

Russell, I.J. 91976). Amphibian lateral line receptors. In R. Llinas W. Precht (Eds.) *Frog neurobiology.* Berlin: Springer-Verlag.

Ryan, M.J. (1980). Female mate choice in a neotropical frog. *Science, 209,* 523–525.

Saunders, J.C., & Johnstone, B.M. (1972). A comparative analysis of middle ear function in non-mammalian vertebrates. *Acta Otolaryngology, 73,* 353–361.

Sedra, S.N., & Michael, M.I. (1959). The ontogenesis of the sound conducting apparatus in salientia. *Journal of Morphology, 104,* 359–375.

Shofner, W.P., & Feng, A.S. (1981). Post-metamorphic development of the frequency selectivities and sensitivities of the peripheral auditory system of the bullfrog, *Rana catesbeiana. Journal of Experimental Biology, 93,* 181–196.

Shofner, W.P., & Feng, A.S. (1983). A quantitative light microscopic study of the bullfrog amphibian papilla tectorium: Correlation with the tonotopic organization. *Hearing Research, 11,* 103–116.

Shofner, W.P., & Feng, A.S. (1984). Quantitative light and scanning electron microscopic study of the developing auditory organs in the bullfrog: Implications on their functional characteristics. *Journal of Comparative Neurology, 224,* 141–154.

Shumway, W. (1940). Stages in the normal development of *Rana pipiens*. *Anatomical Record, 78,* 139–147.

Spaeti, U. (1978). Development of the sensory systems in larval and metamorphosing European grass frog (*Rana temporaria L*). *Journal for Hirnforschung, 19,* 543–575.

Straughan, I.R. (1975). An analysis of the mechanisms of mating call discrimination in the frogs *Hyla regilla* and *H. cadaverina*. *Copeia 1975,* 415–424.

Streeter, G.L. (1907). Some factors in the development of the amphibian ear vesicle and further experiments on equilibration. *Journal of Experimental Zoology, 4,* 431–445.

Streeter, G.L. (1921). Migration of the ear vesicle in the tadpole during normal development, 21, 115–126.

Strother, W.F. (1959). The electrical response of the auditory mechanism in the bullfrog (*Rana catesbeiana*). *Journal of Comparative Physiological Psychology, 52,* 157–162.

Sullivan, B.K. (1982). Sexual selection in woodhouse's toad (*Bufo woodhousei*). I. Chrous organization. *Animal Behavior, 30,* 680–686.

Sullivan, B.K. (1983a). Sexual selection in the great plains toad (*Bufo cognatus*). *Behavior, 84,* 258–264.

Sullivan, B.K. (1983b). Sexual selection in woodhouse's toad (*Bufo woodhousei*). II. Female choice. *Animal Behavior, 31,* 1011–1017.

Taylor, A.C., & Kollros, J.J. (1946). Stages in the normal development of *Rana pipiens* larvae. *Anatomical Record, 94,* 7–23.

van Bergeijk, W.A. (1957). Lung volume of amphibian tadpoles. *Science,* 126, 120.

van Bergeijk, W.A. (1967). The evolution of vertebrate hearing. In W.D. Neff (Ed.), *Contributions to sensory physiology* (vol. 2). New York: Academic Press.

Waldman, B. (1981). Sibling recognition in toad tadpoles: The role in experience. *Zeitschrift für Tierpsychology, 56,* 341–358.

Waldman, B., & Adler, K. (1979). Toad tadpoles associate preferentially with siblings. *Nature, 282,* 611–613.

Walkowiak, W. (1980). The coding of auditory signals in the torus semicircularis of the fire-bellied toad and the grass frog: Responses to simple stimuli and to conspecific calls. *Journal of Comparative Physiology, 138,* 131–148.

Weiss, B.A., Stuart, B.H., & Strother, W.F. (1973). Auditory sensitivity in the *Rana catesbeiana* tadpole. *Journal of Herpetology, 7,* 211–214.

Wells, K.D. (1977). Territoriality and male mating success in the green frog (*Rana clamitans*). *Ecology, 58,* 750–762.

Wever, E.G. (1973). The ear and hearing in the frog, *Rana pipiens*. *Journal of Morphology, 141,* 461–478.

Wilbur, H.M., Rubenstein, D.I., & Fairchild, L. (1978). Sexual selection in toads: the roles of female choice and male body size. *Evolution, 32,* 264–270.

Wilczynski, W., & Capranica, R.R. (1984). The auditory system of anuran amphibian. *Progress in Neurobiology, 22,* 1–38.

Wilczynski, W., Zakon, H., & Brenowitz, E. (1983). A sexual difference in basilar papilla tuning in the *Hyla crucifer* auditory system and its behavioral significance. *Society for Neuroscience Abstract, 9,* 531.

Willis, Y.L., Moyle, D.L., & Baskett, T.S. (1956). Emergence, breeding, hibernation, movements and transformation of the bullfrog, *Rana catesbeiana,* in Missouri. *Copeia,* pp. 30–41.

Witschi, E. (1949). The larval ear of the frog and its transformation during metamorphosis. *Zeitscrift für Naturforschung, 4b,* 230–242.

Witschi, E. (1950). The bronchial diverticula of *Xenopus laevis* Daudin. *Anatomical Record, 108,* 590.

Witschi, E. (1955). The bronchial columella of the ear of larval Ranidae. *Journal of Morphol-*

ogy, 96, 497–511.

Witschi, E. (1956). *Development of vertebrates.* Philadelphia, PA: Saunders.

Wright, A.J. (1914). *North American anura. life histories of the anura of Ithaca, New York.* Washington, DC: Carnegie Institution of Washington.

Wright, M.R. (1951). The lateral line system of sense organs. *Quarterly Review of Biology, 26,* 264–280.

Zakon, H.H. (1983). Reorganization of connectivity in amphibian central auditory system following VIIIth nerve regeneration: Time course. *Journal of Neurophysiology,* 31, 1410–1427.

Zakon, H., & Capranica, R.R. (1981). Reformation of organized connections in the auditory system after regeneration of the eighth nerve. *Science, 213,* 242–244.

4 Development of the Auditory Nerve

John F. Brugge
Department of Neurophysiology and Waisman Center on
Mental Retardation and Human Development
University of Wisconsin, Madison, WI 53705

INTRODUCTION

Over the past two decades there has been a virtual avalanche of data on the physiology of the auditory nerve in the normal and hearing-impaired adult mammal. From these data we have gained considerable insight into the mechanisms by which acoustic energy is transduced into action potentials by the mechanical and neural elements of the organ of Corti and by which acoustic information is then transmitted from the inner ear to the brain. The experimental approaches used so successfully in studies in the adult animal have, in recent years, been employed in the young animal whose peripheral auditory system is undergoing maturational changes. Most of the work has been carried out in the kitten, mainly because much of the adult data to which the kitten results are compared have been obtained from the cat and because the kitten's peripheral auditory system continues to mature rather gradually for a month or more after birth. Anatomical studies on the developing peripheral auditory system are providing information on the structural bases for the functional development revealed in auditory nerve recordings. This chapter reviews the progress made in understanding the development of the peripheral auditory system from the discharge properties of single eighth-nerve fibers. Other approaches to understanding functional auditory development have been employed, and some of these are reviewed in other chapters in this volume. More direct studies on the development of the middle ear and cochlea will not be covered here in great detail; those descriptions can be found in other reviews on these subjects (Romand, 1983; Rubel, 1975; Saunders, Kaltenbach, & Relkin, 1983). The mechanisms that regulate the development of hair cells and guide the distal processes of spiral ganglion cells to their target sites at the bases of the hair cells are only partially understood. Discussion of these mechanisms is also outside the scope of this chapter, but reviews of the subject have been written recently by Sobkowicz and Rose (1983) and Van de Water (1983).

STRUCTURAL MATURATION OF THE AUDITORY NERVE AND COCHLEAR INNERVATION PATTERNS

In the newborn kitten, spiral ganglion cells and auditory nerve fibers are small, densely packed, and poorly myelinated (Javel, Walsh, & McGee, this volume; Romand & Romand, 1982; Romand, Sans, Romand & Marty, 1976; Romand, Romand, Mulle, & Marty, 1980; Walsh, McGee, Wagahoff, & Scott, 1985). The onset of myelination of the processes of spiral ganglion cells seems to precede that of the perikaryon. At this time the distal processes of spiral ganglion cells and the terminals of olivocochlear neurons contact hair cells, although the innervation patterns are quite different from the ones observed in the adult animal (Pujol & Marty, 1970; Pujol, Carlier, & Devigne, 1978, 1979). Immature afferent and efferent endings make direct contact with the bases of inner hair cells (IHCs). At the bases of outer hair cells (OHCs) only immature afferent synapses are recognized; apparently efferent axons that make up the tunnel-crossing fibers have not yet reached their final destinations. Nonetheless, from the time of birth when a strong acoustic stimulus evokes a cochlear response, electrical stimulation of the crossed olivocochlear bundle results in an increase in amplitude of the cochlear microphonic and summating potentials and a decrease in the N1 component of the eighth-nerve compound action potential (Carlier & Pujol, 1976). These effects are even stronger in the young kitten than in the adult cat. Just what role this highly developed, yet changing, efferent projection system plays in early cochlear development is unknown.

During the first week or two after birth in the cat, around the time of onset of hearing and shortly thereafter, some remarkable changes take place in the auditory nerve and its connections with hair cells. Myelination of auditory nerve fibers and the perikarya of the spiral ganglion cells is now well underway. Compared to the newborn, a greater proportion of afferent synapses appear to contact IHCs, and efferent endings are recognized at the bases of OHCs. Pujol et al. (1978) suggested that during this time afferent and efferent axonal endings compete for synaptic space at the base of the hair cell. This hypothesis was tested in kittens by surgically sectioning the efferent axons that course through the dorsal brainstem prior to the time they reach OHCs and observing the resultant innervation pattern (Pujol & Carlier, 1982). In cochleas of animals reared with their olivocochlear bundles sectioned, normal adult OHCs were found, even though the efferent terminals were not present at their bases. On the other hand, a relatively high number of afferent synapses remained in touch with the OHCs, many of them making contact with the OHC membrane that had developed structurally in apparent anticipation of an efferent contact. Two conclusions were drawn from these results. First, the final stages of OHC differentiation seem to occur in the absence of efferent input, including the formation and retention of postsynaptic specializations normally associated with efferent endings. Second, the afferent axons do not retract unless forced to do so by incoming efferent terminals. The physiological roles of the afferent axons that remain under such conditions are not clear. By three weeks of age the organ of Corti of the cat looks perfectly mature from a synaptic point of view. Myelination of the auditory nerve is not complete, on the other hand, until some 3–6 months postpartum (Romand et al., 1976; Walsh et al., 1985).

The organs of Corti of the mouse (Kikuchi & Hilding, 1965; Shnerson, Devigne, & Pujol, 1982), rat (Lenoir, Shnerson, & Pujol, 1980), hamster (Pujol & Abonnenc, 1977), and guinea pig (Pujol & Hilding, 1973) are also very immature at birth, although both IHCs and OHCs and their synaptic contacts are recognized at that time. The spiral ganglion neurons, including their processes, are not myelinated in the hamster at birth. In this animal, the process begins 3 days after birth and is completed during the third postnatal week (Pujol & Abonnenc, 1977). It is also reported that IHCs of the newborn mouse and rat, like those of the newborn cat, receive both afferent and efferent endings, whereas OHCs are contacted by afferent terminals only. Over the next 3 weeks of postnatal life there is considerable change in the structure of the hair cells and in sculpting of synaptic space, mainly at the bases of OHCs. The arrival of efferent endings at the bases of OHCs during the second postnatal week coincides with the onset of hearing and, in the mouse at least, the subsequent maturation of the efferent synapses on OHCs is correlated with functional maturation of the cochlea (Shnerson & Pujol, 1982).

Less is known about the development of the central terminals of auditory nerve fibers than about the development of their peripheral innervation patterns. In the kitten, the terminals of the ascending branches of the auditory nerve, the end bulbs of Held, undergo considerable remodeling during the first few weeks of postnatal life (Ryugo & Fekete, 1982), which may account for some of the functional changes recorded in neurons of the anteroventral cochlear nucleus (AVCN) during that early postnatal period (Brugge, Javel, & Kitzes, 1978; Brugge, Kitzes, & Javel, 1981; Romand & Marty, 1975).

In the newborn hamster, cochlear nerve fibers are seen entering the ventral but not the dorsal cochlear nucleus (DCN; Schweitzer & Cant, 1984). The ingrowth of fibers to the DCN occurs during the first 10 days or so of postnatal life and follows a spatial gradient; the dorsomedial region, which receives afferent fibers from the cochlear base, is invaded before the ventrolateral area which is connected with the cochlear apex. Thus, the maturational gradient of cochlear afferent innervation of the DCN may parallel, in the hamster at least, the base-to-apex developmental gradient of the organ of Corti.

A similar picture emerges from studies of the development of afferent innervation of the DCN of the gerbil (Schwartz & Ryan, 1985). Synaptic structures are sparse in this area until a few days prior to the onset of hearing. Development is then rapid and synaptic morphology is essentially adultlike by the end of the third postnatal week.

DEVELOPMENT OF THRESHOLD

The pure-tone threshold for an auditory nerve fiber is related both to the fiber's characteristic frequency (CF) and postnatal age (Dolan, Teas, & Walton, 1985; Kettner, Feng, & Brugge, 1985; Romand, 1983). This is illustrated in Figure 1 where threshold values at the CF are plotted as a function of CF for auditory nerve fibers in young kittens and adult cats. The solid line on each graph estimates the lowest thresholds obtained in adult nerve fibers in this particular study (see also Liberman, 1978).

Within the first week of postnatal life in the cat, threshold responses of auditory nerve fibers to tonal stimulation typically require intensities greater than 100 dB SPL and are rarely obtained at frequencies greater than about 8 kHz. With advancing age, thresholds fall, reaching adult values sometime during the third to fifth weeks postpartum. By the second postnatal week, the CF representation reaches about 20 kHz or more, and thresholds, while still high, have for many fibers fallen well below 100 dB. The range of thresholds at this time may be 80 dB or more especially in the mid-CF region (Dolan et al., 1985), a region of the cat cochlea in which OHCs develop earliest (Mair, 1973). After the first week of life, the time course of threshold development is, on the average, independent of CF, as can be seen in Figure 2, which plots the average threshold as a function of postnatal age for low-, medium-, and high-CF fibers (corresponding to approximately equal distances along the basilar membrane of the adult cat).

The mechanisms that underlie these changes in threshold are poorly understood, but they likely involve the structural maturation of both the middle and inner ears. During the first week of life the middle ear cavity of the kitten is filled with undifferentiated mesenchymal tissue, the ossicles are not fully calcified, and the tympanic bulla is cartilaginous and small as compared to the adult cat. By the end of the second week most of the mesenchymal tissue is resorbed and the middle ear cavity is largely air filled. Clearing of the middle ear cavity coincides in time with reduced thresholds recorded at the level of the auditory nerve (Dolan et al., 1985; Kettner et al., 1985) and cochlear nuclei (Brugge et al., 1978). While sound transmission loss due to an underdeveloped middle ear may account for much of the threshold elevation observed during the early postnatal period, there is some question whether the subsequent 70–100-dB improvement in threshold can be accounted for on the basis of improved sound transmission alone. A portion of the threshold elevation in kittens can be attributed to immature mechanical mechanisms in the

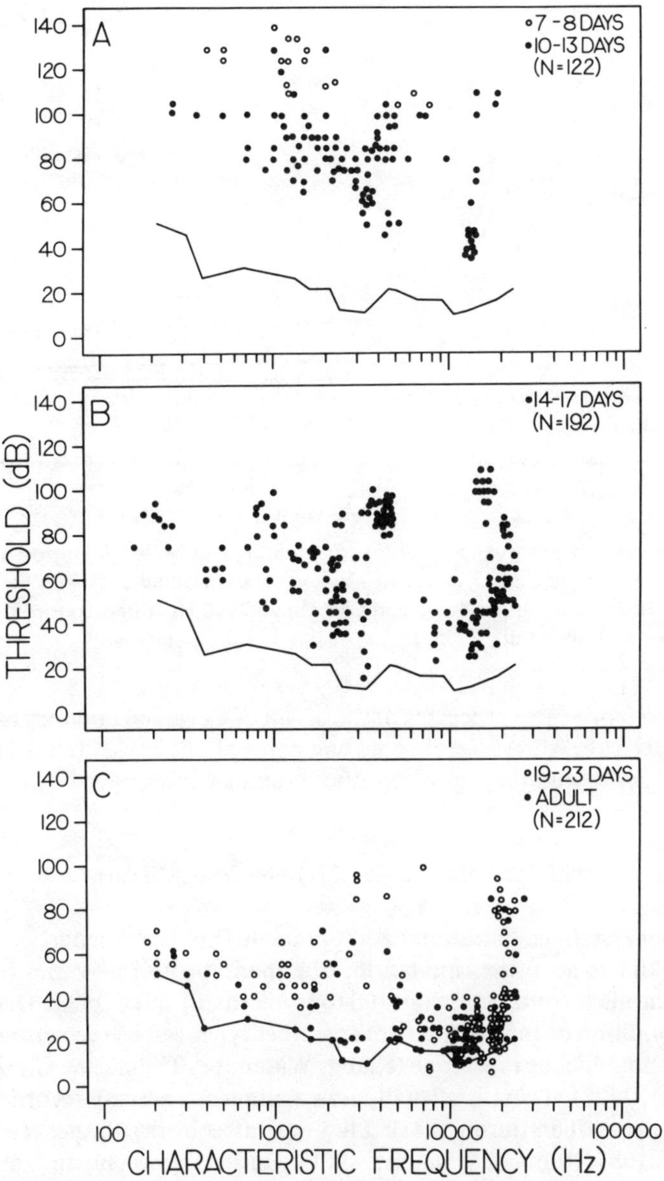

Figure 1. Threshold at CF plotted as a function of CF for auditory nerve fibers in kittens and cats. (A) Thresholds obtained at 7–8 days (open circles) and 10–13 days (filled circles) after birth. (B) Thresholds obtained from kittens 14–17 days of age. (C) Thresholds obtained from 19–23-day-old kittens (open circles) and adult cats (filled circles). The solid line in each graph estimates the lowest thresholds obtained for adult cats. The number of auditory nerve fibers (*N*) studied is shown on each graph. (Reproduced from Kettner et al., 1985, by permission of the publisher.)

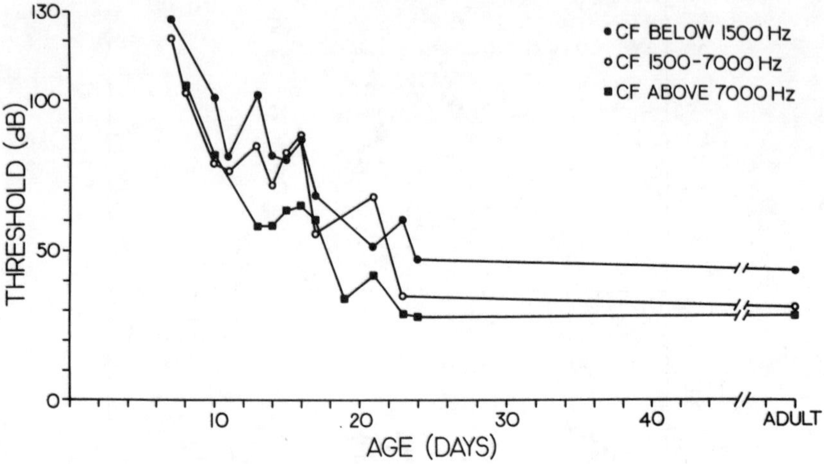

Figure 2. Average threshold values for auditory nerve fibers plotted as a function of age for three ranges of CF: CFs below 1500 Hz (filled circles), CFs between 1500 and 7000 Hz (open circles), and CFs above 7000 Hz (filled squares). (Reproduced from Kettner et al., 1985, by permission of the publisher.)

cochlea and/or neural processes of the organ of Corti and auditory nerve. As we shall see later, threshold changes can come about by age-related changes in the shapes of auditory nerve threshold tuning curves.

DEVELOPMENT OF SPONTANEOUS ACTIVITY

Auditory nerve fibers in normal adult animals fire spontaneously in the absence of known acoustic stimulation. The spontaneous rate varies from one fiber to the next, from more than 100 to fewer than 1 spikes per s. Depending on the condition of the ear, two or three fiber types can be recognized on the basis of spontaneous rate alone (Kiang, Watanabe, Thomas, & Clark, 1965; Liberman, 1978). There is virtually no spontaneous activity recorded in cat auditory nerve fibers during the first few days after birth (Kettner et al., 1985; Romand, 1983; Romand & Dauzat, 1981). During the second and third postnatal weeks only one population of spontaneously active fibers is recognized, and the rates rarely exceed 20 spikes per s. Even as late as 40 days postpartum this rate only increases, on the average, by about 5 spikes per s.

There are perhaps several mechanisms that, together, govern spontaneous activity in the adult auditory nerve, but they are only partly understood. It is apparent that action potentials are triggered near the distal terminals of eighth-nerve fibers by postsynaptic potentials resulting from quantal release of neurotransmitter from presynaptic sites at the bases of the hair cell (e.g.,

Furukawa & Matsuura, 1978). Sewell (1984b) recently showed that intravenous injection of furosemide, an ototoxic diuretic, into anesthetized adult cats results in a simultaneous reduction in the endocochlear potential (EP) and the level of spontaneous activity of single auditory nerve fibers. These results are consistent with the hypothesis that spontaneous activity in the adult cat is the result of voltage-dependent release of the hair cell neurotransmitter. The EP in the kitten is very low at birth and only gradually achieves its adult magnitude during the first postnatal month (Fernandez & Hinojosa, 1974). Thus, one reason for a low spontaneous rate in kitten auditory nerve fibers may be the relatively low flow of resting current through the young hair cell. Indeed, this may also account for the relatively low maximal discharge rate recorded in fibers from very young kittens (Kettner et al., 1985).

In auditory nerve fibers innervating damaged adult cochleas, spontaneous activity is often abnormally low (Kiang, Moxon, & Levine, 1970; Kiang, Liberman, & Levine, 1976; Liberman & Dodds, 1984; Liberman & Kiang, 1978; Robertson & Manly, 1974). Such a decrease in activity has been correlated with a selective loss of the tallest row of stereocilia of IHCs (Liberman & Dodds, 1984; Liberman & Kiang, 1978). It has been suggested that the decrease in spontaneous rate occurs under these conditions because of the reduction in resting current that normally flows through the stereocilia membrane and eventually releases neurotransmitter at the synapse. It is conceivable that in newborn animals the stereocilia membranes are underdeveloped, which, when coupled with a relatively small endocochlear potential, could lead to small resting currents. This, in turn, could result in a low spontaneous discharge rate.

The level of spontaneous activity in the adult auditory nerve is also highly correlated with fiber diameter, synaptic morphology, and synaptic location around the circumference of the IHC (Liberman, 1980a, 1980b, 1982; Liberman & Oliver, 1984). In fact, fibers with the smallest diameters tend to have the lowest spontaneous rates. These structural properties undergo considerable change during development, which may account, in part at least, for changes in the spontaneous activity level in maturing primary afferent neurons.

DEVELOPMENT OF FREQUENCY SELECTIVITY

Auditory nerve fibers are responsive within a restricted range of frequencies and intensities, referred to as the response area of the fiber. The threshold tuning curve, which plots the sound pressure level required to evoke a criterion threshold response as a function of stimulus frequency, outlines the response area. The shape of the tuning curve accurately reflects the shape of the mechanical resonance curve derived from the segment of the basilar membrane contacted by the fiber under study (e.g., Khanna & Leonard, 1982; Rhode, 1978). The frequency to which the fiber is most sensitive, the best or characteristic frequency, corresponds to a restricted locus of resonance along the basilar membrane. Thus, from the shape of the tuning curve alone, it is possible to make inferences about cochlear mechanisms.

During the first postnatal week in the kitten, auditory nerve responses are restricted to stimulus frequencies below about 8 kHz. Tuning curves recorded at this time are characteristically broad and, because of this, it is difficult to assign to them a CF (Dolan et al., 1985; Romand, 1983). Because the cochlear base matures structurally before the apex, some think that the broad low-frequency tuning curves are derived from fibers innervating the cochlear base. Romand (1983) has suggested that such a shallow function represents the tail of what in fact is a tuning curve of a high-CF fiber and that the underdeveloped middle ear so attenuates high-frequency sounds that the more sharply tuned tip of the curve is never seen.

Frequency selectivity in the kitten auditory nerve develops rapidly during the next few weeks of life. As shown in Figure 3, the most striking changes are the deepening of the tip of the tuning curve with the concomitant drop in fiber threshold (the tip-to-tail ratio increases) and the appearance of fibers with progressively higher CFs. By the end of the first postnatal month, tuning curves have the shapes generally attributed to adult animals (Dolan et al., 1985; Romand, 1979, 1983).

It has been suggested that the change in tip-to-tail ratio during development may reflect the changes in relative contributions made by IHCs and OHCs to the shape of the tuning curve (Brugge et al., 1981; Dolan et al., 1985). This notion derives from the fact that, in adult animals with OHCs destroyed by ototoxins or acoustic overstimulation, the tuning curves of auditory nerve fibers innervating the region round the OHC lesions are characteristically broad; they appear as though their tips have been removed (Dallos & Harris, 1978; Evans & Harrison, 1978; Evans & Klinke, 1982; Harrison & Evans, 1979; Kiang et al., 1976; Liberman & Dodds, 1984; Liberman & Mulroy, 1982; Schmiedt, Zwislocki, & Hamernik, 1980). Thus, according to one hypothesis, during the first 2 weeks or so of postnatal life in the kitten, the frequency selectivity of auditory nerve fibers is governed mainly by the output of the IHC with the later developing OHC gradually contributing to frequency sharpening. In support of this hypothesis, Dolan et al. (1985) recently found that fibers with CFs around 5 kHz develop adultlike tuning curves earlier than fibers with higher or lower CFs. According to Mair (1973), it is the region of the cat cochlea representing 5 kHz in which OHCs are first structurally mature. The mechanisms by which IHCs and OHCs might interact are not well understood. One way, postulated by Liberman and Dodds (1984), is that activity of OHCs is transmitted via the tectorial membrane to the tallest row of IHC stereocilia on the IHCs. This mechanism

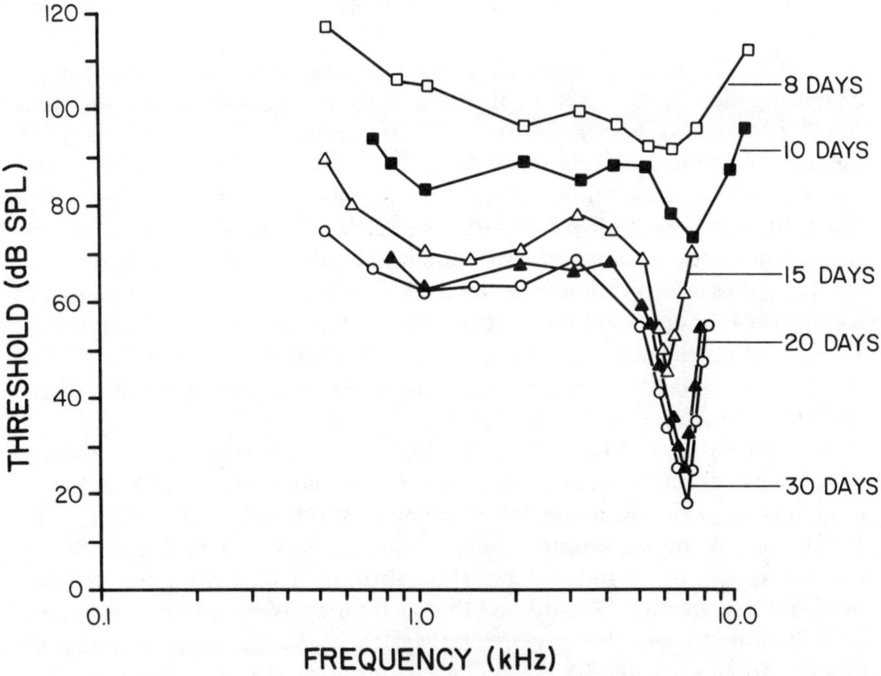

Figure 3. Threshold tuning curves derived from responses of fiber auditory nerve fibers in kittens of different ages. Curves were chosen to compare tuning at the same CF. (Adapted from Romand, 1983, by permission of the publisher.)

is suggested by the observation that blunt tuning curves are recorded from cochleas in which the outer row of stereocilia on IHCs have been damaged.

More recently Sewell (1984a) reported that intravenous administration of furosemide elevates the threshold of auditory nerve fibers and simultaneously reduces the endocochlear potential. Threshold elevation in these experiments occurred mainly at frequencies around the tip of the tuning curve resulting in a decrease in the fibers' frequency selectivity. The correlation between EP and threshold at CF is high; there is approximately 1 dB of threshold elevation for every millivolt (mV) decrease in EP. In the newborn kitten thresholds are high, tuning curves are relatively shallow, and the EP is less than 15 mV in amplitude. The EP grows steadily over the succeeding 3–5 weeks when it reaches adult values of some 70–100 mV (Fernandez & Hinojosa, 1974). Thresholds and tuning curve shapes become adultlike during this same time period. Applying Sewell's (1984a) formula to the developing kitten, the growth of the EP would correspond to a threshold shift of some 80 dB, which is close to that recorded during the first few weeks of postnatal life.

RATE VERSUS INTENSITY

As a rule in auditory nerve fibers of the adult cat, spike count is an increasing monotonic function of sound pressure level over a range of some 20–40 dB (Sachs & Abbas, 1974); this is referred to as the dynamic range of the fiber. At stimulus levels above those that result in saturation firing, spike count usually changes little or may fall slightly. In some cases, however, when the levels reach 80–95 dB SPL, the discharge rate falls abruptly; with further increases in sound intensity of but a few dB the spike rate just as abruptly returns to saturation firing levels (Kiang & Moxon, 1972; Liberman & Kiang, 1984). This dip in the function may reach spontaneous firing levels. These relationships hold throughout the fiber's response area, although the slope of the rising phase of the spike-count-versus-intensity-curve may differ on either side of the CF (Sachs & Abbas, 1974).

In auditory nerve fibers of kittens younger than 2 weeks of age, the dynamic range is narrower than that observed in older kittens and adult cats (Dolan et al., 1985; Romand, 1983; Romand & Dauzat, 1981; Walsh et al., 1985). Representative auditory nerve data are shown in Figure 4. At the earliest ages shown, spike count rises abruptly from threshold, reaches maximal firing within 5–10 dB and then, with increasing intensity, levels off or falls dramatically. With advancing age the dynamic range lengthens so that, by about the end of the second week of life, the slope of the steeply rising portion of the rate-versus-intensity function is similar to that derived from such curves from adult auditory nerve fibers. This age-related change in the slope of the rate curve follows a course similar to that exhibited by the input–output function derived from gross auditory nerve action potential (AP) recording from the round window (Carlier & Pujol, 1978).

It has been suggested that in the adult animal the outputs of both IHCs and OHCs contribute to the shape of the input–output function of the auditory nerve (Liberman & Kiang, 1984; Sellick, Patussi, & Johnstone, 1982; Sokolich, Hamernik, Zwislocki, & Schmiedt, 1976; Wang & Dallos, 1972). According to one hypothesis, OHCs contribute the more gradual rising part of the curve, just above threshold, whereas the IHCs provide for the remainder of the function (Carlier & Pujol, 1978). This notion was given support by findings that, in guinea pigs treated with kanomycin which destroyed mainly the OHCs, thresholds were elevated and the input–output functions derived from gross AP (Dallos & Wang, 1974; Wang & Dallos, 1972) and single-fiber (Harrison, 1981) recordings were exceptionally steep.

A different two-component hypothesis (Liberman & Kiang, 1984) also involves the interaction of IHCs and OHCs. Two components to the rate-versus-intensity function are recognized by a dip in the curve (and a simultaneous phase shift) at relatively high stimulus levels (85–100 dB). In acous-

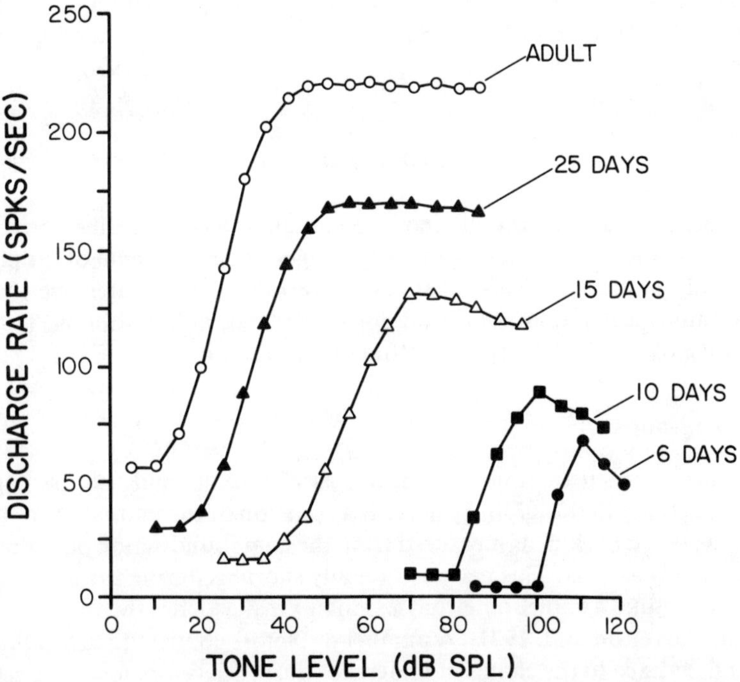

Figure 4. Discharge rate plotted as a function of stimulus intensity at CF for five auditory nerve fibers in kittens and adult cat. (Adapted from Romand, 1983, by permission of the publisher.)

tically traumatized animals in which the OHCs and the tallest stereocilia on IHCs are destroyed, the low-to-moderate intensity component of the function is eliminated as is the tip of the tuning curve. The remaining rate function and tuning curve resemble those derived from auditory nerve discharges in 1-week-old kittens. Liberman and Kiang (1984) speculate that in their adult cats, the low and moderate SPLs which generate one component of the rate function require activity of OHCs to be transmitted mechanically to the tall IHC stereocilia via the tectorial membrane; the second, high threshold, component is dominated by the shorter IHC stereocilia. Recall that during the first few weeks of life the development of the OHC and its innervation pattern, for any given patch of basilar membrane, lag behind that of the IHC, suggesting that, regardless of the mechanisms that might link IHCs and OHCs, in normal newborn kittens the relatively steep rate functions may be governed largely by the more mature IHCs.

The maximal spike count obtained from auditory nerve fibers at CF in week-old kittens is well below that recorded in fibers from older animals and adult cats (Kettner et al., 1985). A week or so later this saturation count has gradually risen to adult levels. Similar observations on the development of firing rates were made in the kitten AVCN (Brugge et al., 1978).

TIMING OF THE DISCHARGE

The time structure of the discharge of an auditory nerve fiber undergoes some dramatic changes during the latter stages of development of the peripheral auditory system. These changes are reflected in the latent period, the peristimulus distribution of action potentials, and, at low stimulus frequencies, the positions of the spikes within the stimulus cycle.

Latent Period

The time between the onset of an acoustic stimulus and the first sign of evoked activity in the auditory nerve is a function of the animal's age. In kittens, the latent period, as measured from the compound action potential, approaches some 3 ms. This period gradually shortens during the next 3 weeks when it assumes a value somewhat less than 1 ms, which is the value recorded in adult cats (Romand, 1971). A number of factors contribute to this time delay and perhaps to the change it undergoes during development. The relative contribution of each of these possible sources of temporal delay is difficult to determine. Although no direct mechanical measurements have been made of the basilar membrane motion in the newborn animal, it may be the case that propagation time is impeded by the mechanical properties of an immature organ of Corti, especially in the apical region of the cochlea where maturation is last to occur. Another possible source of delay may be in the transmission across the hair cell–auditory-nerve-fiber synapse which, as previously mentioned, is not mature until some 3 weeks after birth. Finally, it could be expected that conduction velocity is relatively low in the small, thinly myelinated kitten auditory nerve fibers, although it is difficult to see how a change in conduction velocity alone could, over such a short distance, account for a change in latency of several milliseconds

Peristimulus Time Structure

The peristimulus response profile of the discharge of an auditory nerve fiber undergoes substantial change during the first few weeks of life in the cat (Carlier, Abonnenc, & Pujol, 1975; Romand, 1983; Walsh, McGee, & Javel, 1982). In response to an intense tone of 50-ms duration, auditory nerve fibers during the first few days of life respond with little more than an onset burst of spikes. By about the fifth day of life the discharge takes on the temporal profile of a "primarylike" response which characterizes adult auditory nerve fibers (see also Brugge et al., 1978). As shown in Figure 5, when the tone is lengthened, the response of auditory nerve fibers of very young kittens is not sustained but breaks up into spike bursts which are separated by intervals of around 100–150 ms. The great majority of auditory nerve fibers pass through this bursting stage, which may last until around the end of the second postnatal week. The mechanisms that underlie this burst activity are not known, but they appear not to represent a rhythm inherent in the spiral ganglion cell, because the interburst interval changes with the frequency and intensity of the tone (Walsh et al., 1985). These bursts are seen in the discharges of central auditory neurons as well (Brugge & O'Connor, 1984; Pujol, 1972; Romand & Marty, 1975). By about the third postnatal week, the peristimulus response pattern is indistinguishable from that derived from auditory nerve recordings in adult cats.

Phase Locking

It is a general rule in adult animals that, in response to suprathreshold low-frequency sounds below about 4 kHz, the discharge of an auditory nerve fiber is locked to a particular phase of the stimulus waveform (Brugge, Anderson, Hind, & Rose, 1969; Johnson, 1980; Rose, Brugge, Anderson, & Hind, 1967). Consequently, the nerve impulses within such a discharge train occur at intervals corresponding to integral multiples of the period of the stimulating wave form that arises on the basilar membrane in response to the low-frequency sound. This so-called period–time code is required by the volley theory of hearing that Wever (1949) put forward several decades ago.

Phase locking is best displayed in the period histogram, which plots the distribution of spikes during one stimulus cycle. A measure of phase locking, called the vector strength or synchronization index, may also be derived from the spike distribution (see Goldberg & Brown, 1969, for the derivation) and used for comparing the timing among fibers. This index ranges in value from zero to one; a value of zero is typically associated with a flat period histogram indicating no relationship of spike firing to a particular phase of the stimulus cycle, whereas a value near one is associated with a sharply peaked, unimodal histogram indicating that impulses are tightly grouped around a particular phase angle of the stimulus wave form. Period histograms and the associated synchronization indices are shown in Figure 6 for auditory nerve fibers from kittens and adult cats. The histograms are derived from responses of 16 different auditory nerve fibers to one of four stimulus frequencies placed at or near the fiber's CF at an intensity set 10–30 dB above threshold.

It can be readily seen in Figure 6 that secure phase locking is present at 500 Hz in both young kittens 7 days of age and in the adult cat. As stimulus frequency is raised, the degree of synchrony falls off more rapidly in the young

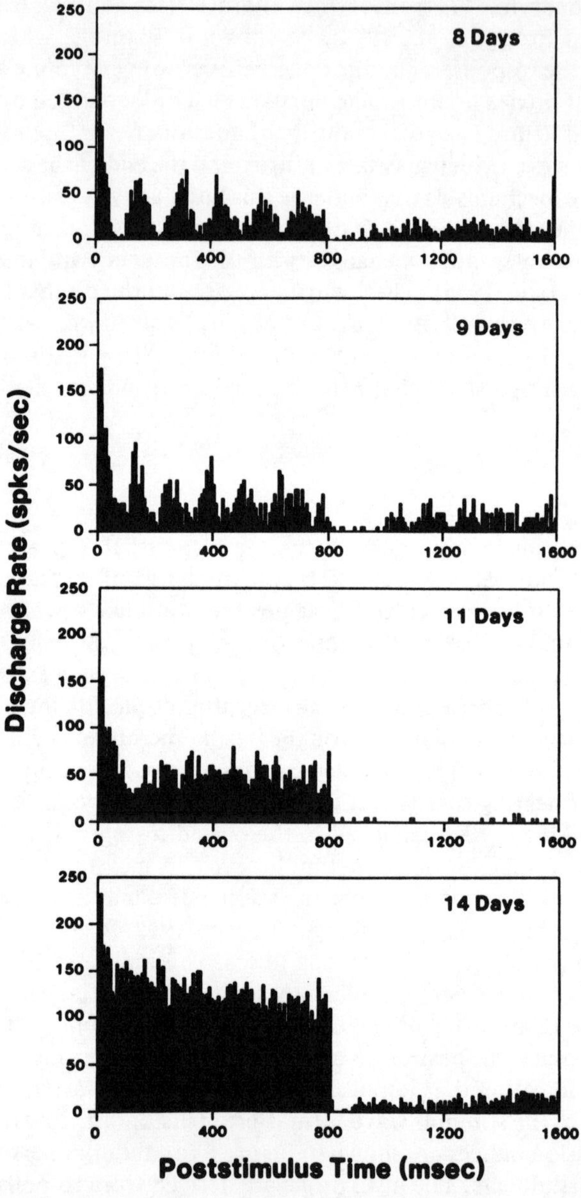

Figure 5. Peristimulus time histograms derived from auditory nerve fiber responses to CF tones at moderate stimulus intensities. Tone duration in all cases is 800 msec (Walsh, McGee, & Javel, 1982).

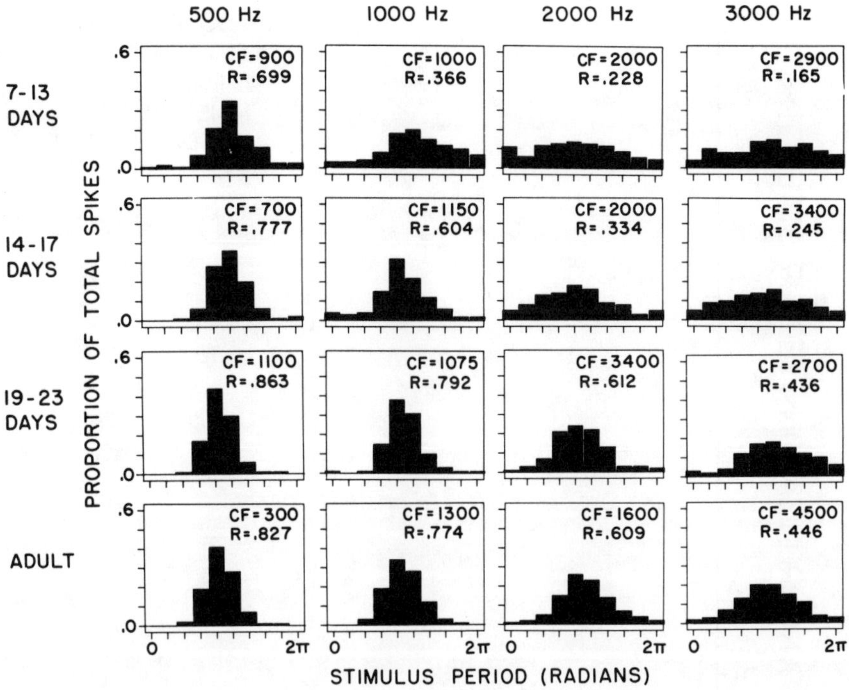

Figure 6. Period histograms derived from discharges of 16 auditory nerve fibers at stimulus frequencies of 500, 1000, 2000, and 3000 Hz. Data presented for cats of different postnatal ages. The CF of the fiber studied and the vector strength of the response are displayed with each histogram. (Reproduced from Kettner et al., 1985, by permission of the publisher.)

kitten than it does in the older kitten or adult cat. The upper frequency limit for phase locking in the adult is reached gradually toward the end of the third postnatal week, a time when thresholds also reach their adult values. The time course of development of the phase locked response is similar for fibers with different CFs. The relationships of synchronization, stimulus frequency, and the age of the animal are shown in Figure 7. At all ages, the maximal phase synchrony at any given low frequency is generally obtained at stimulus intensities less than 20 dB above the rate threshold and some 10–30 dB below the saturation firing level of the fiber.

The factors that limit phase locking in animals of any age are not well understood. In the kitten some or all of them may reside in the cochlea which is undergoing dramatic structural change during the time that phase locking matures. The fact that the cochlear microphonic potential is present over the full audible frequency range by the end of the first postnatal week (Romand, 1971) would seem to indicate that the basilar membrane and other peripheral

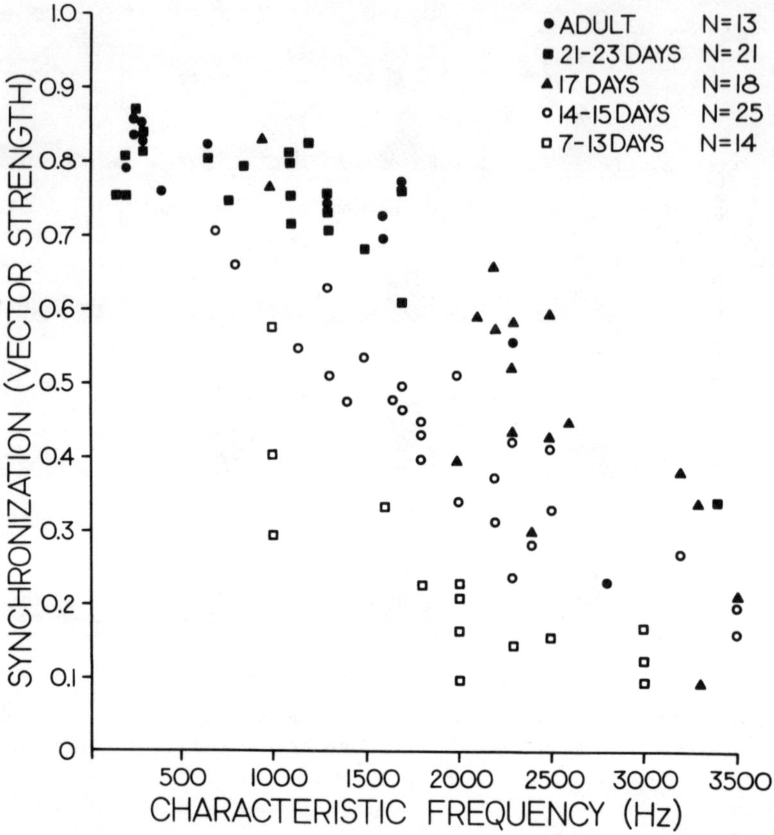

Figure 7. Maximal vector strength at CF plotted as a function of CF for auditory nerve fibers from several postnatal age groups. (Reproduced from Kettner et al., 1985, by permission of the publisher.)

auditory structures are transducing signals normally over a range of frequencies wider than that to which auditory nerve fibers phase-lock. Russell and Sellick (1978) suggest from their results of intracellular recording of adult cochlear IHCs that in the adult the fall in phase synchrony with increasing frequency is due to the passive electrical properties of the hair cell membrane. Assuming that these passive electrical properties of hair cells exert the same control over spike timing in cat and kitten, then age-related changes in synchrony may be the result of changes in the passive electrical properties of developing hair cell membranes.

The underdeveloped synapses between the hair cell and auditory nerve fiber may also contribute to relatively poor phase synchrony in kitten auditory nerve fibers. Recall that the time course of development of synapses on IHCs, from which it is assumed that most, if not all, auditory nerve recordings are made, is highly correlated with that of phase locking ability of auditory nerve fibers.

Developmental changes in the phase-locked response could result from immaturities associated with the auditory nerve fiber itself. It is likely that both conduction velocity and refractory period are influenced by the changes taking place in axonal growth and myelination. If a changed conduction velocity is shared equally by all action potentials in the discharge, it is difficult to see how this factor alone could disrupt synchrony. It is known that the absolute refractory period is not the factor that limits phase locking in the adult animal at moderate discharge rates (Johnson & Swami, 1983; Rose et al., 1967), although at high discharge rates the time of occurrence of the spike may be influenced by nerve conduction time (Gaumond, Molnar, & Kim, 1982). Whatever the mechanisms involved, if a longer refractory period and/or a lower conduction velocity lead(s) to a greater variability ("jitter") in the time at which a spike occurs, then the upper limit for phase locking would be reduced (see also Anderson, 1973).

At all ages, the degree of phase locking is a function of stimulus intensity as well as frequency (Johnson, 1980; Kettner et al., 1985). Locking becomes more pronounced as stimulus intensity is increased above threshold. Maximal synchrony is usually achieved around 20–30 dB above threshold. At higher SPLs the degree of phase locking levels off or decreases slightly. In both the cat (Johnson, 1980) and kitten (Kettner et al., 1985), phase locking reaches a maximum at stimulus intensities below that at which discharge rate saturates. In kitten fibers showing spontaneous activity, phase locking is often demonstrable at sound pressure levels below those needed to raise firing rate, a finding that is common in the adult nerve (Johnson, 1980; Rose et al., 1967).

In both kitten (Kettner et al., 1985) and adult cat (Gibson, Hind, Kitzes, & Rose, 1977), when stimulus frequency is changed at a constant SPL over the range of phase-locking frequencies, there is a systematic shift in the average phase of the discharge. The data points relating changes in stimulus frequency to the cumulative phase shift may be fit with a straight line, although there is additional evidence in adult animals that this relationship may be more complex than a linear fit implies (e.g., Ronkin, 1986). Regardless of the departure from a straight-line relationship, the slope of a linearly fitted curve reflects a time delay, which includes mainly the travel time along the basilar membrane and fixed neural delays between the cochlea and the electrode recording site. For kittens in the third postnatal week, estimates of time delays are close to those derived from similar experiments in adult cats, especially for fibers with CFs above 3 kHz (Kettner et al., 1985). For fibers with lower CFs, delays tend to be somewhat longer and to vary more between fibers as compared to the adult. Ronkin (1986), in a fine-grained study of the phase behavior of discharges from adult gerbil auditory nerve fibers, found rather complicated phase-versus-frequency curves, which he attributed to local properties of the mechanisms that influence normal sensitivity and tuning of auditory nerve fibers. Such detailed studies in newborn animals may give similar clues as to the developing local mechanical properties of the basilar membrane.

SUMMARY AND CONCLUSIONS

The spiral ganglion neuron, which includes its peripheral and central processes, is in all mammals studied so far underdeveloped at birth. During the early postnatal developmental period, which varies from one species to the next, there are dramatic maturational changes in the innervation of the hair cells of the organ of Corti and of the neurons of the cochlear nuclei. The auditory nerve fiber and spiral ganglion cell body grow and acquire a myelin sheath. Furthermore, there are structural changes going on simultaneously in the middle ear and the cochlea. These structural changes are accompanied by equally striking functional changes as revealed in the discharge properties of single auditory nerve fibers.

Thresholds, spontaneous activity, frequency and intensity sensitivity, and timing are properties of auditory nerve fibers that are changing shortly after birth. Many of these changes are attributed not so much to the developing nerve as they are to developing middle and inner ears. This would include changes in the transmission properties of the middle ear, the mechanical properties of the cochlear partition, the passive electrical properties of hair cell membranes, the presumed interactions between inner and outer hair cells, and the afferent and efferent innervation patterns at the bases of the hair cells.

REFERENCES

Anderson, D.J. (1973). Quantitative model for the effects of stimulus frequency on synchronization of auditory nerve discharges. *Journal of the Acoustical Society of America, 54,* 361–364.

Brugge, J.F., Anderson, D.J., Hind, J.E., & Rose, J.E. (1969). Time structure of discharges in single auditory nerve fibers of the squirrel monkey in response to complex periodic sounds. *Journal of Neurophysiology, 32,* 286–301.

Brugge, J.F., Javel, E., & Kitzes, L.M. (1978). Signs of functional maturation of peripheral auditory system in discharge patterns of neurons in anteroventral cochlear nucleus of kittens. *Journal of Neurophysiology, 41,* 1557–1579.

Brugge, J.F., Kitzes, L.M., & Javel, E. (1981). Postnatal development of frequency and intensity sensitivity of neurons in the anteroventral cochlear nucleus of kittens. *Hearing Research, 5,* 217–229.

Brugge, J.F., & O'Connor, T.A. (1984). Postnatal functional development of the dorsal and posteroventral cochlear nuclei of the cat. *Journal of the Acoustical Society of America, 75,* 1548–1562.

Carlier, E., Abonnenc, M., & Pujol, R. (1975). Maturation des responses unitaires a la stimulation tonale dans le nerf cochleaire du chaton. [Maturation of unit response to tonal stimulation in the cochlear nerve of the cat] *Journal de Physiologie (Paris), 70,* 129–138.

Carlier, E., & Pujol, R. (1976). Early effects of efferent stimulation on the kitten cochlea. *Neuroscience Letters, 3,* 21–27.

Carlier, E., & Pujol, R. (1978). Role of inner and outer hair cells in coding sound intensity: An ontogenetic approach. *Brain Research, 147,* 174–176.

Dallos, P., & Harris, D. (1978). Properties of auditory nerve responses in absence of outer hair cells. *Journal of Neurophysiology, 41,* 365–383.

Dallos, P., & Wang, C.-Y. (1974). Bioelectric correlates of kanamycin intoxication. *Audiology, 13,* 277–289.

Dolan, D.F., Teas, D.C., & Walton, J.P. (1985). Postnatal development of physiological responses in auditory nerve fibers. *Journal of the Acoustical Society of America, 78,* 544–554.

Evans, E.F., & Harrison, R.V. (1978). Correlation between outer hair cell damage and deterioration of cochlear nerve tuning properties in the guinea pig. *Journal of Physiol. (London), 256,* 43–44.

Evans, E.F., & Klinke, R. (1982). The effects of intracellular and systemic furosemide on the properties of single cochlear nerve fibers in the cat. *Journal of Physiol. (London), 33,* 409–428.

Fernandez, C., & Hinojosa, R. (1974). Postnatal development of endocochlear potential and stria vascularis in the cat. *Acta Otolaryngologica, 78,* 173–186.

Furukawa, T., & Matsuura, S. (1978). Adaptive rundown of excitatory post-synaptic potentials at synapses between hair cells and eighth nerve fibres in the goldfish. *Journal of Physiol. (London), 276,* 193–209.

Gaumond, R.P., Molnar, C.E., & Kim, D.O. (1982). Stimulus and recovery dependence of cat cochlear nerve fiber discharge probability. *Journal of Neurophysiology, 48,* 856–873.

Gibson, M.M., Hind, J.E., Kitzes, L.M., & Rose, J.E. (1977). Estimation of traveling wave parameters from the response properties of cat AVCN neurons. In E.F. Evans & J.P. Wilson (Eds.), *Psychophysics and physiology of hearing* (pp. 57–68). London: Academic Press.

Goldberg, J.M., & Brown, P.B. (1969). Responses of binaural neurons of dog superior olivary complex to dichotic tonal stimuli: Some physiologic mechanisms of sound localization. *Journal of Neurophysiology, 32,* 613–636.

Harrison, R.V. (1981). Rate versus intensity functions and related AP responses in normal and pathological guinea pig and human cochleas. *Journal of the Acoustical Society of America, 70,* 1036–1044.

Harrison, R.V., & Evans, E.F. (1979). Cochlea fiber responses in guinea pigs with well defined cochlear lesions. In H. Hoke & E. de Boer (Eds.), *Models of the auditory system and related signal processing techniques, Scand. Audiol. Suppl., 9,* 83–92.

Johnson, D.H. (1980). The relationship between spike rate and synchrony in responses of auditory-nerve fibers to single tones. *Journal of the Acoustical Society of America, 68,* 1115–1122.

Johnson, D., & Swami, A. (1983). The transmission of signals by auditory-nerve fiber discharge patterns. *Journal of the Acoustical Society of America, 47,* 493–501.

Kettner, R.E., Feng, J.-Z., & Brugge, J.F. (1985). Postnatal development of the phase locked response to low frequency tones of auditory nerve fibers in the cat. *Journal of Neuroscience, 5,* 275–283.

Khanna, S.M., & Leonard, D.G.B. (1982). Basilar membrane tuning in the cat cochlea. *Science, 215,* 305–306.

Kiang, N.Y.-S., Liberman, M.C., & Levine, R.A. (1976). Auditory nerve activity in cats exposed to ototoxic drugs and high-intensity sounds. *Annals of Otology, Rhinology, and Laryngology, 75,* 1–17.

Kiang, N.Y.-S., & Moxon, E.C. (1972). Physiological considerations in artificial stimulation of the inner ear. *Annals of Otology, Rhinology, and Laryngology, 81,* 714–731.

Kiang, N.Y.-S., Moxon, E.C., & Levine, R.A. (1970). Auditory nerve activity in cats with normal and abnormal cochleas. In G.E.W. Wolsenholme & J. Knight (Eds.), *Sensorineural hearing loss* (pp. 241–273). London: Churchill.

Kiang, N.Y.-S., Watanabe, T., Thomas, E.C., & Clark, L.F. (1965). *Discharge patterns of single fibers in the cat's auditory nerve.* Cambridge, MA: MIT Press.

Kikuchi, K., & Hilding, D.A. (1965). The development of the organ of Corti in the mouse. *Acta Otolaryngologica, 60,* 207–222.

Lenoir, M., Shnerson, A., & Pujol, R. (1980). Cochlear receptor development in the rat with emphasis on synaptogenesis. *Anatomy and Embryology, 160,* 253–262.

Liberman, M.C. (1978). Auditory-nerve response from cats raised in a low-noise chamber. *Journal of the Acoustical Society of America, 63,* 442–455.

Liberman, M.C. (1980a). Efferent synapses in the inner hair cell area of the cat cochlea: An electron-microscopic study of serial sections. *Hearing Research, 3,* 189–204.

Liberman, M.C. (1980b). Morphological differences among radical afferent fibers in the cat cochlea: An electron-microscopic study of serial sections. *Hearing Research, 3,* 45–63.

Liberman, M.C. (1982). Single neuron labeling in the cat auditory nerve. *Science, 216,* 1239–1241.

Liberman, M.C., & Dodds, L.W. (1984). Single-neuron labeling and chronic cochlear pathology. II. Stereocilia damage and alterations of spontaneous discharge rates. *Hearing Research, 16,* 43–53.

Liberman, M.C., & Kiang, N.Y.-S. (1978). Acoustic trauma in cats: Cochlear pathology and auditory-nerve activity. *Acta Otolaryngologica Supplement, 358,* 1–63.

Liberman, M.C., & Kiang, N.Y.-S. (1984). Single-neuron labeling and chronic cochlear pathology. IV. Stereocilia damage and alterations in rate- and phase-level functions. *Hearing Research, 16,* 75–90.

Liberman, M.C., & Mulroy, M.J. (1982). Acute and chronic effects of acoustic trauma: Cochlear pathology and auditory-nerve pathophysiology. In P. Hammernick, D. Henderson, & R. Salvi (Eds.), *New perspectives in noise-induced hearing loss* (pp. 105–135). New York: Raven.

Liberman, M.C., & Oliver, M.E. (1984). Morphometry of intracellularly labeled neurons of the auditory nerve: correlation with functional properties. *Journal of Comparative Neurology, 223,* 163–176.

Mair, I.W.S. (1973). Hereditary deafness in the white cat. *Acta Otolaryngologica, 314,* 1–48.

Pujol, R. (1972). Development of tone-burst responses along the auditory pathway in the cat. *Acta Otolaryngological, 74,* 383–391.

Pujol, R., & Abonnenc, M. (1977). Receptor maturation and synaptogenesis in the golden hamster cochlea. *Archives of Oto-Rhino-Laryngology, 217,* 1–12.

Pujol, R., & Carlier, E. (1982). Cochlear synaptogenesis after sectioning the efferent bundle. *Developmental Brain Research, 3,* 151–154.

Pujol, R., Carlier, E., & Devigne, C. (1978). Different patterns of cochlear innervation during development of the kitten. *Journal of Comparative Neurology, 177,* 529–536.

Pujol, R., Carlier, E., & Devigne, C. (1979). Significance of presynaptic formations in early stages of cochlear synaptogenesis. *Neuroscience Letters, 15,* 97–102.

Pujol, R., & Hilding, D. (1973). Anatomy and physiology of the onset of auditory function. *Acta Otolaryngology, 76,* 1–10.

Pujol, R., & Marty, R. (1970). Postnatal maturation in the cochlea of the cat. *Journal of Comparative Neurology, 139,* 115–126.

Rhode, W. (1978). Some observations on cochlear mechanics. *Journal of the Acoustical Society of America, 64,* 158–176.

Robertson, D., & Manley, G.A. (1974). Manipulation o frequency analysis in the cochlear ganglion of the guinea pig. *Journal of Comparative Physiology, 91,* 363–375.

Romand, R. (1971). *Maturation des potentials cochleaires dans la periode postnatale.* [Maturation of the cochlear potentials during the postnatal period].Unpublished thesis, Université des Science et Techniques du Languedoc, Montpellier, Languedoc, France.

Romand, R. (1979). Development of auditory nerve activity in kitten. *Brain Research, 173,* 554–556.

Romand, R. (1983). Development of the cochlea. In R. Romand (Ed.), *Development of auditory and vestibular systems,* (pp. 47–88). New York: Academic Press.

Romand, R., & Dauzat, M. (1981). Spontaneous activity and signal processing in the cochlear nerve of kittens. *Journal of the Acoustical Society of America, 69,* S52.

Romand, R., & Marty, R. (1975). Postnatal maturation of the cochlear nuclei in the cat: A neurophysiological study. *Brain Research, 83,* 225–233.

Romand, R., & Romand M.-R. (1982). Myelination kinetics of spiral ganglion cells in the kitten. *Journal of Comparative Neurology, 204,* 1–5.

Romand, R., Romand, M.-R., Mulle, Ch., & Marty, R. (1980). Early stages of myelination in the spiral ganglion cells of kittens during development. *Acta Otolaryngologica, 90,* 391–397.

Romand, R., Sans, A., Romand, M.-R., & Marty, R. (1976). The structural maturation of the stato-acoustic nerve in the cat. *Journal of Comparative Neurology, 170,* 1–16.

Ronkin, D. (1985). Anomalous phase relations in threshold-level responses from gerbil auditory nerve fibers. *Journal of the Acoustical Society of America, 79,* 417–425.

Rose, J.E., Brugge, J.F., Anderson, D.J., & Hind, J.E. (1967). Phase-locked responses to low-frequency tones in single auditory nerve fibers of the squirrel monkey. *Journal of Neurophysiology, 30,* 769–793.

Rubel, E.W. (1978). Ontogeny of structure and function in the vertebrate auditory system. In M. Jacobson (Ed.). *Handbook of sensory physiology IX: Development of sensory systems* (pp. 135–237). New York: Springer-Verlag.

Russell, I.J., & Sellick, P.M. (1978). Intracellular studies of hair cells in the mammalian cochlea. *Journal of Physiology (London), 284,* 261–290.

Ryugo, D.K., & Fekete, D.M. (1982). Morphology of primary axosomatic endings in the anteroventral cochlear nucleus of the cat: A study of the endbulbs of Held. *Journal of Comparative Neurology, 210,* 239–257.

Sachs, M.B., & Abbas, P.J. (1974). Rate versus level functions for auditory-nerve fibers in cats: Tone-burst stimuli. *The Journal of the Acoustical Society of America, 56,* 1835–1847.

Saunders, J.C., Kaltenbach, J.A., & Relkin, E.M. (1983). The structural and functional development of the outer and middle ear. In R. Romand (Ed.), *Development of auditory and vestibular systems,* (pp. 3–25). New York: Academic Press.

Schmiedt, R.A., Zwislocki, J.J., & Hamernik, R.P. (1980). Effects of hair cell lesions on responses of cochlear nerve fibers. I. Lesions, tuning curves, two-tone inhibition, and responses to trapezoidal-wave patterns. *Journal of Neurophysiology, 43,* 1367–1389.

Schwartz, I.R., & Ryan, A.F. (1985). Development of neurons and synaptic terminals in the cochlear nucleus of the mongolian gerbil. In *Proceedings of the Association for Research in Otolaryngology, Abstracts.*

Schweitzer, L., & Cant, N.B. (1984). Development of the cochlear innervation of the dorsal cochlear nucleus of the hamster. *Journal of Comparative Neurology, 225,* 228–243.

Sellick, P.M., Patussi, R., & Johnstone, B.M. (1982). Modulation of responses of spiral ganglion cells in the guinea pig cochlea by low frequency sound. *Hearing Research, 7,*

199–222.

Sewell, W.F. (1984a). The effects of furosemide on the endocochlear potential and auditory-nerve fibers tuning curves in cats. *Hearing Research, 14,* 305–314.

Sewell, W.F. (1984b). The relation between the endocochlear potential and spontaneous activity in auditory nerve fibres of the cat. *Journal of Physiology (London), 347,* 685–696.

Shnerson, A., Devigne, C., & Pujol, R. (1982). Age-related changes in the C57BL/6J mouse cochlea. II. Ultrastructural findings. *Developmental Brain Research, 2,* 77–88.

Shnerson, A., & Pujol, R. (1982). Age-related changes in the C57BL/6J mouse. I. Physological findings. *Developmental Brain Research, 2,* 65–75.

Sobkowicz, H.M., & Rose, J.E. (1983). Innervation of the organ of Corti of the fetal mouse in culture. In R. Romand (Ed.), *Development of auditory and vestibular systems* (pp. 27–45). New York: Academic Press.

Sokolich, W.G., Hamernik, R.P., Zwislocki, J.J., & Schmiedt, R.R. (1976). Inferred response polarities of cochlear hair cells. *Journal of the Acoustical Society of America, 59,* 963–974.

Van de Water, T.R. (1983). Embryogenesis of the inner ear: *"In vitro"* studies. In R. Romand (Ed.), *Development of auditory and vestibular systems* (pp. 337–374). New York: Academic Press.

Walsh, E.J., McGee, J., & Javel, E. (1982). Development of auditory nerve fiber responses in kittens. *Neuroscience Abstracts, 8,* 345.

Walsh, E.J., McGee, J., Wagahoff, D., & Scott, V. (1985). Myelination of auditory nerve, trapezoidal, and brachium of the inferior colliculus axons in the cat. In *Proceedings of the Association for Research in Otolaryngology, Abstracts.*

Wang, C.-Y., & Dallos, P. (1972). Latency of whole nerve action potentials. Influence of hair cell normalcy. *Journal of the Acoustical Society of America, 52,* 1678–1686.

Wever, E.G. (1949). *Theory of Hearing.* New York: Wiley.

5 Development of Auditory Evoked Potentials in the Kitten*

Jennifer S. Buchwald
Carl Shipley
Department of Physiology, Brain Research Institute, and
Mental Retardation Research Center
School of Medicine, University of California
Los Angeles, CA 90024

INTRODUCTION

For a number of years we have studied the central processing of auditory information as revealed by scalp recorded evoked potentials in human subjects and in the cats as an experimental model. These potentials, which commence within 1–2 ms of stimulus onset and may last for 500–800 ms, reflect the activation of various brain regions and brain systems. If the primary generator substrate of a particular evoked potential component can be defined, that evoked potential then becomes a convenient analytical electrophysiological probe. Thus, changes in the latency, amplitude, or general morphology of a particular auditory evoked response component can be used to assess the functioning of its generator substrate system during early development, the protracted changes of old age, acute trauma and chronic disease, or simply during physiological stresses imposed by parametric manipulations of the stimulus.

Insofar as the scalp recorded evoked potentials are noninvasive, they provide an ideal tool for studying longitudinal development of auditory function within the same subject while at the same time allowing for comparisons with other anatomical and physiological data obtained at specific periods in development across subjects. This chapter is presented as a brief overview of the experimental data which we have collected in an attempt to define the sequence of auditory evoked potentials that can be recorded from the scalp of normal, awake, adult cats, the neuronal substrate reflected by each of these evoked potential components, and the differential development of certain auditory evoked potential components in the kitten during the first year of life. In general, a prolonged sequence of auditory evoked potentials with latencies ranging from 1–400 msc can be recorded from the vertex of the

*This work has been supported by USPHS Research Grants HD-05958, HD-04612, and AG 04088.

awake restrained cat. This sequence is reproducible within and across subjects and is not altered by complete neuromuscular paralysis. The effects of click rate, pentobarbital anesthesia, sleep, and chronic lesions of a number of different brain areas were evaluated for each of the components, as were depth-recorded field potentials and single unit correlates of the surface recorded responses.

SHORT-LATENCY AUDITORY EVOKED POTENTIALS

ABR Waves 1 to 5

In the cat, a series of five short-latency evoked potentials induced by click stimuli can be recorded by a disc electrode placed on the scalp vertex or by a screw implanted in the skull at the vertex; in most cases, the neck or pinna is used as reference (Jewett, 1970; Lev & Sohmer, 1972). This sequence of waves, each of which is separated by an interval of approximately 1 msc, spans a time period of less than 10 msc following stimulus onset (Fig. 1). As will be discussed, these waves have been shown to originate from brainstem generators and have therefore been termed the auditory brainstem response (ABR).

Parametric Studies. Comparisons of ABR amplitude and latency in the awake cat and in the same cat following injections of sodium pentobarbital or ketamine at anesthetic levels or in the same cat during stages of slow wave sleep or rapid-eye movement (REM) sleep show no significant differences (Buchwald, 1983; Chen & Buchwald, 1986). The effects of varying stimulus parameters upon the latency and amplitude of waves 1 to 5 have been extensively studied (Buchwald, 1983). Click rates of 1, 2, 5, 10, 20, 50, 100, and 200/s produce parallel decrements in the amplitudes of all five waves in the cat at rates above 10/s or more, i.e., ABR waves 1 to 5 show similar recovery cycles; only small (0.1 to 0.2 ms) increases in latency occur at the fastest rates (Huang & Buchwald, 1978). With increasing stimulus intensity, amplitudes increase and latencies decrease. These data indicate that waves 1 to 5 are similarly affected by systematic changes in stimulus parameters of rate or intensity.

Depth Recordings of Local Field Potentials and Single Unit Responses Correlated with the ABR. Single units, multiple units, and evoked potentials were recorded from the auditory nerve and cochlear nucleus (CN) and their excitability-recovery functions studied during rates of click stimulation which extended from 1/10 s to 100/s (Huang & Buchwald, 1978, 1979, 1980). Evoked potentials in the auditory nerve and cochlear nucleus showed virtually identical recovery cycles with no change in response amplitude until stimulus rates exceeded 10/s. Some single units likewise showed time-locked "on" responses with no change until stimulus rates exceeded 10/s. Other units, with variable response latencies, showed marked decrements to click rates as low as 1/5 s. Such data suggested that a subpopulation of "timekeeper" neurons, i.e., neurons with little or no latency jitter and recovery cycles that accommodated click rates of 10/s , might correlate in latency with the ABR peaks, and this led to the more extensive study of brainstem nuclei described below.

In this series of experiments, single units and evoked potentials were recorded from the CN, superior olivary complex (SOC), nucleus of the lateral lemniscus (LL), and inferior colliculus (IC), while concurrent recordings of the ABR were made from the vertex (Huang & Buchwald, 1977). The largest component of the depth evoked potential recorded in each successive nucleus was found to occur at a latency which corresponded to the latency of successive ABR wave components. Single units at each relay nucleus showed a wide range of response latencies; however, a subgroup of cells was found in each nucleus which showed exact latencies, i.e., the neuronal latency showed less than ± 0.1ms *SD* over 10 trials. In all cases, these time-locked, "timekeeper" cells showed the shortest latencies. Their average latency in each successive nucleus was essentially the same as the average latency of the successive ABR wave components, i.e., timekeeper units in the CN showed the same average latency as wave 2, in the SOC the same as that of wave 3, and in the LL the same as that of wave 4. The IC units were more variable but still overlapped wave 5 latency. The timekeeper cells were resistant to rapid rates of stimulation and showed no change in click response until rates exceeded 10/s. Thus, a high level of synaptic security distinguished these timekeeper cells from adjacent cells with more variable latencies and longer recovery cycles. Recovery cycles for waves 1 to 5 of the ABR, as already noted, mirrored those of timekeeper neurons.

Lesion Studies. In the adult cat ABR, waves 1 to 5 remained essentially unchanged after complete precollicular decerebration, indicating that the brain rostral to the level of the IC is not essential for an intact ABR (Buchwald & Huang, 1975). In this series of lesion studies, it was also shown that wave 5 disappeared after complete bilateral aspiration of the IC. When the CN were bilaterally isolated from the brainstem, only waves 1 and 2 remained; and when the auditory nerve was bilaterally isolated from the CN, only wave 1 remained, indicating that the CN was essential for wave 2 and the brainstem between the CN and IC was essential for waves 3 and 4. After the auditory nerve was isolated from the CN, only wave 1 remained, but it disappeared at death, indicating peripheral activation of the auditory nerve was essential for wave 1. A mid-sagittal section of the brainstem from the level of the IC to the caudal pole of the CN abolished or markedly diminished wave 3, indicating that crossed projections were essential for normal wave amplitude. Waves 4 and 5 were reduced by 50% or more with this lesion, indicating that crossed and uncrossed projections converged almost equally upon the generator substrate. Lesions of the periolivary and ventral nuclei of the LL abolished wave 4. Chronic lesion effects were studied with regard to the contribution of the IC to wave 5 (Buchwald, 1983). Following extensive bilateral IC lesions in the adult cat, which encompassed the lateral and ventral extent of the nucleus, postoperative recordings were carried out over a 1-week period. No distinguishable potential was recorded after wave 4, which lends support to an IC origin for wave 5.

Overview of ABR Generators

On the basis of current electrophysiological and anatomical data as well as parametric and correlative studies of the ABRs, we have proposed a number of hypotheses regarding ABR generation (Buchwald, 1983). Our general hypotheses are that (a) ABRs reflect graded postsynaptic potentials (PSPs) rather than action potentials (APs) discharged at the cell soma or transmitted along the axon; (b) ABR latencies and amplitudes reflect interactive but essentially different physiological processes; and (c) ABR waves reflect substrate systems which are functionally separable. Hypotheses specific to the generation of each ABR wave are that: (a) generator potentials in the unmyelinated terminal dendrites of the auditory nerve are the substrate of wave 1; (b) PSPs in the ventral cochlear nucleus are the generators of wave 2; (c) ventral CN projections to the medial SOC (of both sides) produce dendritic PSPs, and resultant bilateral field potentials of equal latency and mirror image polarity comprise the generator substrate of wave 3; (d) ventral CN projections to the ventral LL (of both sides) produce bilateral field potentials which comprise the generator substrate for wave 4; (e) bilateral field potentials in the ventrolateral central nucleus of the IC, produced by projections from the ventral LL region of binaural interaction, comprise the generator substrate of wave 5 (Fig. 1).

Waves 6 and 7

In a series of studies on awake restrained cats, ABR waves 1–5 were shown to be followed by smaller and less well defined waves 6 and 7, with peak latencies in the 6–8 and 10–12 ms range, respectively (Fig. 1) (Buchwald, Hinman, Norman, Huang, & Brown, 1981). These potentials were not abolished by fast click rates (i.e., up to 30/s) nor by moderate levels (35 mg/kg) of pentobarbital. Correlative extra- and intracranial studies (Buchwald et al., 1981) indicated that wave 6 occurred in the same latency range as the poten-

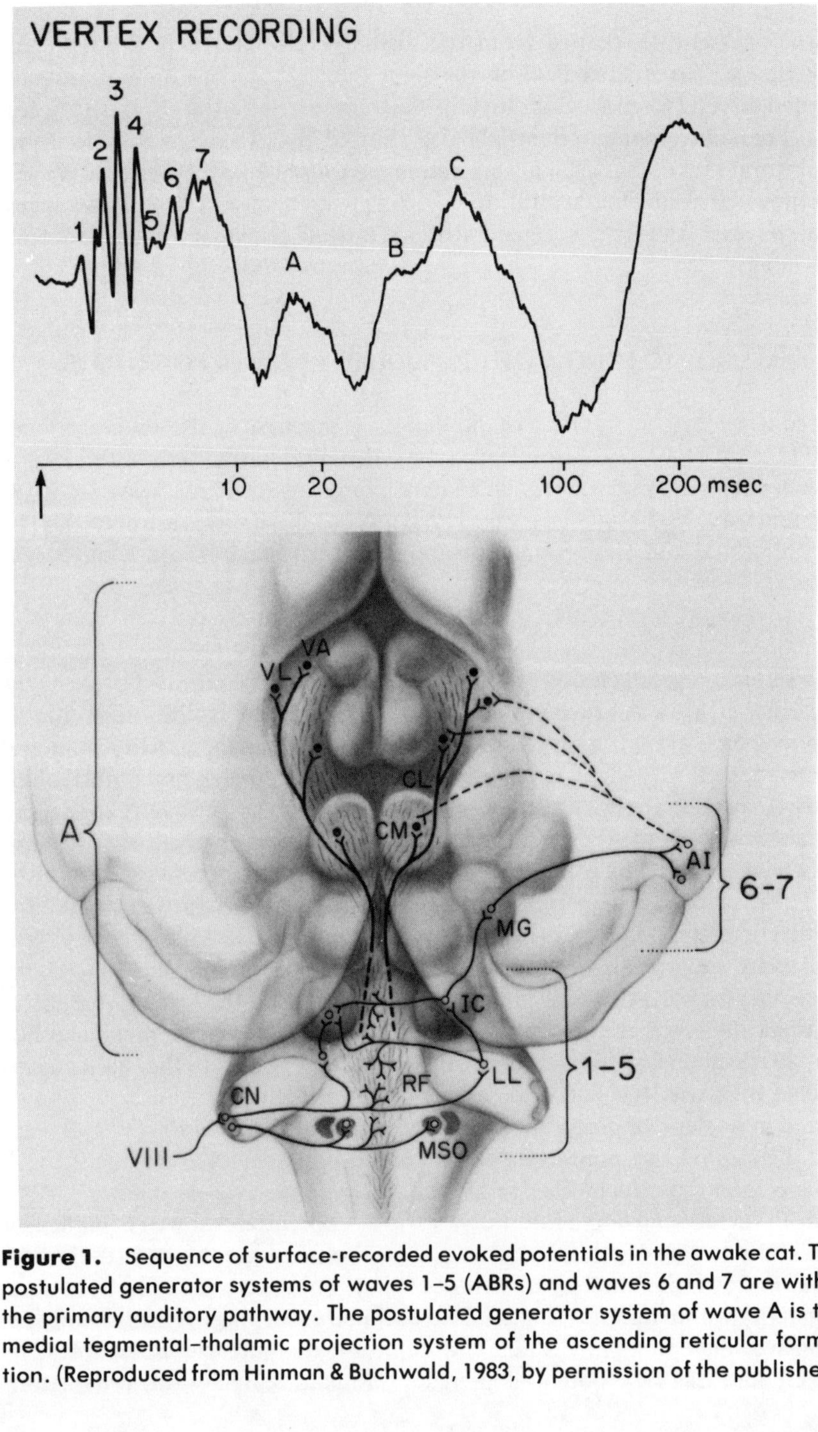

Figure 1. Sequence of surface-recorded evoked potentials in the awake cat. The postulated generator systems of waves 1–5 (ABRs) and waves 6 and 7 are within the primary auditory pathway. The postulated generator system of wave A is the medial tegmental–thalamic projection system of the ascending reticular formation. (Reproduced from Hinman & Buchwald, 1983, by permission of the publisher.)

tial concurrently recorded from the medial geniculate body (MGB), pars principalis. Wave 7 occurred in the same latency range as the potential recorded directly from the middle ectosylvian gyrus, i.e., primary auditory cortex. These intracranial potentials also showed click recovery functions and barbiturate resistance which were similar to those of waves 6 and 7. Wave 7 disappeared following aspiration of ectosylvian cortex. These data suggest that waves 6 and 7 reflect generators in medial geniculate body and ectosylvian gyrus.

MIDDLE- TO LONG-LATENCY AUDITORY EVOKED POTENTIALS

In contrast to the stability of potentials 1 through 7, the longer latency waves were relatively unstable. We have become particularly interested in three of these waves: wave A, in a latency range of 20–25 ms; wave C, 50–75 ms; and wave E, 200–400 ms (Fig. 1, 2, 3). All of these waves are abolished by pentobarbital and diminish and disappear as click rates exceed 2/s.

Wave A

In a series of chronic lesion studies, vertex recordings continued to show the presence of wave A (20–25 ms latency) after bilateral aspiration of middle suprasylvian gyrus, ectosylvian gyrus, or frontal lobes. After bilateral hemispherectomy, which removed all cortex, basal ganglia, and limbic lobes, wave A was not abolished. Thus, the generator system of wave A appears to be largely independent of auditory cortex and adjacent association cortex but may be modulated by other forebrain systems.

The rostral brainstem and thalamus of awake cats were further studied for depth correlates of wave A (Hinman & Buchwald, 1983). Mid-latency potentials were recorded from the level of the cuneiform nucleus (14–15 ms latencies) forward through the medial tegmentum to the level of the intralaminar thalamic nuclei centralis lateralis (CL) and centre median (CM) (17–20 ms latencies). While this medial projection system to the thalamus involved primarily CL and CM, slightly longer latency responses were also found in nucleus ventralis anterior (VA) and ventralis lateralis (VL). A ventral diencephalic response was characterized by latencies averaging 0.5–1.2 ms less than those from the dorsal thalamic regions.

Both surface and depth mid-latency wave A potentials showed comparable sensitivity to rate of stimulation and were abolished at rates greater than 5–10/s. Following 35 mg/kg of pentobarbital, both were replaced by a deep negativity within minutes (Fig. 2). Extracellular recordings of acoustically responsive single units in CL and CM demonstrated latencies comparable to the CL and CM field potential latencies (Hinman & Buchwald, 1983). Both

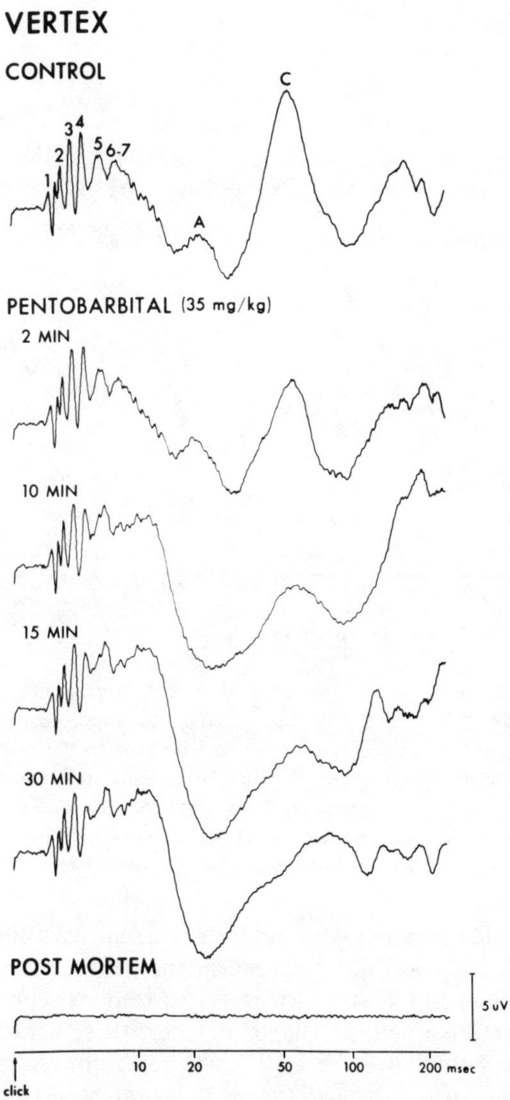

Figure 2. Effects of pentobarbital on vertex recorded evoked potentials. After 30 min, there is little effect on the shorter latency potentials, except for an increased positivity at 10–12 ms. In contrast, waves A and C disappear, and a deep negative through appears at 20 ms. After a lethal dose of barbiturate, postmortem recordings were carried out under identical conditions as a control for possible artifacts in the recordings. (Reproduced from Buchwald et al., 1981, by permission of the publisher.)

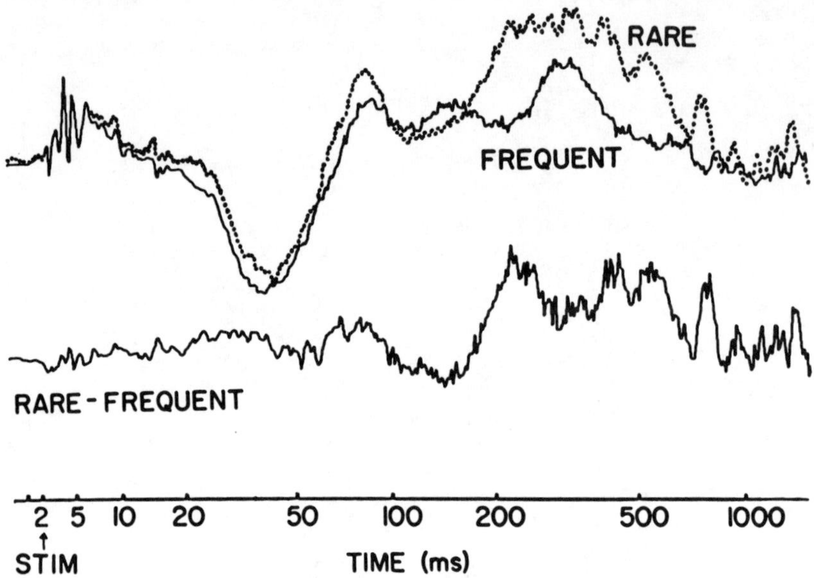

Figure 3. Typical data from one young adult cat show a positive endogenous potential with a latency of 200–400 ms, as shown in this example. The top traces (positivity up) represent averaged responses to frequent (80%) and rare (15%) loud clicks. The bottom trace represents the difference potential resulting from subtraction of the frequent from the rare response. The most consistent rare–frequent difference potential across cats occurred between 200 and 400 ms. (Reproduced from Harrison & Buchwald, 1985, by permission of the publisher.)

the units and field potentials were similarly rate sensitive. Bilateral aspiration of the inferior colliculus did not abolish the depth or surface responses. Rather, recordings in CL and CM suggested response enhancement over a 2-week postoperative period. Taken together, these data suggest that the 20–25 ms vertex potential, wave A, reflects a generator system which projects from cuneiform nucleus through the medial tegmentum to the medial thalamus, particularly to CL and CM (Fig. 1). While the functional significance of this medial auditory projection system remains to be determined, it is now known to be intimately related to sleep–arousal behavior (Chen & Buchwald, 1986). When the waking cat becomes drowsy and then goes into slow-wave sleep, as indicated by behavioral observations with concurrent EEG, EMG, and EOG recordings, wave A becomes progressively smaller in amplitude and disappears. If the sleep pattern shifts from slow-wave to paradoxical (REM) sleep, wave A increases and may become as large or larger in amplitude than in the waking state. Concurrent recordings of waves 1–7 showed no change in these waves across the sleep-wakefulness spectrum.

Wave C

Wave C appears as a broad positivity, usually larger in amplitude than wave A, with a peak latency in the 50–100 ms range (Fig. 1). Wave C is the largest, most uniformly present of the longer latency potentials and was observed in all cats studied. Like wave A, it disappears under pentobarbital anesthesia and during click presentation rates of 5–10/s. Wave C continued to appear after aspiration of suprasylvian and ectosylvian gyri and after frontal lobectomy, but disappeared after bilateral hemispherectomy (Buchwald et al., 1981). Thus, wave C reflects a generator system which differs from that of wave A, but which also appears to be largely independent of the primary geniculo-cortical auditory pathway. The functional significance of this system differs from that of wave A insofar as the amplitude of wave C during slow-wave sleep and REM was not tightly coupled to alterations in wave A amplitude.

Wave E ("P300-like" response)

In the human, the "P300" response, which occurs at a latency of approximately 300 ms, appears to be a measure of stimulus discrimination, of sequential information processing and of short-term memory (Donchin, 1981; Ford, Mohrs, Pfefferbaum, & Kopell, 1980; Squires, Donchin, Herning, & McCarthy, 1977). In the cat, wave E appears to be correlated with similar parameters. In an attempt to study endogenous potentials in the cat that might resemble those in the human, e.g., the P300, we utilized loud and soft clicks as rare and frequent stimuli and a third tonal conditioning stimulus to provide auditory focus and an objective measure of attention by virtue of behavioral conditioned responses (Buchwald & Squires, 1982). Each recording session consisted of 4 runs of 500 stimulus presentations at 1.5 s interstimulus intervals. In 2 runs, the loud click occurred frequently ($p = 80\%$) and the soft click rarely ($p = 15\%$). In the other 2 runs the probabilities were reversed, and the loud click occurred rarely ($p = 15\%$) and the soft click frequently ($p = 80\%$). The target conditioning stimulus, a 4kHz tone followed by eyelid shock, also occurred rarely ($p = 5\%$) and resulted in conditioned blink responses. All three stimuli were randomly ordered. In normal adult cats, comparison of responses to the "rare" loud click with responses to the "frequent" click indicated a significantly greater "rare response" positivity in the 200–400 ms latency range (Fig. 3). Similarly, when responses to the rare soft clicks were compared with responses to the frequent soft clicks, a larger positive response in this time period occurred to the rare stimuli.

Data from a number of studies (Wilder, Farley, & Starr, 1981; Buchwald & Squires, 1982; Harrison & Buchwald, 1985; Harrison, Buchwald, and Kaga, 1986) indicate that the cat endogenous, wave-E response resembles the human P300 in several respects: (a) it occurs only when the stimuli are task relevant, i.e., during acoustic conditioning but not during habituation procedures; (b) it depends upon the probability of the stimuli, i.e., it does not appear when the stimulus occurs with an 80% probability but does appear when the stimulus probability drops to 15%; (c) it is not dependent upon a particular stimulus parameter, i.e., intensity; (d) it is produced by stimulus omission and is not, therefore, simply an arousal response to an unexpected stimulus; (e) principal components analysis (PCA) shows a factor in the 300 ms range, with significant differences in the factor scores to rare and frequent stimuli (Harrison & Buchwald, 1985), similar to the human PCA factor obtained during P300 procedures; (f) it changes functionally with old age in the cat as the P300 does in the human (Harrison & Buchwald, 1985).

As noted for waves A and C, wave E generation was abolished by moderate doses of pentobarbital (Buchwald & Squires, 1982). In 4 adult cats in which wave E was demonstrated, the primary auditory cortex was ablated bilaterally with subsequent histological verification (Harrison, Buchwald, & Kaga, 1986). After 12 postoperative sessions, statistical analyses demonstrated that the 300 ms endogenous potential was still present. While the generator system of this P300-like response is currently under investigation, we conclude from this study that the primary auditory cortex is not necessary.

OVERVIEW OF MIDDLE- TO LONG-LATENCY EVOKED POTENTIAL GENERATORS

Based on these studies, the following conclusions are suggested: vertex waves 1 through 7 show high fidelity, rate-resistant, barbiturate-insensitive, auditory transmission which is unaffected by sleep versus arousal and appears to reflect activation of the primary auditory system from auditory nerve to auditory cortex. In contrast to the stability of waves 1 through 7, the subsequent waves are relatively unstable. Wave A, in a latency range of 20–25 ms, and wave C, 50–75 ms, disappear at click rates of 5–10/s, are abolished by moderate levels of pentobarbital and show marked but different amplitude changes as a function of sleep versus arousal. Wave E, in a 200–400 ms latency range, resembles the human P300 endogenous response, is also abolished by pentobarbital anesthesia and, like Waves A and C, continues to be elicited after aspiration of primary auditory cortex. These potentials thus appear to be generated by forebrain systems which process auditory information very differently than the primary geniculo-cortical system. They appear to function in parallel with the primary system rather than serially, insofar as auditory information is relayed up from the brain stem to these systems rather than relayed back from auditory cortex.

DEVELOPMENTAL STUDIES: SHORT-LATENCY POTENTIALS

Auditory Brainstem Response Development

In our initial study of ABR development (Shipley, Buchwald, Norman, & Guthrie, 1980), 28 kittens from 7 litters were recorded over a postnatal period ranging from birth to 60 days. Repeated longitudinal observations on particular kittens were supplemented with observations on additional kittens during the first and second postnatal week to determine the age of onset of ABRs. The position of the animal and sound source within the recording chamber were held constant across recording sessions, as was click intensity, except during recordings in which intensity effects were specifically studied. Click rates of 1, 10, 50, and 100/s were routinely presented. Reference electrodes at the tongue, pinna, and neck showed volume-conducted responses to the click stimuli and resulted in considerable distortion of the activity recorded by the vertex electrode; the forepaw, in contrast showed no activity and a vertex-forepaw electrode configuration provided good resolution of the ABRs across development.

While Jewett and Romano (1972) first noted the appearance of cat ABRs at 12–14 days, in our study evoked potentials to the loud free-field click stimuli were recorded from the vertex of kittens 4–6 days after birth, approximately the same age at which acoustic stimuli first induce behavioral responses (Foss & Flottorp, 1974; Villablanca & Olmstead, 1979) and at which depth evoked potentials are first recorded in brainstem auditory nuclei of kittens (Pujol, 1972). Initially, the ABRs were acutely sensitive to both rate and intensity of the stimulus, and the earliest responses were detectable only with relatively loud stimuli and slow click repetition rates (Fig. 4). These ABRs were diffuse, high threshold, and fatigued rapidly, characteristics shared by the earliest evoked potentials in the auditory relay nuclei (Pujol, 1969, 1972; Pujol & Hilding, 1973; Romand, Granier, & Marty, 1973). Moreover, as a function of age, all ABR components showed exponential decreases in latency similar to those of the depth recorded evoked potentials.

Over the first 2 postnatal weeks, the ABR potentials showed a marked decrease in threshold, increased resistance to fast click rates, and better definition of wave forms (Fig. 5). Because all of the brainstem evoked potentials could be recorded concurrently and longitudinally in the same subject, a number of developmental comparisons were possible among the ABR components. The absolute values for ABR wave 1 latency were very similar to those for the auditory nerve N1 potential, e.g., at 10 days the mean latency for wave 1 was 1.8 ms and for N1 was 1.6 ms (Romand, 1971). Both wave 1 and N1 latencies attained similar adult values of 0.8–0.9 ms by about 30 days. The second and third waves were initially composed of two components. The

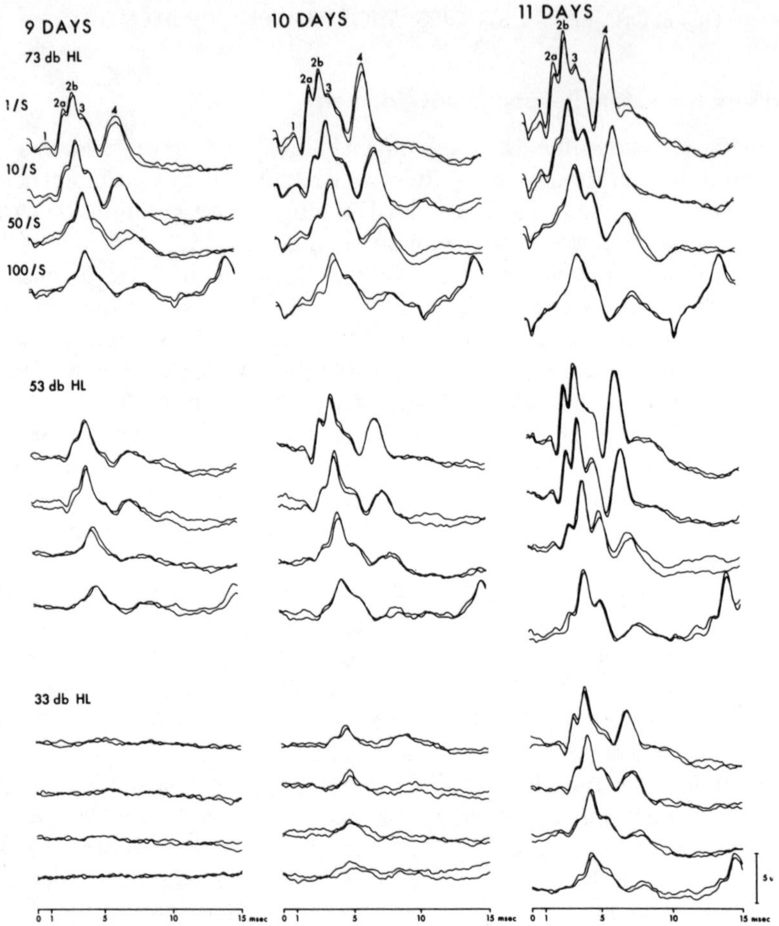

Figure 4. Effects of stimulus intensity and click rate in one kitten on the first 3 days that ABRs were evoked by the 73 HL stimulus. (Reproduced from Shipley et al., 1980, by permission of the publisher.)

2a and 2b components of wave 2 tended to merge during the second month, although they did not fuse entirely, so that 2a could still be discerned as a leading shoulder on the more prominent 2b. On the basis of similar latencies between wave 2a and a maximum voltage field in the cochlear nucleus area of auditory nerve termination, the unmyelinated central terminals of the auditory nerve have been suggested as the generator of wave 2a (Achor & Starr, 1980a). Comparisons between wave 2b and evoked potentials recorded from the ventral CN (Pujol, 1972; Romand & Marty, 1975) indicate that at about the same postnatal age both of these responses reached the same adult

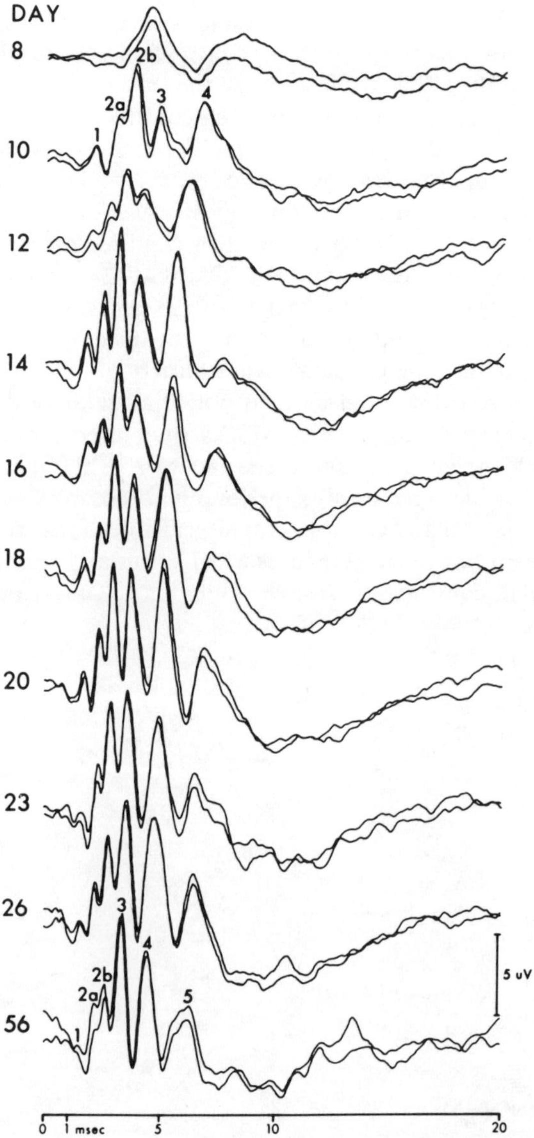

Figure 5. ABR developmental sequence from one kitten across the first 2 months of life. The stimulus (46 db HL, 10/s clicks) occurs at the trace onset. (Reproduced from Shipley et al., 1980, by permission of the publisher.)

latencies of 2–3 ms. In contrast, dorsal CN responses were longer in latency and slower to reach adult values (Romand & Marty, 1975). This developmental correlation of wave 2b with the ventral and not dorsal CN is consistent with the finding that aspiration of the entire CN abolishes wave 2 (Buchwald & Huang, 1975), but aspiration confined to the dorsal CN does not affect ABR wave 2 in the adult cat (Achor & Starr, 1980b). The wave 3 bimodality was more transient than that of wave 2, and the 3a and 3b components were less discrete. The development of wave 3 was complex in that it was initially smaller than wave 2 and then acquired a second component which was observed in most, but not all, kittens at 12–19 days of age (Fig. 6). These components merged by 18–25 days of age, and wave 3 amplitude often showed a marked and rapid increase during the third postnatal week.

In addition to the adult cat data cited, a variety of other data link the medial superior olive (MSO) and its field potentials with wave 3 (Buchwald, 1983). Brainstem levels rostral to the MSO are not important for the integrity of wave 3, while the MSO and its crossed and uncrossed trapezoid body input are essential. The MSO is the only superior olivary complex nucleus which receives both ipsilateral and contralateral direct projections from the cochlear nucleus and displays evoked responses which occur at the same latency to either ipsilateral or contralateral stimuli. Thus, wave 3 meets the requirement,

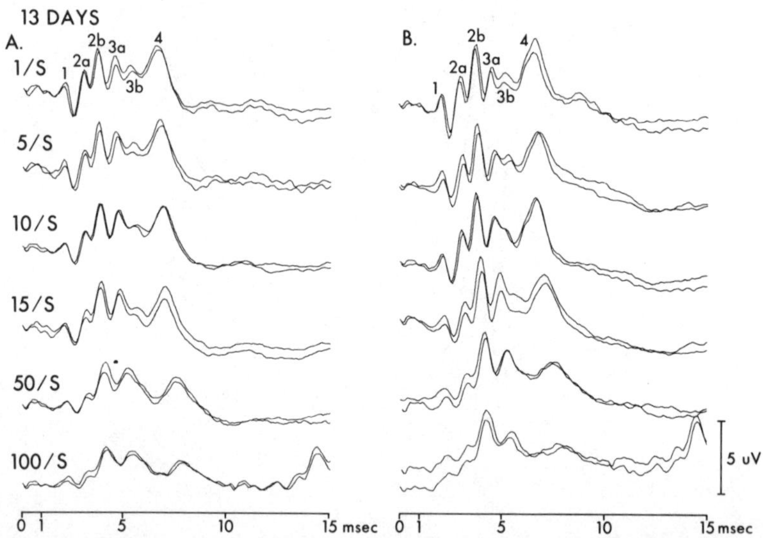

Figure 6. ABRs from 2 kittens of the same litter at 13 days of age. Note bimodality of wave 3, which is transiently present only at this stage of development. (Reproduced from Buchwald, 1983, by permission of the publisher.)

in the adult, for evoked potential contributions from ipsilateral and contralateral generators which temporally superimpose. The kitten data suggest that immature ipsilateral and contralateral projections from the ventral CN to the MSO produce responses of slightly different latencies during the second postnatal week, waves 3a and 3b, whereas by the third postnatal week an adult pattern of temporally synchronous ipsilateral and contralateral projections to the MSO has developed, and the unimodal wave 3 shows an adult peak latency value.

Wave 4, which reflects activation of the ventral nuclei of the lateral lemniscus (Buchwald, 1983), was undifferentiated in the earliest records (Fig. 5) but was large and well defined by the end of the second week. The development of binaural interaction effects, as shown by this wave, will be discussed in more detail.

Wave 5 appeared later than waves 1–4, i.e., not until approximately 14 days postnatally, and was small and unstable until the end of the third week (Fig. 5). It is difficult to attribute the absence of wave 5 prior to this time to peripheral factors, since all other waves were present. Rather, the data suggest that the generator of wave 5 is not mature enough to respond initially. Moreover, the effect of click rate on amplitude was especially evident in wave 5, which disappeared at rates of 100/s up to 4 weeks of age. Overall, these data indicate that the neural substrate of wave 5 develops more slowly than do the generator substrates of waves 1–4. The age of onset of wave 5 corresponds to the period between 11 and 21 days in which evoked responses were first recorded in the IC with free-field stimulation (Maruseva & Malysheva, 1970) and during which a marked drop in IC unit response thresholds also occured (Aitkin & Moore, 1975). Thus, wave 5, with a postulated generator in the IC, as previously summarized, shows a time course of development which agrees well with IC responses during the early postnatal period.

With regard to the neuronal substrate most relevant to the ABRs, the role of timekeeper "on" response neurons has been previously discussed. Such synchronized, stimulus-locked "on" potentials are essential for computer-averaged responses induced by multiple stimulus trials. In the early development of neuronal response patterns, "on" responses are the first type recorded in the auditory brainstem nuclei, e.g., in CN (Pujol, 1972; Romand & Marty, 1975), the SOC (Romand et al., 1973), the IC (Aitkin & Moore, 1975; Maruseva & Malysheva, 1970; Pujol, 1969, 1972), the MGB (Pujol, 1972). Other more complex response patterns, e.g., rhythmical, sustained, and patterned, appear at later postnatal ages (Pujol, 1969, 1972; Romand et al., 1973; Romand & Marty, 1975). Thus, the ABRs seem to reflect activation within the auditory brainstem nuclei of neurons which function earliest, in an ontogenetic sense, and indicate differential developmental changes and maturational interactions across these neuronal pools.

Wave 6 Development

Wave 6 first appeared between 30 and 45 days of age, at least 2 weeks after waves 1–5 (Figs. 7 & 8). In order to determine the approximate age at which wave 6 developed, kittens were studied at intervals of 5 to 10 days between the ages of 20 and 40 days (Shipley, Strecker, & Buchwald, 1984). In 3 kittens wave 6 was first noted at 30 days and was present in 3 other kittens by 37 days. While it is possible that wave 6 would have been observed at an earlier age with louder stimulation, the absolute intensity of stimulation should not affect the relative order of appearance of the waves during development. Moreover, wave 6 initially could be recorded only with rates of stimulation reduced to 2/s, while the ABRs showed virtually no affect of 10/s versus 1/s click rates. Thus, regardless of stimulus intensity, wave 6 initially appeared and developed mature latency and recovery cycle functions only some time after the earlier ABR potentials. Since wave 6 is thought to be generated rostral to the IC, as previously discussed, its relatively late appearance extends to forebrain levels the caudal-rostral gradient of brainstem auditory pathway maturation indicated by wave 1–5 development.

Wave 7 Development

Wave 7 first appeared between 30 and 50 days of age, at least 2 weeks later than waves 1–5 (Fig. 7). The wave indicated as number 7 in Figure 7 has, by day 75, assumed the 10–12 ms latency of the primary auditory potential recorded directly from the middle ectosylvian cortex. In the kitten this vertex potential was much clearer and more prominent than in the adult cat; it was also much more easily "fatigued" by rapid rates of stimulation. Even at 75 days of age, wave 7 was almost totally abolished at click rates of 10/s, whereas the ABR responses were completely stable. Thus, as in the case of wave 6, both the initial appearance of wave 7 and the development of its adult recovery cycle lagged significantly behind the ABRs. While cautious interpretation is important in relating evoked potentials in the kitten to the waves which occur within the same time windows in the adult, the causal relation which has been shown between wave 7 and the primary auditory cortex in the adult (Buchwald et al., 1981) provides a basis for suggesting that the kitten wave 7 may reflect functional development of primary auditory cortex. Studies of this wave in the kitten are still in progress in our laboratory.

Development of Binaural Interaction Effects

Binaural interactions are reflected by differences between the ABRs obtained from binaural stimulation and the ABRs constructed by adding the results of separate monaural stimulation to each ear. Typically in the adult cat,

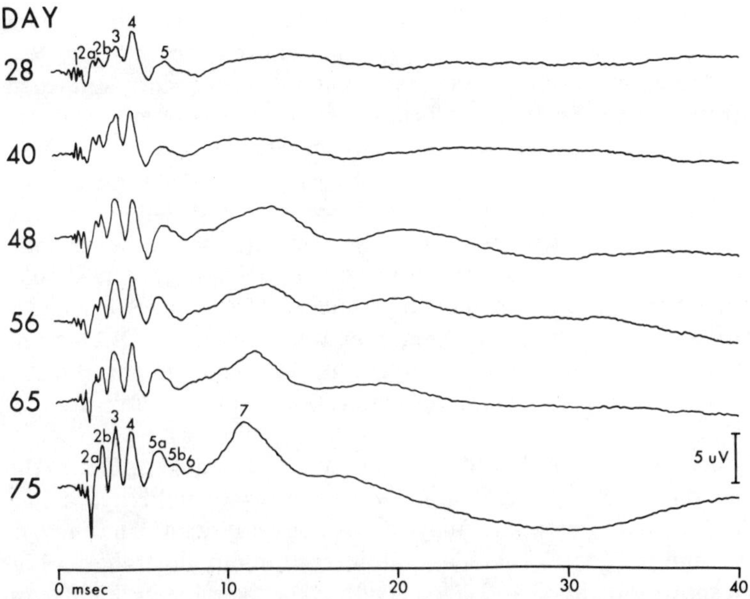

Figure 7. Short-latency evoked potential developmental sequence across the first 11 weeks of life. The 1/s click stimulus occurs at the trace onset. (Reproduced from Shipley & Buchwald, 1985, by permission of the authors.)

the summed monaural response is larger than the binaural response for some waves of the ABR, indicating that differences exist between monaural and binaural signal processing in the neural generators of these waves. Our earlier observations showed binaural interactions on ABR waves 4 and 5 but not on waves 1–3 (Huang & Buchwald, 1978; Buchwald, 1983). These observations were confirmed in experiments in which monaural click intensity was below threshold for ABRs evoked by air or bone conducted sound to the opposite ear. This threshold was determined by surgically deafening the kitten monaurally, stimulating the deafened ear, and observing what click intensity produced an ABR by air or bone conduction to the normal contralateral ear. Binaural interactions which were not attributable to air- or bone-conducted acoustic crossover were reliably observed in adults at the latencies of ABR waves 4, 5, and 6 (Shipley et al., 1984). In addition, a small but reliable positivity was seen at a latency intermediate between ABR waves 4 and 5 that was consistently larger for monaural than for binaural stimulation. A ratio reflecting the percent of binaural interaction was calculated by dividing the amplitude of the summed monaural response associated with each peak in the ABR by the amplitude of that peak in the binaural stimulation condition. The average value of this ratio was, for wave 4, 1.46, for wave 5, 1.60, and for wave 6, 1.56. In summary, binaural interaction in the adult cat is not observed for ABR waves 1–3, but is pronounced for waves 4, 5, and 6.

The development of binaural interaction was subsequently studied in 6 kittens from 3 litters beginning at 20 days of age, shortly after the age at which ABR wave 5 appears in a well-defined form (Shipley et al., 1984). Insofar as waves 4, 5, and 6 developed later than waves 1–3, we hypothesized that functional maturation of binaural convergence upon the generator neurons of waves 4, 5, and 6 might occur at a different rate than the development of monaural activation. Such a functional developmental gradient should be reflected by different degrees of binaural interaction for waves 4, 5, and 6 in the kitten versus the adult cat. Differences between the rate of ABR development and the rate of ABR binaural interaction development might, thereby, provide a sensitive index of functional maturation within the brainstem auditory pathway.

Typical ABRs from a 20-day-old kitten are presented in Fig. 8. Binaural interactions were clearly present for waves 4, 4′, and 5 at this age, as indicated by the difference potentials. Wave 6 was not yet present. The emergence of wave 6 and the form of its binaural interaction are illustrated in Figure 9, which shows data at 30 and 40 days of age for the same kitten illustrated in Figure 8. From the first day that wave 6 was observed, a binaural interaction "difference potential" was present at the latency of wave 6.

In order to test the hypothesis that binaural processing might develop at a different rate than purely monaural processing, one-way analyses of variance were carried out on the binaural interaction ratios for waves 4 and 5 in the kitten and the adult cat. These tests could not be carried out for wave 6 since it was not present at 20 days. No significant effect of age was found for the binaural interaction effect of either wave 4 or 5 at any of the rates of click stimulation used in this study, i.e., 10, 50, and 100/s. The developmental sequence observed, therefore, indicates that binaural interactions are present at an adult level by 20 days of age. It is possible that developmental changes might have been observed had we been able to study binaural interaction at an earlier age, e.g., 10 to 15 days, when wave 4 is first reliably present. However, it was difficult to compare monaural and binaural responses in younger kittens because of relatively high thresholds and differences between the thresholds of each ear.

There is presently little direct information on the neural substrate of these ABR binaural interaction effects. Sagittal section of the brainstem at the level of the trapezoid body has been reported to eliminate binaural interactions in cats (Fullerton & Hosford, 1979), while lesions at the level of the inferior colliculus eliminated the wave 5, but not the wave 4, binaural interaction components in several species including the cat (Huang, 1980). Two early studies (Kemp & Robinson, 1937; Rosenzweig & Sutton, 1958), using depth recordings of local field potentials, examined binaural convergence in the nu-

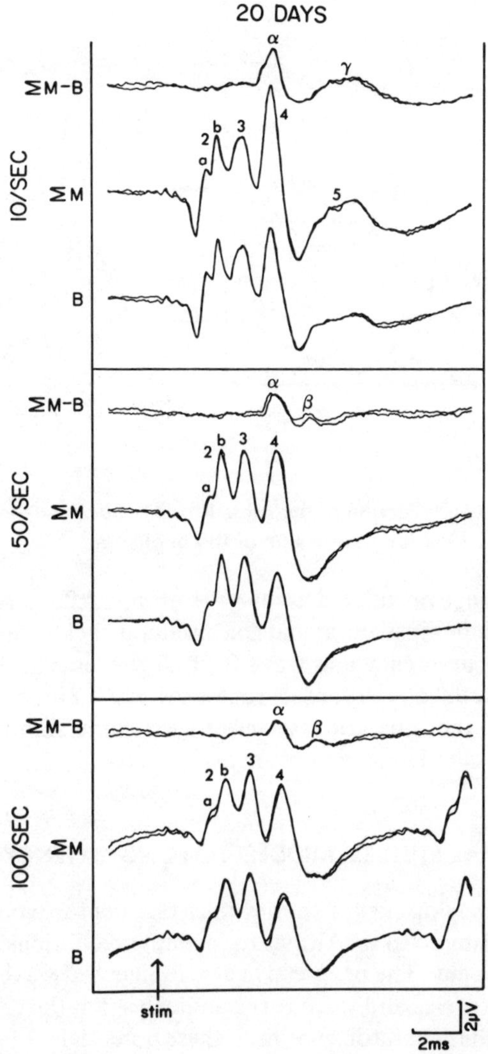

Figure 8. Binaural interaction for a 20-day-old kitten at 10, 50, and 100 clicks/s. Odd and even stimulus presentations were averaged on separate channels and superimposed to determine wave-form reliability. ABR evoked by summed monaural responses (Sigma M) are shown above the ABR evoked by the same stimuli presented binaurally. The summed monaural wave form was constructed by digitally summing the responses from each ear. The difference wave form, or Sigma M-B, was derived by digitally subtracting the binaural from the summed monaural response, and qualitatively illustrates the effect of binaural interaction. (Reproduced from Shipley et al., 1984, by permission of the publisher.)

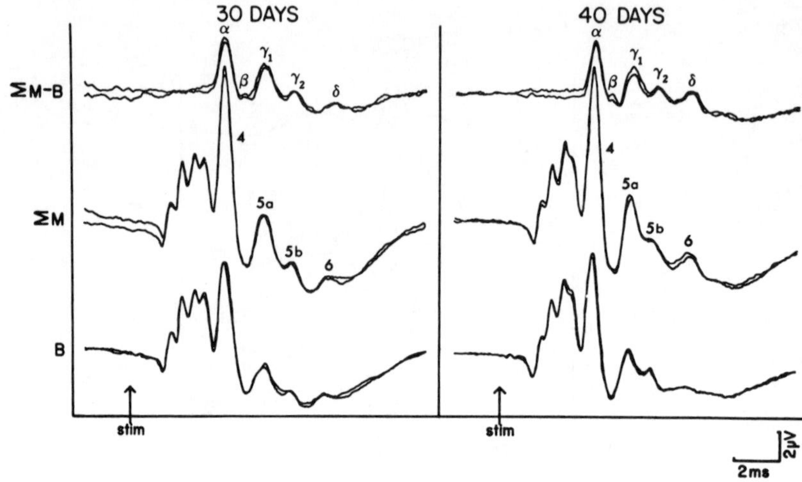

Figure 9. Binaural interaction of the same kitten at 30 and 40 days. (Reproduced from Shipley et al., 1984, by permission of the publisher.)

cleus of the LL, since postulated as the generator of ABR wave 4 (Buchwald, 1983). In both studies ipsilateral and contralateral click stimuli produced responses of identical latency and wave form at the lemniscal recording site. The sum of these locally recorded responses was, moreover, consistently greater than was the binaural response to the same stimuli presented together.

DEVELOPMENTAL STUDIES: MIDDLE- TO LONG-LATENCY POTENTIALS

In most of our developmental studies thus far, pentobarbital or ketamine have been administered to the kittens to facilitate recordings in the free-field stimulus environment. The progressive development of waves 1–7 in the kittens to mature latencies and wave forms indicates that the drugs did not significantly affect the generator systems of these potentials, a fact that is generally accepted for the adult cat.

In contrast, auditory evoked potentials with latencies in excess of 15 ms disappear or are markedly reduced in the adult cat following injections of pentobarbital or ketamine. Thus, it is reasonable to postulate that a similar situation prevails in the kitten. We have not observed the emergence of middle- to long-latency potentials in kittens up to 75 days of age under the drugged condition, even with rates of stimulation as slow as 1/s (Fig. 7). Until these recordings can be extended to a series of undrugged kittens, it is not possible to make any statements about the relative rate of development of these later waves and their generator systems. As summarized earlier, our work on the adult cat indicates that wave A (20–25 ms latency), wave C (50–75-ms latency), and wave E (200–400-ms latency) each reflects a different generator system with a markedly different function relative to central processing of auditory information. Studies of the development of these later waves will provide us with a means of determining the time course over which their generator systems emerge and mature and whether the later waves originating from nonprimary neural substrates will show precocious or retarded development when compared with the concurrently recorded brainstem waves 1–5 and forebrain waves 6 and 7 of the primary auditory pathway.

SUMMARY

This chapter has been presented as a progress report of laboratory work directed toward sorting out the ways in which auditory signals are centrally processed in the adult and in the developing kitten. The sequence of surface-recorded auditory evoked potentials which range from 1–400 ms in the awake, adult cat provides an intriguing indication that the brain is processing auditory signals in time domains that far exceed the 10–12 ms transmission time from cochlea to auditory cortex. Moreover waves 1–7, which reflect activation of the primary auditory pathway from auditory nerve to cortex, are unaltered by deep sleep or surgical levels of anesthesia. The subject is unresponsive to sound, even though the signal continues to ascend normally to cortical levels. Thus, it is clear that "hearing" requires more than the activation of this primary system.

Indeed, after complete bilateral aspiration of primary auditory cortex, none of the later auditory evoked potentials, i.e., waves A, C, and E, are significantly changed. These later waves, however, do change and disappear as a function of sleep or anesthesia, conditions in which the subject no longer "hears." The relatively long recovery cycles shown by the later waves also suggest a kind of "short-term memory" for the preceding stimulus. In the case of wave E, more complex discrimination and sequential processing functions seem to be occurring. These later waves appear to reflect several different generator systems, each receiving input from the auditory brainstem and functioning in parallel with the primary auditory system.

We have, thus far, focused on the development of the short-latency, primary pathway potentials 1–7 in the kitten. A caudal–cephalic developmental gradient was demonstrated: Wave 5 appeared later and attained adult latency and recovery cycle functions significantly later than did waves 1–4, while waves 6 and 7 appeared markedly later and attained adult latencies later than wave 5. The postulated generator substrate for wave 5, in the ventral lateral

IC, thus appears to develop more slowly than do the postulated generators in CN, SOC, and LL for waves 2, 3, and 4. The MGB, pars principalis, and middle ectosylvian gyrus, postulated as generator substrates for waves 6 and 7, develop subsequently with a time course that lags behind all of the brainstem nuclei, including the IC.

The demonstration of binaural interaction effects on waves 4, 5, and 6 in the adult indicated binaurally convergent input on the generator neurons of these waves. Kittens were tested for the presence of this phenomenon in order to determine whether a developmental gradient also occurred in the function of monaural versus convergent binaural projections. The binaural interaction effects were found to be present at adult values as early as the waves could be recorded in the kitten, which suggests ontogenetic importance for this kind of binaural convergence.

We are only now beginning to focus on the development of the waves subsequent to the 1–7 sequence. The postulated generator system of wave A, the medial tegmental-intralaminar thalamic component of the ascending reticular formation, is a phylogenetically ancient system and might be expected to function quite early in development. In general, the later waves reflect complex cognitive aspects of central auditory information processing. Their differential ontogeny, particularly in relation to the entire sequence of evoked potentials, should indicate to what extent there are developmental gradients among these various generator systems.

REFERENCES

Achor, L.J., & Starr, A. (1980a). Auditory brain stem responses in the cat, I. Intracranial and extracranial recordings. *Electroencephalography and clinical Neurophysiology, 48,* 154–173.

Achor, L.J., & Starr, A. (1980b). Auditory brain stem responses in the cat. II. Effects of lesions. *Electroencephalography and clinical Neurophysiology, 48,* 174–190.

Aitkin, L.M., & Moore, D.R. (1975). Inferior colliculus. II. Development of tuning characteristics and tonotopic organization in central nucleus of neonatal cat. *Journal of Neurophysiology, 38,* 1208–1216.

Buchwald, J.S. (1983). Generators. In E.J. Moore (Ed.), *Bases of auditory and brain-stem evoked responses.* New York: Grune & Stratton.

Buchwald, J.S., Hinman, C., Norman, R.J., Huang, C.M., & Brown, K.A. (1981). Middle- and long-latency auditory evoked responses recorded from the vertex of normal and chronically lesioned cats, Brain Research, 205, 91–109.

Buchwald, J.S., & Huang, C.M. (1975). Origins of the far-field acoustic response in the cat. *Science, 189,* 382–384.

Buchwald, J.S., & Squires, N.S. (1982). Endogenous auditory potentials in the cat. In C.D. Woody (Ed.), *Conditioning: Representation of involved neural function.* New York: Plenum Press.

Chen, B., & Buchwald, J.S. (1986). *Middle latency auditory evoked responses:* Differential effects of sleep in the cat. *Electroencephalography and Clinical Neurophysiology.*

Donchin, E. (1981), Surprise! Surprise?. *Psychophysiology, 18,* 493–513.

Ford, J.M., Mohrs, R.C., Pfefferbaum, A., & Kopell, B.S. (1980). On the utility of P3 latency and RT for studying cognitive processes. *Progress in Brain Research, 54,* 661–667.

Foss, I., & Flottorp, G. (1974). A comparative study of the development of hearing and vision on various species commonly used in experiments. *Acta-oto-laryngology (Basel), 77,* 202–214.

Fullerton, B.C., & Hosford, H.L. (1979). Effects of midline brainstem lesion on the short-latency auditory evoked response. *Neuroscience Society Abstracts, 5,* 20.

Harrison, J., and Buchwald, J. (1985). Aging changes in the cat P300 mimic the human. *Electroencephalography and Clinical Neurophysiology, 62,* 227–234.

Harrison, J., Buchwald, J., & Kaga, K. (1986). Cat P300 present after primary auditory cortex ablation. *Electroencephalography and Clinical Neurophysiology, 63,* 180–187

Hinman, C.L., & Buchwald, J.S. (1983). Depth evoked potential and single unit correlates of vertex midlatency auditory evoked responses. *Brain Research, 264,* 57–67.

Huang, C.A. (1980). A comparative study of the brain stem auditory response in mammals, *Brain Research, 184,* 215–219.

Huang, C.M., & Buchwald, J.S. (1977). Interpretation of the vertex short-latency acoustic response: A study of single neurons in the brain stem, *Brain Research, 137,* 291–303.

Huang, C.M., & Buchwald, J.S. (1978). Factors that affect the amplitudes and latencies of the vertex short latency acoustic responses in the cat. *Electroencephalography and Clinical Neurophysiology, 44,* 179–186.

Huang, C.M., & Buchwald, J.S. (1979). Single unit response in the cochlear nucleus to slowly repeated tones. *Brain Research, 1973,* 562–566.

Huang, C.M., & Buchwald, J.S. (1980). Changes of acoustic nerve and cochlear nucleus evoked potentials due to repetitive stimulation. *Electroencephalography and Clinical Neurophysiology, 49,* 15–22.

Jewett, D.L., (1970). Volume-conducted potentials in response to auditory stimuli as detected by averaging in the cat. *Electroencephalography and Clinical Neurophysiology, 28,* 609–618.

Jewett, D.L., & Romano, M.N. (1972). Neonatal development of auditory system potentials averaged from the scalp of rat and cat, *Brain Research, 36,* 101–115.

Kemp, E.H., & Robinson, E.H. (1937). Electric responses of the brainstem to bilateral auditory stimulation. *American Journal of Physiology, 120,* 316–322.

Lev, A., & Sohmer, H. (1972). Sources of averaged neural responses recorded in animal and human subjects during cochlear audiometry (electrocochleogram). *Archiz Fur Klinische Und Experimentelle Ohren, Nasen–Und Kehlkopfheilkunde, 201,* 79–90.

Maruseva, A.M., & Malysheva, V.I. (1970). Effect of acoustic stimulation on unit activity of inferior colliculus in cats. *Zhurnal Ezoliutsionnoi Biokhimii i Fiziologii, 6,* 225–234.

Pujol, R. (1969). Development des responses a la stimulation sonore dans le colliculus inferieur chez le chat. [Development of responses to auditory stimuli in the inferior colliculus of the cat]*Journal of Physiology (Paris), 61,* 411–421.

Pujol, R. (1972). Development of tone-burst responses along the auditory pathway in the cat. *Acta oto-laryngology (Basel), 74,* 383–391.

Pujol, R., & Hilding, D. (1973). Anatomy and physiology of the onset of auditory function. *Acta oto-laryngology (Basel), 76,* 1–10.

Romand, R. (1971). Maturation des potentiels cochleaires dans la periode perinatale chez le chat et chez le cobaye. [Maturation of the cochlear potential in the perinatal period of the cat and the guinea pig] *Journal de Physiologie (Paris), 63,* 763–782.

Romand, R., Granier, M.R., & Marty, R. (1973). Development postnatal de l'activité provoquee dans l'olive superieure laterale chez le chat par la stimulation sonore [Postnatal development of evoked activity in the lateral superior olive with stimulation in the cat]. *Journal de Physiologie (Paris), 66,* 303–315.

Romand, R., & Marty, R. (1975). Postnatal maturation of the cochlear nuclei in the cat: a neurophysiological study. *Brain Research, 83,* 225–233.

Rosenzweig, M.R., & Sutton, D. (1958). Binaural interaction in lateral lemniscus of cat. *Journal of Neurophysiology, 21,* 1–23.

Shipley, C., Buchwald, J.S., Norman, R., & Guthrie, D. (1980). Brainstem auditory evoked response development in the kitten. *Brain Research, 182,* 313–326.

Shipley, C., Strecker, G., & Buchwald, J.S. (1984). Binaural interaction effects on the auditory brainstem response of the cat and kitten. *Brain Research, 321,* 299–309.

Squires, K.E., Donchin, E., Herning, R., & McCarthy, G. (1977). On the influence of task relevance and stimulus probability on ERP components. *Electroencephalography and Clinical Neurophysiology, 42,* 1–14.

Villablanca, J.R., & Olmstead, C.E. (1979). Neurological development of kittens. *Developmental Psychobiology, 12,* 101–127.

Wilder, M.B., Farley, G.R., & Starr, A. (1981). Endogenous late positive component of the evoked potential in cats corresponding to P300 in humans. *Science, 211,* 605–607.

6 Development of Auditory Evoked Potentials*

Eric Javel
Edward J. Walsh
JoAnn D. McGee
The Boys Town National Institute for Communication Disorders in Children
Omaha, NE 68131

MATURATION OF AUDITORY EVOKED POTENTIALS

Introduction

Evoked potentials (EPs) originating in the central auditory nervous system were first investigated in the 1930s (e.g., Davis, Davis, Loomis, Harvey, & Hobart, 1939). They have been used since the mid-1950s to study the postnatal development of hearing in several mammalian species (e.g., Grossman, 1955; Rose, Adrian, & Santibanez, 1957; Ellingson & Wilcott, 1960). The early studies determined that auditory EPs are highly replicable and relatively easy to record using noninvasive techniques. Because of this, routine recording of EPs has emerged as one of the primary evaluative tools for assessing clinical auditory function in cases where standard behavioral or audiometric techniques cannot be used.

Early studies of far-field auditory evoked potentials were limited for technological reasons to recordings of low-frequency, event-related responses that originated primarily from cortical areas. These responses have come to be known as the averaged electrical response (AER). An example of the AER wave shape is shown in Figure 1. Typically, each voltage deflection is given a name, with P1 referring to the first positive peak, N1 to the first negative peak, and so on. These voltage deflections are of relatively high amplitude and originate in the cortex. The early AER peaks almost certainly arise from

---

* This work was supported in part by an NINCDS research grant awarded to E. Javel, by an NINCDS program project grant awarded to the Boys Town National Institute, and by a grant from the Deafness Research Foundation awarded to E. J. Walsh.

Send correspondence to: Eric Javel, Boys Town National Institute, 555 N. 30th St., Omaha, NE 68131. E. Walsh's present adress is: Dept. of Surgery (Otolaryngology), Southern Illinois University, Springfield, IL 62708, and J. McGee's present address is: Dept. of Pharmacology, Southern Illinois University, Springfield, IL 62708.

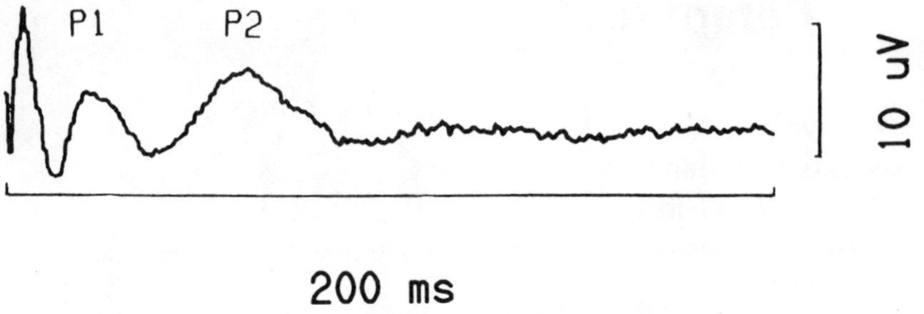

Figure 1. Example of the averaged electrical response (AER) in a mature cat. Stimuli were rarefaction clicks presented at 100 dB p SPL, and active and reference electrodes were attached to the vertex and nose, respectively.

the auditory cortex, but the later peaks probably do not (Starr & Farley, 1983).

Reproducible event-related potentials with very long latencies can also be obtained. These include a positive-going response that in humans has a latency of approximately 300 ms. This is the P300 wave, and it occurs when a novel stimulus is detected within a sequence of repetitive stimuli. Also observable is a negative-going wave that accompanies detection of a task-dependent event (the contingent negative variation, or CNV). These late potentials have been used with reasonable success in research on attention and learning. Middle-latency EPs also exist, and these have been shown to be related to motor and orienting responses to sound. Neither the middle-latency nor the very-long-latency potentials will be discussed here.

AERs are relatively large in amplitude and are generally reproducible, but the ability to record them is greatly influenced by the attentional state of the subject. This limits the utility of the AER in assessing auditory function clinically. In the early 1970s, improvements in digital and analog technology led to the discovery of low-amplitude auditory EPs arising in the first 10 ms following acoustic stimulus onset. It was determined that these are of subcortical origin. Also, it was found that they are relatively insensitive to the state of the subject, they are very reproducible, and they can be elicited at lower stimulus intensities than any of the later EPs (Sohmer & Feinmesser, 1967; Jewett & Williston, 1971). These EPs have been named the auditory brainstem response (ABR). Figure 2 shows an example of an ABR wave form recorded from a mature cat using an active electrode at the cranial vertex and a reference electrode at the nose.[1]

Typically, each positive ABR peak is assigned a Roman numeral. A given peak can be thought of as representing the arrival of the "wavefront" of synchronous, stimulus-elicited impulses at a particular nucleus or major fiber tract of the ascending auditory system. In this scheme, wave I of the ABR arises from the auditory nerve, wave II from the cochlear nucleus, wave III

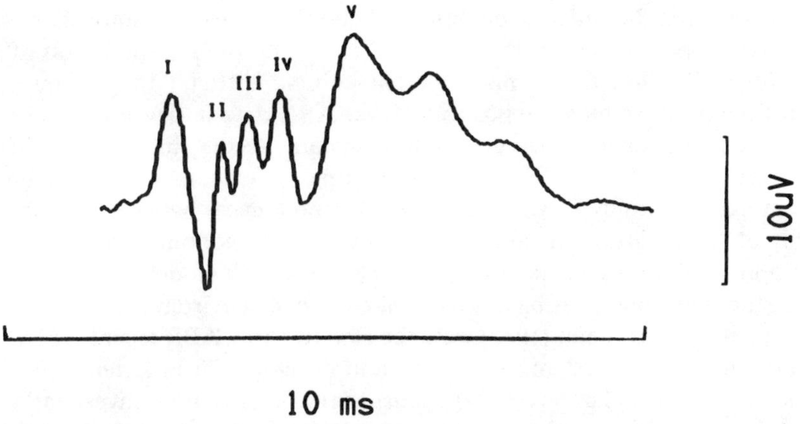

Figure 2. Example of a click-evoked auditory brainstem-evoked response (ABR) from a mature cat. Signal intensity was 100 dB p SPL, the active electrode was at the vertex, and the reference electrode was at the nose.

from the superior olive, and so on. While this way of describing the sources of the ABR waves has been shown to be technically incorrect because waves after wave I likely are derived from neural responses from multiple sites (Buchwald & Huang, 1975; Achor & Starr, 1980; Moller, Jannetta, & Moller, 1982), the simple view is accurate enough for the purposes of this discussion.

Several investigations have established that the ABR, as well as providing a gross measure of auditory system function, could also be used as an indicator of general neurological function in both developing and mature organisms (e.g., Starr & Hamilton, 1976; Starr, 1976; Galambos & Hecox, 1978). Even though its accuracy for diagnostic purposes is often limited (Stockard & Westmoreland, 1981), ABR screening of high-risk newborns has nonetheless been put into routine clinical use. A more recently employed use of ABRs is in assessing the survival of the auditory nerve in cases of profound deafness, so that the preoperative feasibility and postoperative performance of implantable cochlear prostheses can be examined (Black, Clark, O'Leary, & Walters, 1983; Gardi & Schindler, 1983; Waring, Don, & Brimacombe, 1983).

Since the developing auditory system undergoes considerable change in its ability to respond to acoustic stimuli, any use of ABRs for clinical assessment of human infants requires that age-dependent norms for latency and threshold be established and that ABRs be characterized for the various pathological conditions that may be encountered. ABR norms for premature infants are difficult to establish for several reasons, the most prominent of which is the difficulty of securing ABRs from sufficient numbers of infants. Also, humans with neurological and other abnormalities are often poor subjects for

ABR research, because the pathological conditions being examined are usually accompanied by other factors that confound the interpretation of the findings. Because these important data are so difficult to procure, it is worthwhile examining the possibility that ABR data in developing animals could be substituted for the desired human data, keeping in mind that different species mature at different rates and that differences in auditory brainstem neuroanatomy exist. If reliable correspondences between human and animal ABR maturation could be established, then not only would early developmental norms be made available, but a research model would also exist for studying clinical problems in a well-controlled environment.

Jewett and Romano (1972) were the first to apply ABR techniques to the study of auditory system maturation and development in kittens and rats, and Hecox and Galambos (1974) published the first extensive investigation of early maturation of ABRs in human infants. Numerous other studies of physiological, anatomical and behavioral development have also been performed (see Rubel, 1978 or 1984, for a review). Taken together, these investigations form the basis for the current understanding of early auditory system development.

The major portion of auditory system development occurs prenatally in humans and in some animals such as guinea pigs. These organisms are born with functioning sensory systems; hence, they are termed *precocious organisms*. However, for many other animals, among which are cats and rats, a substantial portion of sensory system development occurs after birth. These animals are known as *altricious organisms*. As will be shown, postnatal development of hearing does not depend on the maturity of animals' auditory systems at birth. This means that it is valid to compare data from precocious animals with data from altricious animals.

Neural responses to high-intensity acoustic stimuli can be elicited from human infants as early as the sixth postconceptional month (Starr, Amlie, Martin, & Sanders, 1977). At this time, the external and middle ears are poorly differentiated, the middle ear is filled with a dense mesenchymal gel, and the three bones of the middle ear are incompletely ossified. Because of this, sound conduction through the external and middle ears is probably impaired (Relkin & Saunders, 1980). More importantly, the cells and mechanical structures of the cochlea are morphologically immature at this age. Furthermore, it has been shown that a gradient exists wherein basal cochlear regions are more mature at any given developmental stage than apical regions (Retzius, 1884; Bredberg, 1968). Also relevant is the fact that myelin, whose presence affects the conduction velocity of neuronal impulses, is almost totally lacking from auditory nerve fibers and brainstem auditory tracts at this time (Romand, Sans, Romand, & Marty, 1976; Romand & Romand, 1982; Walsh, McGee, Wagahoff, & Scott, 1985).

All morphological aspects of the human auditory system undergo rapid development between the fifth and seventh gestational months. Maturation appears to occur sequentially, however, so that structures in the lower levels of the system mature earlier than those in higher levels. The last part of the system to complete its maturation is the cortex. Myelination studies (e.g., Yakovlev & Lecours, 1967) have shown that human association cortices require up to 12 years, i.e., until puberty, to attain adult morphological status.

Cats undergo essentially the same sequence of developmental events as humans, but the time frame is greatly compressed. At birth, the cat cochlea is poorly differentiated, more so in the apex than in the base (Pujol & Marty, 1970). While weak cochlear microphonics can be elicited from kittens at birth, compound action potentials are entirely lacking (Pujol & Hilding, 1973). In general, reproducible auditory responses can be elicited only after the first few days postpartum, and then only in the presence of stimuli presented at very high intensities.

Studies of cochlear potentials (e.g., Crowley & Hepp-Reymond, 1966; Romand, 1971; Fernandez & Hinojosa, 1974; Carlier, Lenoir, & Pujol, 1979) and single-neuron responses (e.g., Pujol, 1972; Brugge, Javel, & Kitzes, 1978; Romand, 1979; Walsh, McGee, & Javel, 1982) have shown that anatomical maturation is accompanied by physiological maturation, affecting common measures of auditory function such as thresholds and slopes of input–output functions. Maturational effects can also be observed in responses of single neurons. Some aspects of neuronal response that change with advancing age are spontaneous and maximum discharge rates, frequency selectivity or tuning properties, and the ability to synchronize discharges with the cycle of the stimulating waveform (see Brugge, this volume). It appears that the limiting factor in early auditory function at all levels of the system is the development of the hair-cell/auditory-nerve synapse (Pujol, 1972).

As stated earlier, the postnatal maturation of EPs has been studied off and on since the mid-1950s. Grossman (1955) and Rose et al. (1957) were among the first to study the ontogeny of cortical EPs. Jewett and Romano (1972) were the first to study the development of ABRs in animals, and Hecox and Galambos (1974) and Salamy and McKean (1976) were among the first to apply ABR techniques to the question of functional hearing development in human infants. The first extensive longitudinal study of ABR development in cats was performed by Shipley, Norman, Buchwald, & Guthrie (1980). They investigated the age at which ABRs were first elicited, and they followed the maturation of ABR wave-form structure and wave latencies as a function of postnatal age (see Buchwald & Shipley, this volume). This was complemented by one performed by Walsh (1983), who verified the earlier findings and extended them to include the development of ABR wave amplitudes, interwave time intervals, and various aspects of AER maturation. Much of the data that follow are drawn from Walsh's study.

Initial Auditory Evoked Potentials and the "Onset" of Auditory Function

The issue of inception of hearing is an old one, dating at least from the 1940s (e.g., Larsell, McCrady, and Larsell, 1944). As a general rule, it seems that the appearance of far-field auditory evoked potentials is a better indicator of the ability of an animal to sense its acoustic environment than is the appearance of near-field potentials such as the cochlear microphonic. This view stems from the findings that near-field potentials can be elicited at high stimulus intensities at earlier ages than those at which evoked potentials appear and that the near-field potentials do not necessarily correlate with behavioral data. The data of Ehret (1976), Ehret and Romand (1981), and Gray and Rubel (1981) on behavioral thresholds all support the contention that the functional onset of hearing coincides with the appearance of evoked potentials.

Since responses to sound can be elicited at early ages from the cochlea and from single CNS cells only at very high stimulus intensities, that is, above 120 dB sound pressure level (SPL, re 20 μPa), it may be somewhat misleading to speak of auditory function as having a distinct onset. This is because "onset" implies a response criterion, and the criterion depends on the intensity of the stimulus, the type of the stimulus, and the response being measured. We can circumvent this issue simply by referring to hearing "onset" (in quotes) as it relates to the ability of the system to respond to sounds that would be encountered environmentally. As we shall see from EP data, we can point to the end of the first postnatal week as the time when kittens probably have their first auditory experiences and, by inference, the sixth or seventh gestational month as the time when human infants are capable of hearing their first sounds.

Intact kittens do not produce a reliable ABR or AER waveform at any time prior to the end of the first postnatal week, even for stimuli presented at 140 dB SPL (Walsh, McGee, & Javel, 1986a). In addition to the morphologic and neural immaturity of the cochlea and CNS, another reason why evoked potentials are not seen stems from the fact that the kitten's external auditory meatus is collapsed and the pinna is folded over the ear canal at this age. This is not to say, however, that responses cannot be obtained. Mair, Elverland, and Laukli (1978), for example, obtained ABRs from a 2-day-old kitten when the sound source was brought in contact with the skull, and we obtained reproducible ABRs at 4 days of age after surgically exposing the tympanic membrane and presenting click stimuli at 120–130 dB SPL (Walsh, McGee, & Javel, 1983). It must be borne in mind, however, that these recording situations are unnatural. While these and other data (cf. Marty &

Thomas, 1963) indicate that the central auditory system is capable of functioning at this age, it is highly improbable that intact animals will encounter stimuli that are sufficiently intense to activate the auditory system.

There is poor definition to ABR waveforms elicited at very high stimulus intensities from young animals who have had their external ears resected to the tympanic membrane. What is curious about the waveforms is that they are essentially constant between postnatal days 2 and 6. That is, the latencies and amplitudes of the two discernible waves (which, as we shall see, correspond to ABR waves I and V) have approximately the same values, regardless of the age of the animal. Thus, it appears that the first postnatal week, which is a time when cochlear structures are grossly immature, provides only primitive ABR waveforms. The characteristics of these waveforms are presumably governed by the excessively high mass and low stiffness properties of the immature basilar membrane and the excessively poor generation and transmission of neural impulses up the chain of auditory nuclei.

Virtually all normal kittens produce ABR responses to intense clicks as well as to mid- and high-frequency tones by the end of the first postnatal week. The ABR waveforms, however, are very immature in that they possess only two recognizable waves, the wave latencies are prolonged, and the wave amplitudes are small. Reproducible AERs cannot be elicited at this time. While middle- and high-frequency tones can elicit ABRs in kittens at the end of the first postnatal week and cochlear microphonics can be recorded for tones up to 10 kHz at the same age, low-frequency tones produce no recognizable ABRs. In contrast, single auditory nerve fibers and cells of the anteroventral cochlear nucleus respond only to low- and mid-frequency tones at this age (Brugge et al., 1978; Brugge, Kitzes, & Javel, 1981; Walsh et al., 1982)

Maturation of EP Waveforms and Response Threshold

A series of ABR and AER waveforms obtained at various ages from the same kitten for clicks presented at 95–100 dB peak SPL is shown in Figure 3. By following a given wave in time, one can see that there is an age at which the wave first appears. The wave then grows in amplitude and decreases in latency as age increases. We have obtained longitudinal data like these from 44 kittens in 8 litters, collecting examples of ABR and AER waveforms for both clicks and tones presented at intensities ranging from below threshold to, wherever possible, 70–80 dB above threshold at each age. Analyses of data both from individuals and from litters indicate that although considerable variability exists across the entire sample for any measure at any age, there is always a clear mean or median to any aspect of the response. Having established that each ABR measure is distributed approximately normally around a mean, we pooled our data with the idea of studying "average" EPs. Our descriptions, of course, refer only to maturational trends averaged across sev-

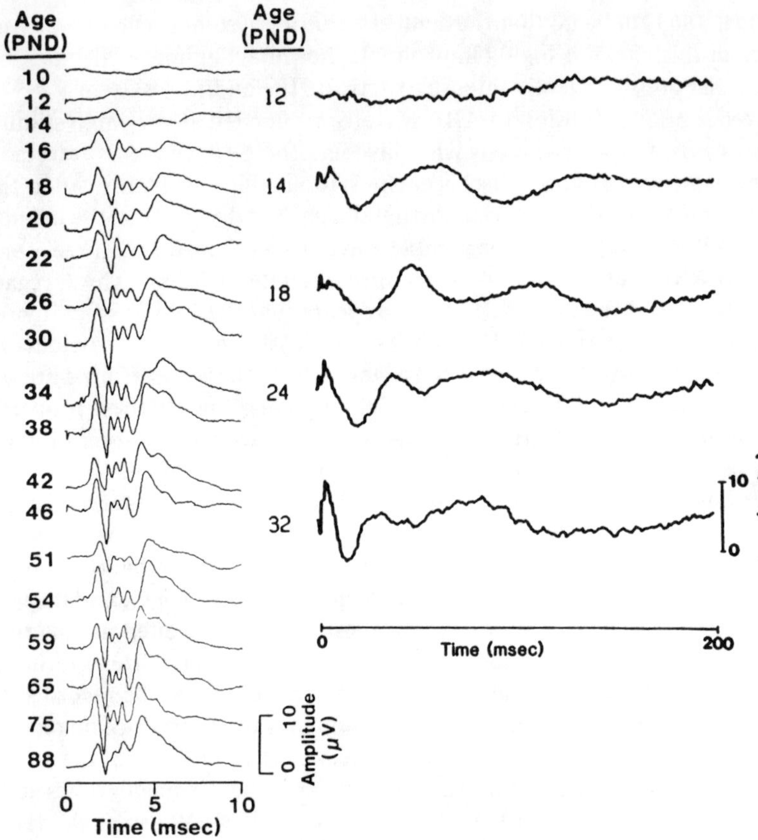

Figure 3. Examples of ABR and AER waveforms obtained in response to 95–100 dB pSPL clicks at several ages following birth.

eral animals. As such, they do not necessarily describe exactly the maturation of auditory EPs in individual animals.

The reason that EPs "appear" at certain ages is simply that structural and neural maturation has enabled the auditory system and, in particular, the cochlea, to begin responding to stimuli presented at some experimenter-selected intensity. The age of initial response, then, depends both on the rate at which hearing thresholds mature and on stimulus intensity. As will be shown, thresholds in kittens mature as quickly as 10 dB per day. And, while initial responses may be seen at 8–9 days of age for stimuli presented at, say, 120 dB SPL, responses may be observed at earlier ages if yet higher intensity stimuli are employed.

By collecting EPs in response to stimuli whose intensities are varied stepwise across a wide range, it is possible to measure wave amplitudes and determine the intensity at which an EP wave just appears. If we assume that this procedure provides an accurate estimate of response threshold, we can follow threshold maturation by employing the same procedure to estimate thresholds for the same animal at several ages. Because AERs were more variable, particularly in very young animals, and because they did not provide threshold estimates that were as sensitive as those derived from ABRs, our description of the maturation of response thresholds will be based only on ABR data.

Plots of thresholds for clicks and tones at 0.25, 2, and 16 kHz as functions of kittens' postnatal ages are shown in Figure 4. It can be seen that there is a period of time prior to 20 days of age during which thresholds improve rapidly. The intensity range over which improvements occur exceeds 100 dB,

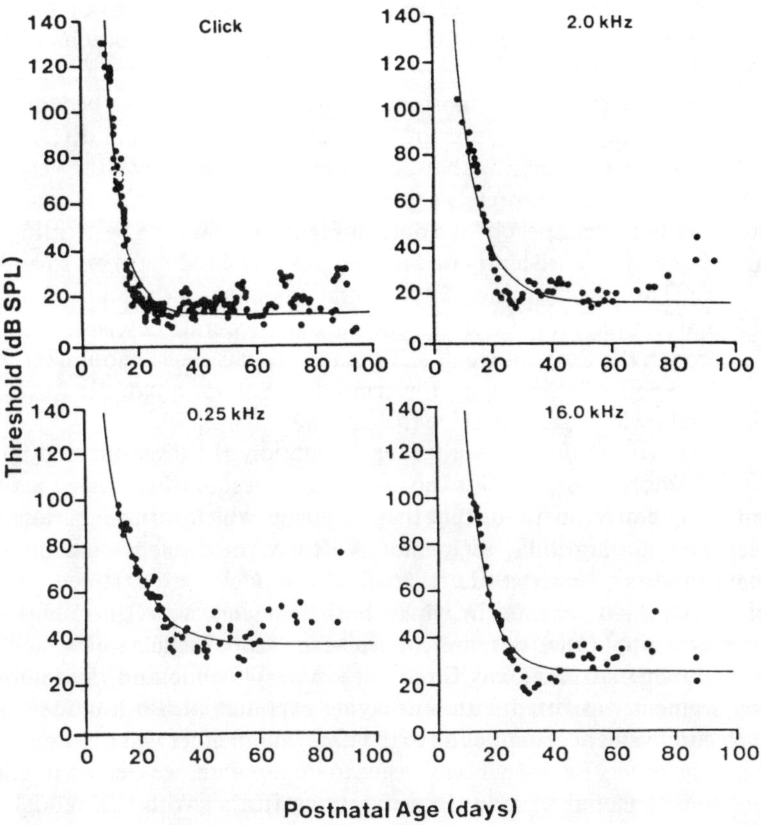

Figure 4. ABR thresholds as a function of age in kittens for clicks and for tones at 250 Hz, 2000 Hz, and 16000 Hz. Data have been fitted with decaying exponential functions of the form $Y = a + b \exp(-cX)$.

which is considerably greater than the amount that can be accounted for by improvements in mechanical transmission of sound through the external and middle ears. The period of rapid improvement in ABR threshold is followed by a period of slower improvements in threshold, with adult values attained by 60 days of age for all stimuli and all EP waves.

Best-fitting expotentials of the form $Y = a + b \exp(-cX)$ are also plotted in Figure 4. The fitted curves show that thresholds for different stimuli mature at somewhat different rates. Thresholds for clicks mature fastest, thresholds for 16-kHz and 2-kHz tones mature next fastest, and thresholds for 0.25-kHz tones mature least quickly. This gradient is consistent with data on the morphological development of the cochlea, where the basal turn structures, which ultimately are maximally sensitive to high-frequency stimuli, attain maturity earlier than the apical turn structures.

The data in Figure 4 also indicate two other important aspects of auditory maturation. First, thresholds for clicks improve at a rate of more than 10 dB per day during the early postnatal period. This is the time when the ear canal opens, the ossicles calcify, the substance in the middle ear is resorbed, and the mechanical and neural structures of the cochlea undergo rapid differentiation. While it is not surprising that thresholds should improve, the very fast rate of improvement is impressive.

The other notable aspect of the data in Figure 4 is that the best-fitting decaying exponential consistently underestimates threshold between 15 and 30 days of age. Thus, while a single exponential accounts for the major features of ABR maturation, it does not provide the most accurate description of the data. Although the time course of ABR maturation is clearly nonlinear, neither single-exponential fits (e.g., Eggermont, 1982) nor quadratic fits (e.g., Fawer & Dubowitz, 1982) describe the data well.

It occurred to us that a two-stage representation of EP maturation might fit the data more closely. With this in mind, we established, using a computer-based iterative method, that there is an age which forms a breakpoint between two maturational segments. We then fitted each segment with alternate models (Walsh et al., 1986a). The models we examined were a double-exponential scheme, in which both segments were fitted with decaying exponential functions, and a linear-exponential scheme, in which the earlier-occurring segment was fitted with a straight line and the later-occurring segment was fitted with a decaying exponential. Both models produced accurate and acceptable fits to the data, and neither was obviously superior to the other. Because it was easier to manipulate, we elected to adopt the linear-exponential scheme. Experimenting further with this model, we found that the best fit occurred when the breakpoint between the linear and exponential segments was taken to be postnatal day 18. Although each EP wave possesses a separate breakpoint, these were so close to one another that we simply took 18 days as the breakpoint for all waves in order to reduce confusion. An example of the results of the linear-exponential model is shown in Figure 5, in which click thresholds are described as a function of age.

It should be kept in mind that although the accuracy in fitting maturational ABR data is improved when a two-stage model is employed, this does not prove that two separate stages of development exist or even that the same structures contribute to the overall response at all times during development. Indeed, there are several factors that contribute to overall maturation. In ad-

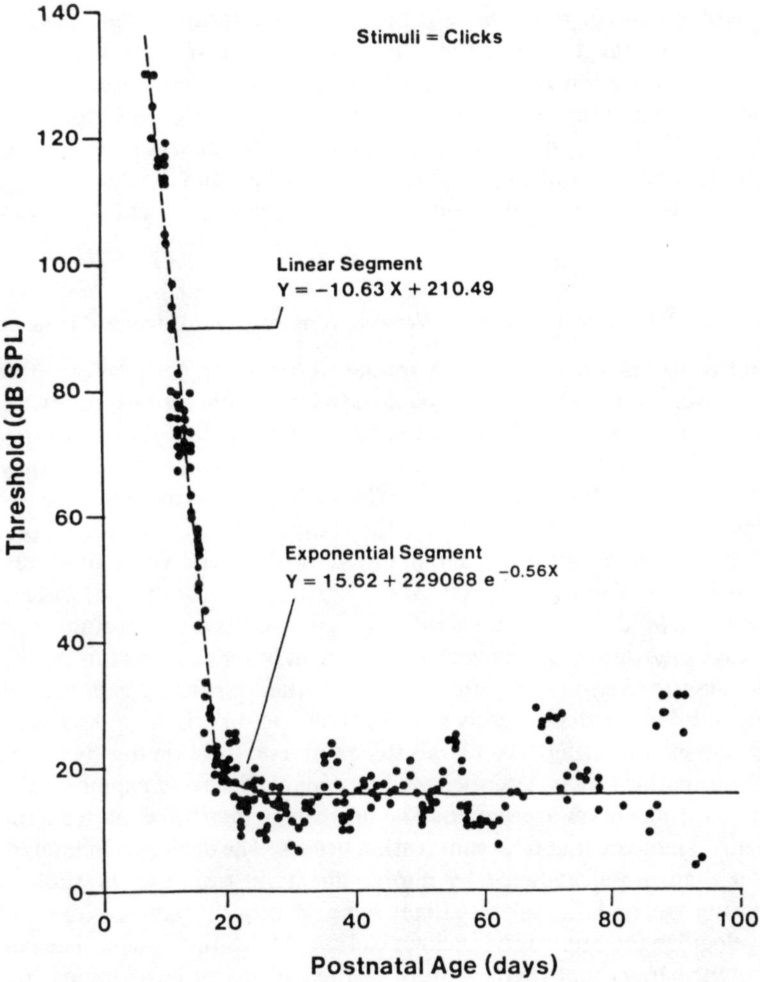

Figure 5. ABR thresholds for 100 dB pSPL clicks as a function of postnatal age in kittens. Data prior to 18 days of age were fitted with a straight line, and later data were fitted with a decaying exponential.

dition to the morphologic development of the external and middle ears and of the cochlea mentioned earlier, we also have to consider the contributions of myelination, neural response synchrony, synaptic efficacy in the CNS, and cell growth. These can and probably do proceed at different rates during postnatal development. Also, as Relkin and Saunders (1980), Rubel and Ryals (1983), and Harris and Dallos (1984) have shown, the immature middle ear and cochlea undergo dramatic change in the way they analyze incoming sound. These changes can affect both the transfer function that governs which frequencies are allowed to enter the cochlea and the mechanical response properties or resonances of the basilar membrane. Regardless of the source of the change, the fact is that a two-segment scheme is necessary if threshold maturation is to be described accurately. For reasons to be described, we can consider the early, fast-maturing phase to be primarily a function of maturation of the peripheral auditory apparatus, including the middle ear and mechanical structures of the cochlea and the late, slowly maturing phase to be primarily a function of maturation of neural elements in the cochlea and CNS.

Maturation of Evoked Potential Wave Latencies and Interwave Intervals

Neural transmission through the immature auditory pathway is substantially slower than it is in mature systems. In 20-day-old kittens, for example, ABR and AER wave latencies are prolonged by factors that can range to three or four, and interwave time intervals are nearly twice as long as they are in adults (Walsh, McGee, & Javel, 1986b). Representative data are shown in Figure 6, where mean latencies for the various EP waves have been plotted as a function of postnatal age, and in Figure 7, where interwave time intervals have been plotted as a function of age. The stimulus in both cases was a click presented at 90-dB peak-equivalent SPL. Two points are important: First, a two-stage maturational sequence is evident. In order to stress this point, the model described earlier was used to provide the best-fitting exponentials in Figure 6. It is clear that an early phase of maturation exists. And second, the interwave intervals (Fig. 7) undergo substantial maturation during postnatal life. This maturation is described well by a single decaying exponential, and the best-fitting curves are shown. The decreasing interwave intervals shown in Figure 7 indicate that CNS maturation occurs. The decreases in latency are greater than those predicted by improvements in response threshold with increasing age, and they are also likely to be influenced by increasing conduction velocities and improved synchronization in CNS fiber tracts. The important point here is that there is more to the functional development of the auditory system than is accounted for by the maturation of its peripheral structures.

Some of the effects of maturation in the peripheral auditory system can be

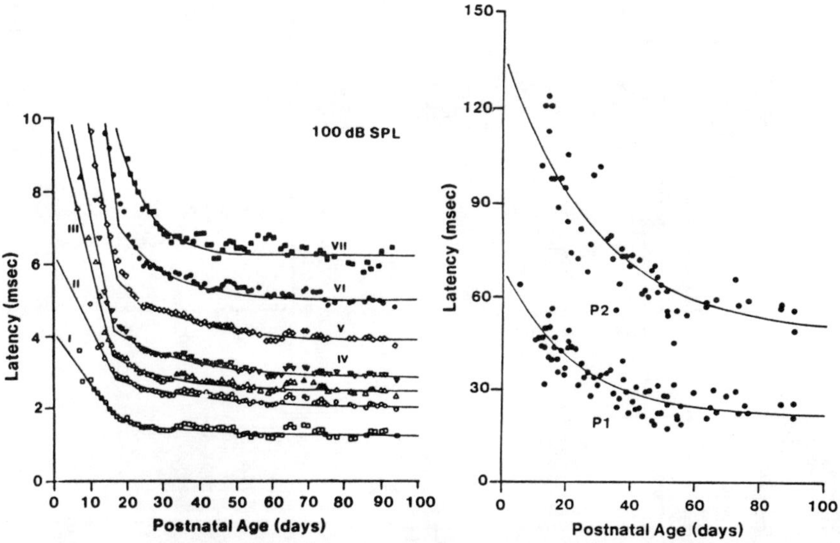

Figure 6. AER and ABR wave latencies as a function of kittens' ages for clicks presented at 100 dB pSPL. Latencies have been corrected for conduction delays. Data are fitted with decaying exponentials, and for ABRs only, the data after 18 postnatal days were used for the fit.

factored out by considering EP data obtained at similar suprathreshold stimulus intensities. That is, we can take changes in absolute threshold sensitivity into account by analyzing data in terms of sensation level, wherein stimulus intensity is expressed in terms of some number of decibels above the response threshold obtained at that age. This procedure removes the confounding factor of improving thresholds, which, as we have already seen, is particularly pronounced in the early postnatal period. Longitudinal ABR data obtained at 70–dB sensation level are shown in Figure 8. The actual stimulus intensities, of course, changed with the kitten's age, being much higher at early ages than at later ages.

The data in Figure 8 provide evidence that substantial maturation of wave latencies exists even when threshold is taken into account. Unlike the data shown in Figures 5 and 6, however, the data in Figure 8 possesses no steeply decreasing linear segment at early ages and are described well by a single decaying exponential. This observation supports the notion that the early stage of auditory development is governed primarily by maturation of mechanical elements in the middle ear and cochlea and that continued improvements in auditory system performance are determined by maturation of neural elements.

Inspection of Figure 6 reveals that although EP wave latencies mature systematically, they seemingly mature at different rates, with ABR wave I

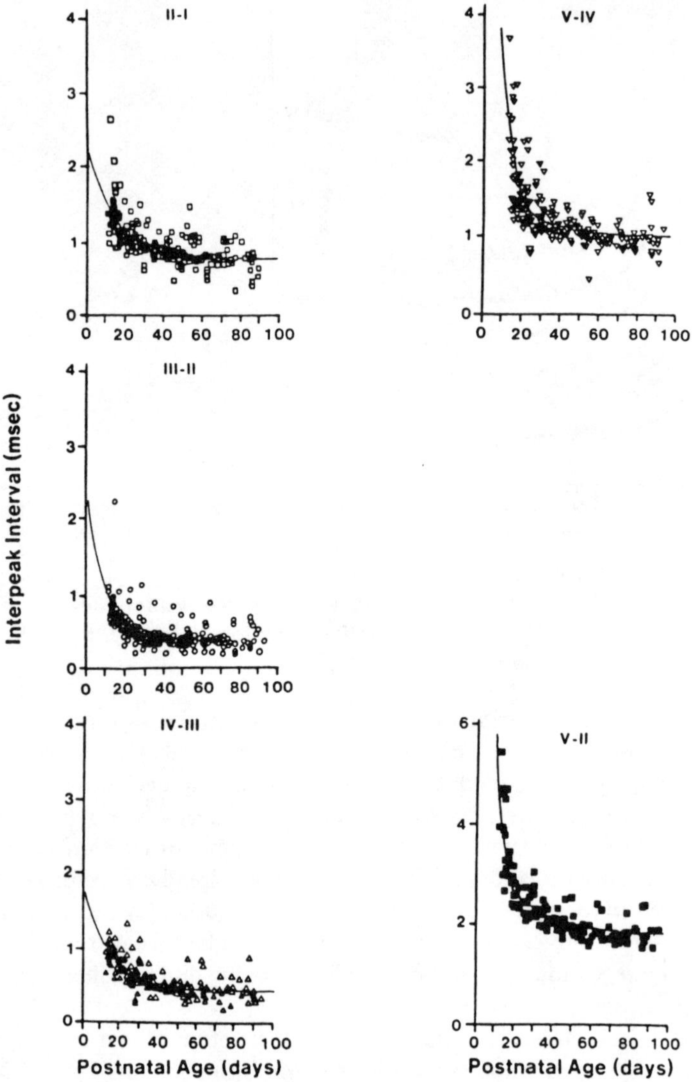

Figure 7. Maturation of ABR interpeak intervals in response to clicks presented at 90 dB pSPL.

maturing earliest and AER wave P2 maturing latest. By normalizing the data for each wave with regard to its asymptotic or adult value, we can show that this is not exactly the case. The results of this normalization are shown in Figure 9, where EP wave latencies at different ages have been expressed as percentages of their adult values. It can be seen, now that absolute latency has been taken into account, that all ABR waves mature at somewhat the same

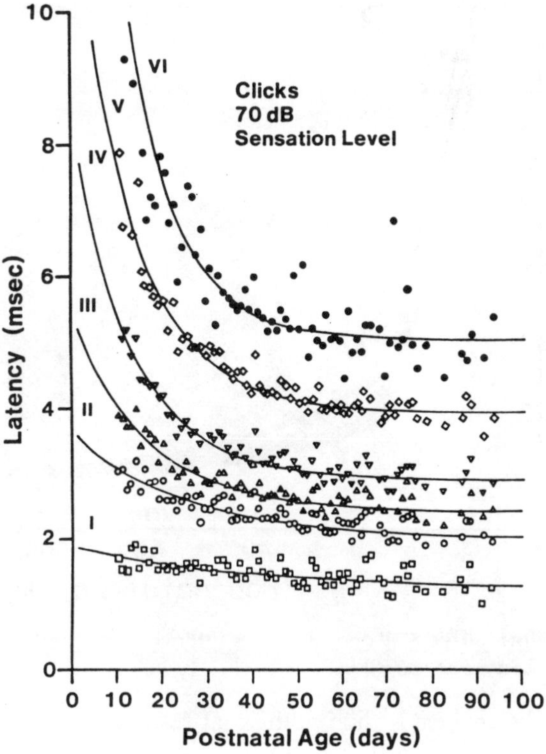

Figure 8. Latencies of ABR waves I through V as a function of age, for clicks presented at 70 dB above threshold at each age.

rate, with substantial differences in maturational rate existing only at very early ages. The normalized data indicate that, prior to 20 days of age, ABR waves I and II mature at nearly the same rate, and that ABR waves III, IV, and V form a group that lags behind these. After 20 days of age, all of the ABR waves mature at approximately the same rate. The AER waves mature slower than the ABR waves, even when their absolute latencies are taken into account.

EP latency data for tonal stimuli were basically the same as those obtained for clicks. In Figure 10 are shown mean latencies for ABR waves I and V as a function of postnatal age in kittens, obtained in response to tone bursts at 0.25, 2, and 16 kHz presented at 100 dB SPL. The data have been fitted with linear and exponential segments according to the model described earlier. Tones at 2 kHz provided the earliest-occurring responses, followed by responses at 16 kHz and 0.25 kHz, respectively. Differences among the rates of maturation of AER wave latencies at these three frequencies were minimal.

What might be termed curious in the light of data on the anatomic devel-

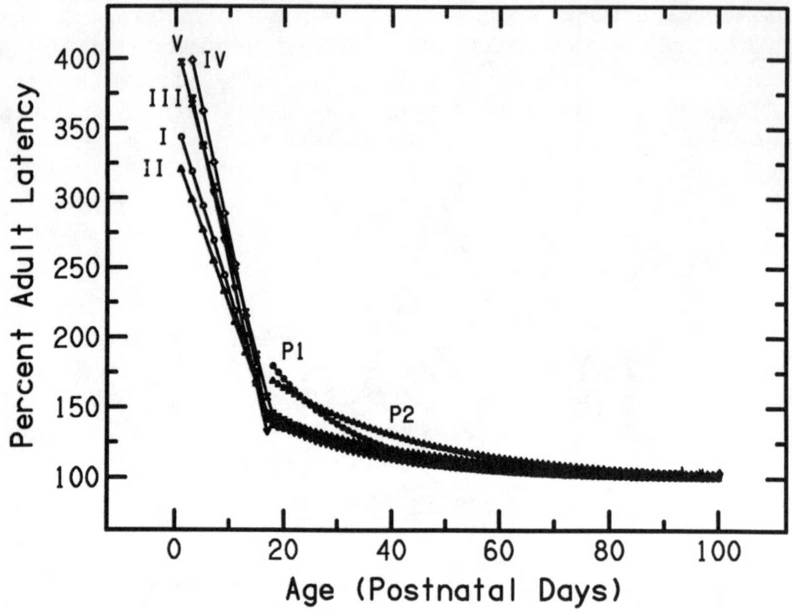

Figure 9. Normalized ABR and AER wave latencies as a function of age in kittens, for clicks presented at 100 dB pSPL.

opment of the cochlea is the finding that responses to 2-kHz tones appear earlier than responses to 16-kHz tones. We have already mentioned the fact that cochlear development proceeds in a base-to-apex direction. If so, then why don't responses to 16-kHz tones appear first? The answer to this question has been alluded to earlier. It has been documented that the band of frequencies capable of producing cochlear microphonics and single-neuron responses is limited to low and middle frequencies during the early postnatal period in rats (Crowley & Hepp-Reymond, 1966) and cats (Pujol, 1972; Brugge, et al., 1978, 1981; Walsh et al., 1982), and that this bandwidth enlarges rapidly with increasing age to encompass the entire audible frequency range. Furthermore, experiments performed by Rubel and Ryals (1983) in chicken hatchlings showed that the cochlear region undergoing damage from exposure to high-intensity, low-frequency tones is not the same region that responds to these frequencies in adult life (see Lippe, Ryals, & Rubel, this volume). Rather, it is the regions that ultimately respond to high frequencies that are damaged. These data have been interpreted to imply that the immature cochlea possesses different mass and stiffness properties along its basilar membrane (relative to those in mature animals) and that the mechanics of the immature basilar membrane are such that basal positions respond to increasingly higher frequencies as maturation proceeds. Further evidence supporting the idea that the cochlea changes its frequency analytic properties in

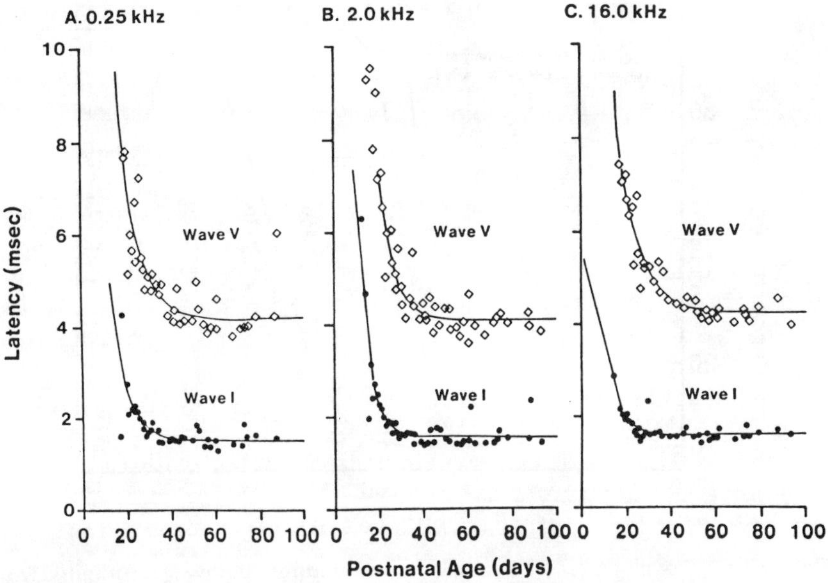

Figure 10. Maturation of ABR wave latencies in response to 100-dB pSPL tones at 250 Hz, 2000 Hz, and 16000 Hz. Data have been fitted with straight lines for ages less than 18 days and with decaying exponentials thereafter.

early life has been provided by Harris and Dallos (1984). They showed with cochlear microphonic tuning curves that the basal turn of the gerbil cochlea undergoes shifts in early postnatal life with regard to the frequencies to which it is most sensitive. Given these changes, it is entirely reasonable that ABR responses to tones should be obtained earliest at middle frequencies and that they should precede responses to high frequencies.

Myelination of Auditory Pathways

The preceding data clearly show that AER wave latencies mature more slowly than ABR waves, and that maturation of AER wave P2 is slightly slower than maturation of wave P1. The differences between ABR and AER maturation may be due to differences in the maturational rates of cortical neurons relative to the maturational rates of brainstem neurons. This view is supported by the anatomic findings of Yakovlev and Lecours (1967), who showed that myelination of cortical fiber tracts in humans is substantially slower than myelination in brainstem tracts. A representation of the development of myelin in primary auditory pathways in humans, taken from the data of Yakovlev and Lecours, is given in Figure 11. The time course of myelination shown in this figure is not meant to be exact.

The data in Figure 9 can be interpreted to indicate that ABR waves mature

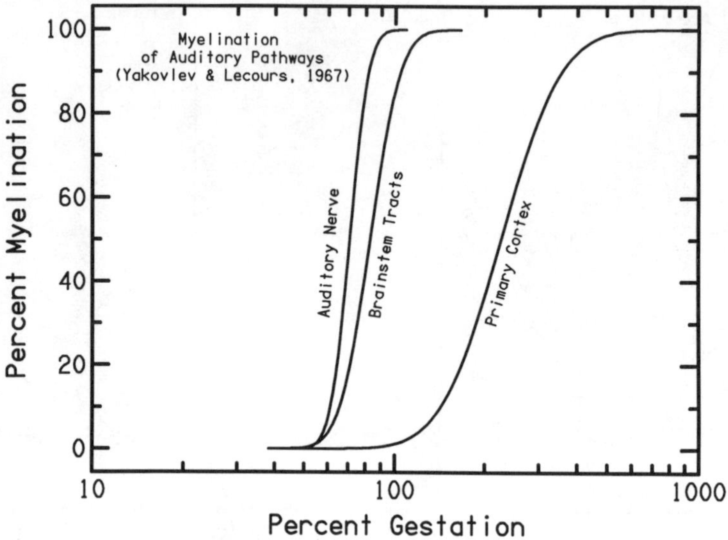

Figure 11. Development of myelin in human auditory pathways. (Adapted from Yakovlev & Lecours, 1967.)

as a single group. A somewhat different view of maturation, however, is obtained when myelination of brainstem auditory tracts is considered. We performed experiments in which myelinated axons in major auditory fiber tracts were stained and photographed at several kittens' ages. Figure 12 shows axonal cross-sections of representative tissue at three ages in the auditory nerve, the trapezoid body (which is one of the output tracts of the cochlear nucleus), and the brachium of the inferior colliculus (which forms the auditory projection from the inferior colliculus to the medial geniculate nucleus of the thalamus). The myelin surrounding individual axons appears as darkly staining ellipses.

Figure 12 shows a relatively clear developmental gradient for myelin. In order to quantify this, similar sections were studied under the electron microscope, and the number of myelin lamellae found around axons of several representative neurons in these three fiber tracts at these ages were counted. The number of myelin lamallae was distributed approximately normally, and the mean counts at each age are shown in Figure 13. It is clearly evident that axons in the auditory nerve become fully myelinated earlier than axons in the trapezoid body, which, in turn, probably mature earlier than axons in the brachium of the inferior colliculus. There is even a suggestion that the upper brainstem tract is not fully myelinated at 6 months of age.

The data shown in Fig. 7 to 13 can be reconciled in the following manner: Morphologic maturation in the CNS is slower than maturation in the peripheral system, and there exists a gradient whereby successively higher levels of

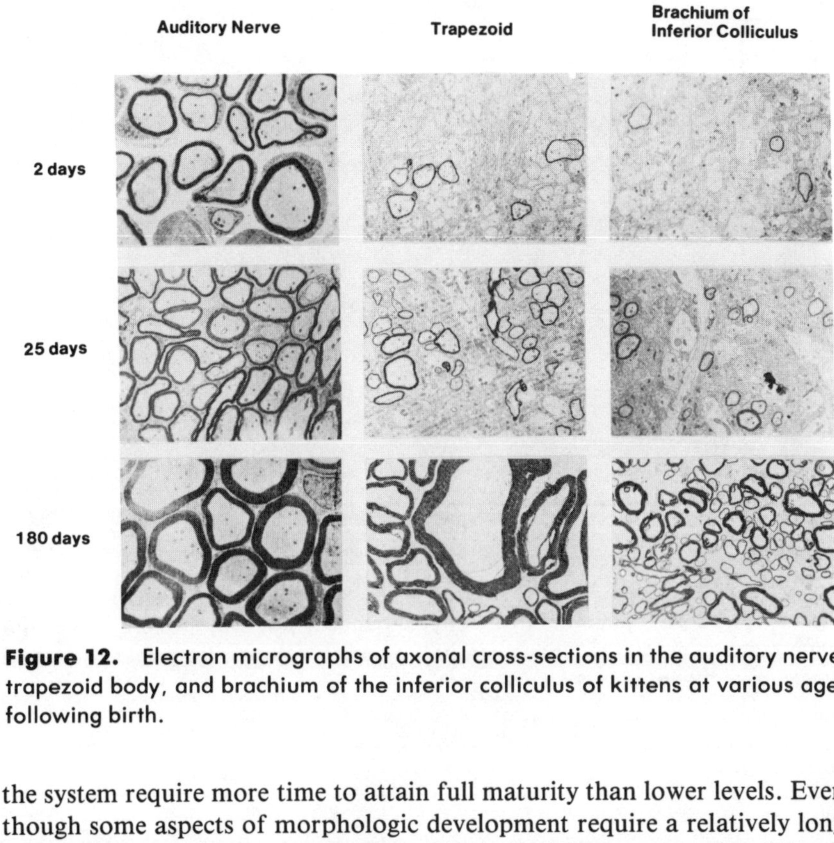

Figure 12. Electron micrographs of axonal cross-sections in the auditory nerve, trapezoid body, and brachium of the inferior colliculus of kittens at various ages following birth.

the system require more time to attain full maturity than lower levels. Even though some aspects of morphologic development require a relatively long time to mature fully, the factors that govern physiologic or functional development in cats are sufficiently developed by the middle of the second postnatal month to produce near-adult wave latencies.

Maturation of Evoked Potential Wave Amplitudes

ABR and AER wave amplitudes in kittens mature in general concordance with the maturation of response thresholds and latencies, with one exception. The exception is that wave amplitudes increase in size with advancing age up to 40–60 days after birth, after which they decline as they approach their adult values (Walsh, McGee, & Javel, 1986c). Mean data on wave amplitudes of ABR wave I and V in kittens are shown in Figure 14. ABR and AER wave amplitudes are uniformly small during the first 2 or 3 postnatal weeks, and they grow systematically and nearly linearly until about 40 days of age. After this, wave amplitudes decline. The time course of amplitude growth during the first 40 postnatal days is slower than the time course of threshold and wave latency maturation.

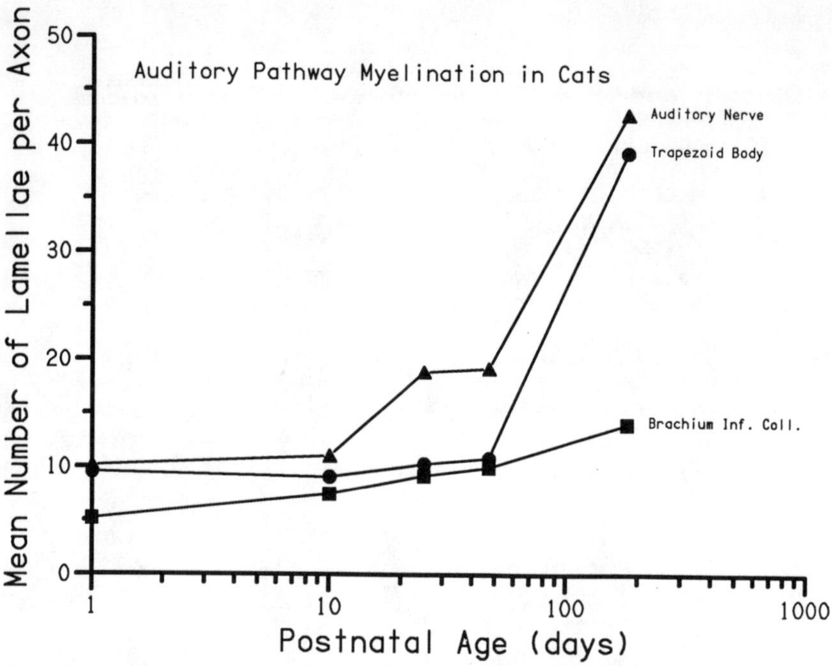

Figure 13. Development of myelin in cat auditory pathways, expressed as the mean number of lamellae per axon in the auditory nerve, trapezoid body, and brachium of the inferior colliculus.

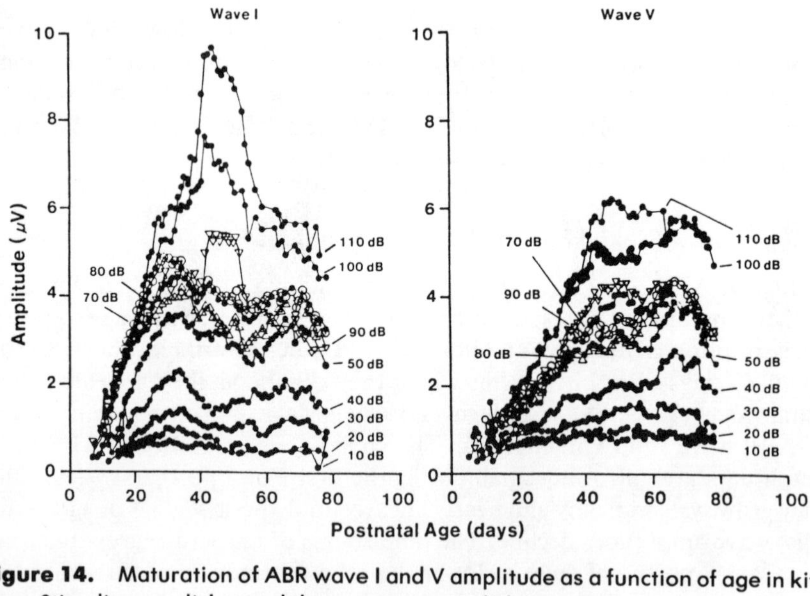

Figure 14. Maturation of ABR wave I and V amplitude as a function of age in kittens. Stimuli were clicks, and the parameter is click intensity.

ABR waves possess different amplitudes. Waves I and V are relatively large, and the other ABR waves are relatively small. In order to observe differences in maturation of amplitudes of individual waves, mean amplitudes of selected ABR waves were normalized. The normalization consisted of scaling each wave amplitude so that it possessed a normalized value of 100 at 43 days of age. This is shown in Figure 15. It can be seen that wave I amplitude matures earliest and that waves II, IV, and V form a group whose amplitudes matures at approximately the same time. Wave VI, which probably arises from the thalamus, lags behind the earlier waves. These findings are qualitatively consistent with the latency and myelination data presented earlier.

The decline in kittens' EP wave amplitude after 40 days of age may be attributed to changes in head and brain size, which, in turn, affect the proximity of the recording electrodes to the wave generators and the orientation of current dipoles relative to the positions of the electrodes. The changing nature of the recording situation during development is indicated in Figure 16, which consists of drawings of kittens' skulls and brains at various ages following birth. In particular, note the relationship of the cranial vertex to the positions of the brainstem and auditory cortex at various ages, and note the increasing complexity of the cortical convolutions as kittens age.

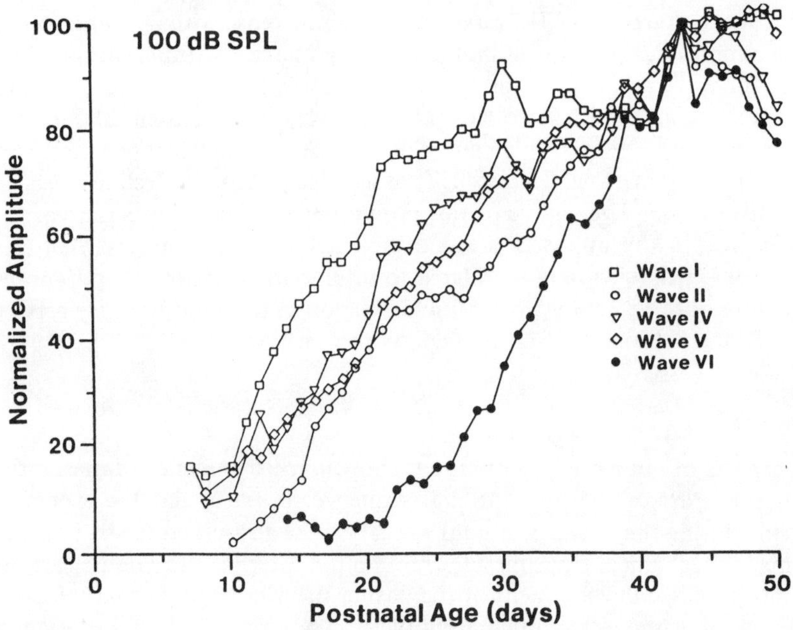

Figure 15. Kitten ABR wave amplitudes as a function of age, expressed as a percentage of adult wave amplitude.

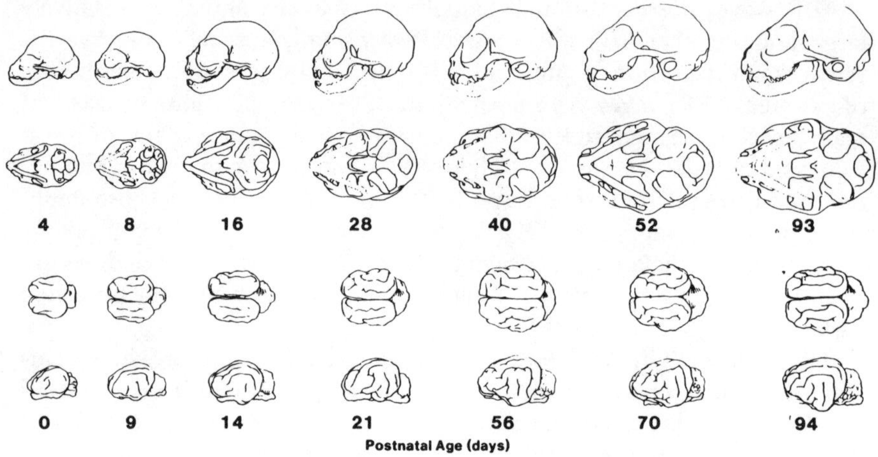

Figure 16. Gross morphologic development of skulls and brains in kittens at various ages.

Input–output functons for ABR wave amplitudes at given ages can be constructed by making vertical cuts through the data shown in Figure 14 and connecting the points. This has been done in Figure 17. Two points are notable. First, rates of growth of EP wave amplitudes increase with age; and second, wave amplitudes grow as stimulus intensity increases. Input–output functions for wave amplitudes show some interesting phenomena. Wave amplitudes tend to grow with increasing intensity over a certain range, above which wave amplitudes reach a plateau or decline. At yet higher intensities, wave amplitudes again grow. The intensity at which a plateau or decline is reached depends on age. The source of this nonmonotonic behavior is unclear, but similarities in the intensity range over which it occurs suggest that nonmonotonic behavior may be related to nonmonotonicities in input–output functions observed at high intensities in responses to single auditory nerve fibers (Kiang & Moxon, 1972; McGee, Walsh, & Javel, 1981).

Summary

All aspects of auditory EPs in kittens show marked evidence of maturation with age. Part of the maturational sequence, in particular the events occurring during the first 3 postnatal weeks, can be accounted for by improvements in mechanical transmission through the external and middle ears and by morphologic development of the basilar membrane and organ of Corti. These are not the only contributing factors, however. CNS maturation, as evidenced by myelination of CNS axons and improvements in EP thresholds and wave latencies at constant sensation levels, is also involved. Improvements in EP thresholds and wave latencies with advancing age are described

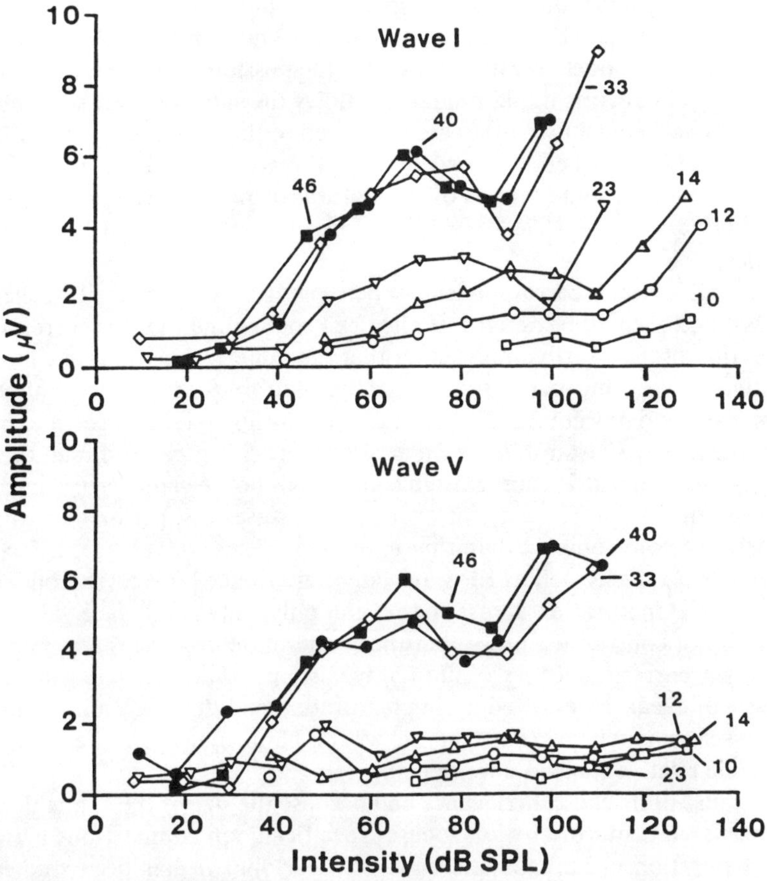

Figure 17. Plots of mean ABR wave I and V amplitude as a function of intensity at several postnatal ages in kittens.

well by a two-stage model. The earlier stage is roughly linear and, in cats, ends during the third postnatal week. The later stage follows a decaying exponential function and ends during the third postnatal month. All ABR waves mature at approximately the same rate, except during the early postnatal period, and maturation of AER waves is slower.

COMPARATIVE ANALYSES OF ABR MATURATION

Introduction

The preceding discussion has centered on EP maturation in developing kittens. We have seen that EPs are first elicited in response to high-intensity stimuli toward the end of the first postnatal week, that their thresholds, wave latencies, and wave amplitudes all improve as the animal approaches functional maturity, and that the time course of EP maturation is described well by a two-stage model. We have suggested the possibility that EP maturation in other animals, including humans, follows the same general sequence of events. The following analyses are addressed to this question. In particular, we want to know whether knowledge of EP maturation in cats might allow the prediction of some aspects of EP maturation in humans and whether we can derive a "generalized" function for EP maturation in mammalian species.

Even if certain correspondences between EP maturational sequences across species could be derived, it must be kept in mind that the correspondences do not necessarily imply either that the same events occur at the same relative times during maturation or that the auditory pathways are similar anatomically and physiologically. For example, owing to larger head and brain size, the average distance between auditory nuclei is greater in man than in cats. Also, some differences exist in connections between nuclei and intrinsic makeup of nuclei. The cat, for example, possesses a superior olive that is somewhat more complex than that in humans. These differences affect EP waveform shape as well as EP wave latencies. Hence, any correspondences between EP maturation across species can only be taken at face value, and they do not constitute a proof that the species develop in the same manner. What the correspondences would imply is simply that the same general sequence of events is followed during maturation and that the examination of one species might provide insight into what is happening in another species at the same relative stage in development.

Because of its clinical relevance and because the size of the available data base is largest, our discussion focuses specifically on comparisons between EP maturation in humans and cats. EP development has been studied in other animals, of course, but when the data on EPs are combined with the data on anatomic development, maturation of cochlear potentials, single-cell responses, etc., there is little doubt that the information available for cats and humans is much more extensive then the information available for other species. Also, since ABRs form a substantial amount of the data base on physiological development of hearing in human infants and since ABRs are relatively insensitive to contamination by artifacts, we will limit the following discussion to the analysis of these EPs.

ABR Measures in Newborns

An orientation to the maturation of ABRs in cats and humans is given in Figure 18, which shows average data on the maturation of the latencies of ABR wave I and wave V (or its homologue) in response to clicks as a function of age in humans and cats. The human data were taken at 55–65 dB nHL

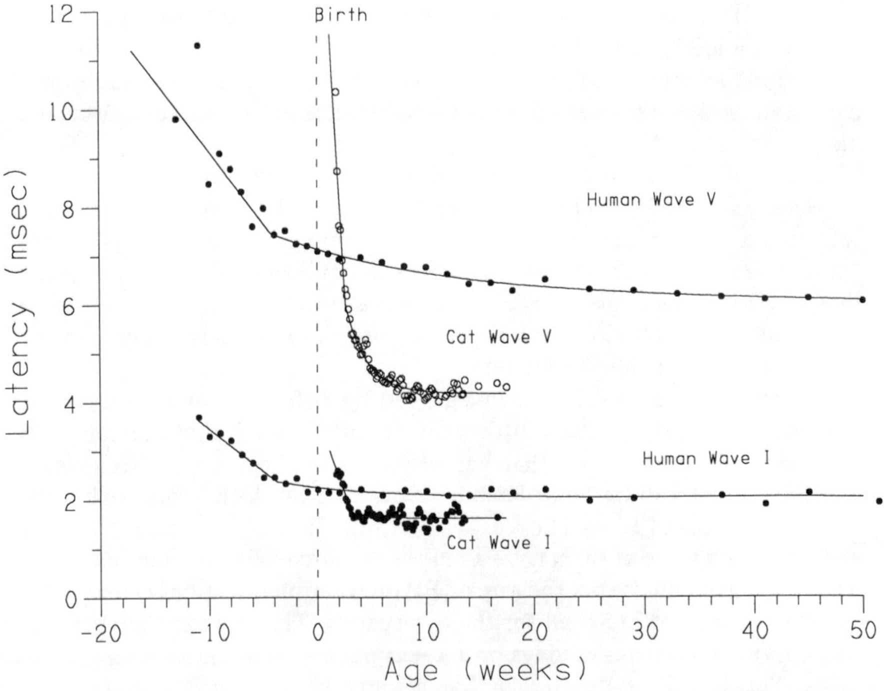

Figure 18. Maturation of ABR wave I and V latency in cats and humans.

(normal hearing level, that is, relative to average adult behavioral thresholds for clicks). The data represent a weighted and corrected average of findings by Hecox (1975), Schulman-Galambos and Galambos (1975), Salamy and McKean (1976), Starr et al. (1977), Goldstein, Krumholz, Felix, Shannon, and Carr (1979), Harris, Mollerstrom, Reimer, and Grennert (1981), Cox, Hack, and Metz (1981), Jacobson, Morehouse, and Johnson (1982), Fawer and Dubowitz (1982), and Teas, Klein, and Kramer (1982). Although data from yet more studies are available, we have included only the ones listed, because they were performed using similar stimulus intensities and similar electrode configurations, namely, an active electrode at the vertex and a reference electrode at the mastoid or earlobe.

Variations in asymptotic ABR wave latencies existed across the human studies. These may have arisen from one or more of a number of sources, among which are acoustic delays resulting from different earphone positions, differences in click polarity, electrical delays in the equipment, the application or nonapplication of corrections, and differences in reference intensities. To compensate for these variations, we applied correction factors to the data from some studies in order to bring wave latencies into registration at functional adulthood. The exact value used for any one study was computed from the asymptotic value obtained for wave I latency and that value was added to or subtracted from all of the data from that study. The correction factors ranged from −0.6 ms to +0.5 ms. Because the addition of a constant to the data does not affect standard deviations, these were carried along without correction.

Data from all of the studies involving humans were tabulated on a week-by-week basis, and *M*s and *SD*s were computed. These were appropriately weighted to take into account differences in sample sizes across studies. The cat data are our own, sampled at 60-dB peak-equivalent SPL. Although this intensity is too low to provide accurate estimates of wave latencies during the early maturational period, it was used because it most closely matches the intensities used in the human studies.

The data in Figure 18 reveal some interesting differences and some equally interesting similarities. The most prominent difference is that human ABRs mature considerably slower than cat ABRs. While the human ABR requires at least a year to attain adult latency values, the cat ABR is approximately mature in 2 months' time. The reasons for the difference in maturational rate are many, and some of them have already been discussed. A potentially noteworthy observation is that the rate of EP maturation might be related to the gestation period or life span for the two species. The average time between conception and birth is 63 days or 9 weeks in cats, and it is 39 weeks in humans. This is a somewhat larger than a fourfold difference. Cats typically live for 12 to 15 years and humans live for 65 to 70 years, which is again a factor of 4 or 5.

A second difference between ABR data from cats and humans is that EP responses from cats can be obtained only after birth, but EP responses from humans can be obtained prior to birth. This relates to differences in sensory system development at birth discussed previously. Curiously, the time at which birth occurs has no apparent effect on EP development. Thus, the transition during birth from a fluid-filled intrauterine environment to a self-sustaining extrauterine environment does not influence EP development in any obvious manner.

Finally, equivalent ABR waves from cats and humans possess different asymptotic or final values. ABR wave V in cats, for example, has an adult latency of about 4.1 ms, while wave V in humans has a longer latency. This discrepancy comes about partly as a result of differences in the lengths of brainstem fiber pathways, and it may also be due to differences in fiber diameters.

The data in Figure 18 were fitted according to the two-stage, linear-exponential model presented earlier, with the breakpoints between the linear and exponential segments taken to be 2.6 weeks of age (or 11.6 weeks postconceptional age) for cats and −4 weeks of age (or 35 weeks postconceptional age) for humans. These breakpoints were computed on the basis of providing the lowest sums of squares of deviations between the predicted and the observed data. The fitted curves are also shown in Figure 18. The linear-exponential model appears to describe the human data as well as it describes the data from cats, and the acceptability of the fits allows us to perform further analyses.

Complete data sets for maturation of ABR waves I and V latencies and the wave I–V time interval in cats and humans are shown in Figure 19, this time expressed as a function of postconceptional age. Also provided are the standard deviations of the data, except for the human I–V time interval, which has no indications of standard deviations, because not all of the studies that contributed findings to this graph provided these measurements. Also shown in Figure 19 are the best-fitting curves according to the linear-exponential model described earlier. The average time of birth is indicated by the vertical dashed line. Again, although the devlopmental stage at the time of birth is vastly different in the two species, the ABR data possess essentially the same features. Since the gestation periods and final values are different, however, the parameters of the best-fitting curves differ.

The wave I–V time interval, commonly called the central conduction time (CCT), provides information on neural transmission in the lower brainstem. In simple terms, it can be thought of as the amount of time it takes for a neural impulse to travel from the auditory nerve to the inferior colliculus. As such, the CCT is a measure derived solely from the CNS. In its mature form, the CCT has no aspects that depend on mechanical or neural transduction of sound. The CCT data in Figure 19 indicate that, even though the asymptotic values differ (2.5 ms for cats, 3.8 ms for humans), the maturation of neural transmission times in the CNS of humans resembles that in cats.

Normalizations

The raw data on ABR wave latencies and interpeak time intervals in cats and humans (Figs. 18 and 19) are too different to compare directly. We can normalize them, however, to take into account differences in maturational rate and asymptotic latency values between the two species. One way to do this is simply to express wave latency or interwave interval as a percentage of the adult value and to express age as a percentage of the average length of gestation. This has been done in Figure 20. Birth, of course, occurs at 100% gestation, and the asymptotic latency or interwave interval is 100% of the adult value. Plotting the data this way makes cross-species differences smaller. There is an indication that expressing postconceptional or postnatal age in terms of gestation length brings the relative time course of human maturation into good registration with the time course of cat maturation. Also, this normalization improves relationships between the ranges of latency and interwave interval values obtained during maturation. Since the normalized data

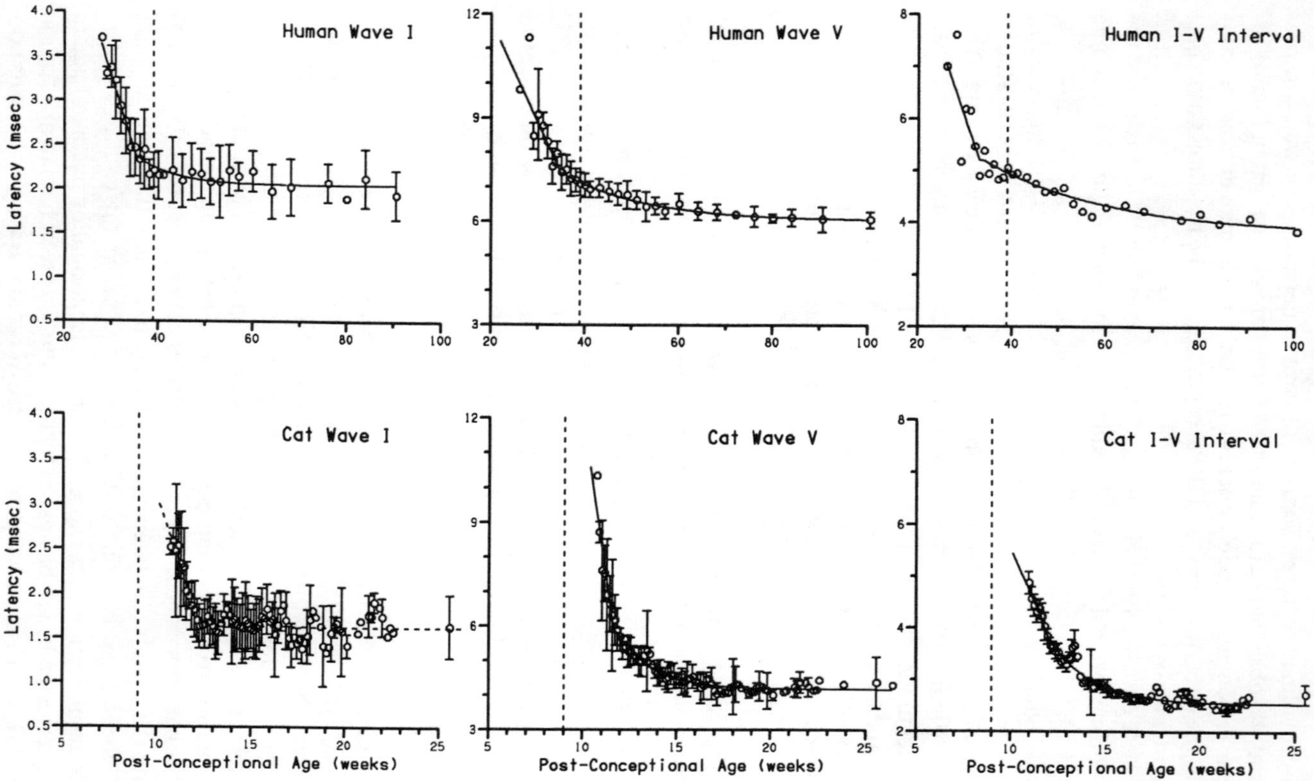

Figure 19. Latency of ABR waves I and V and the wave I–V time interval in humans and cats as a function of age following conception. Bars indicate +/− 1 *SD*. Data from humans were taken from several studies and were adjusted so that final latency values were similar (see text).

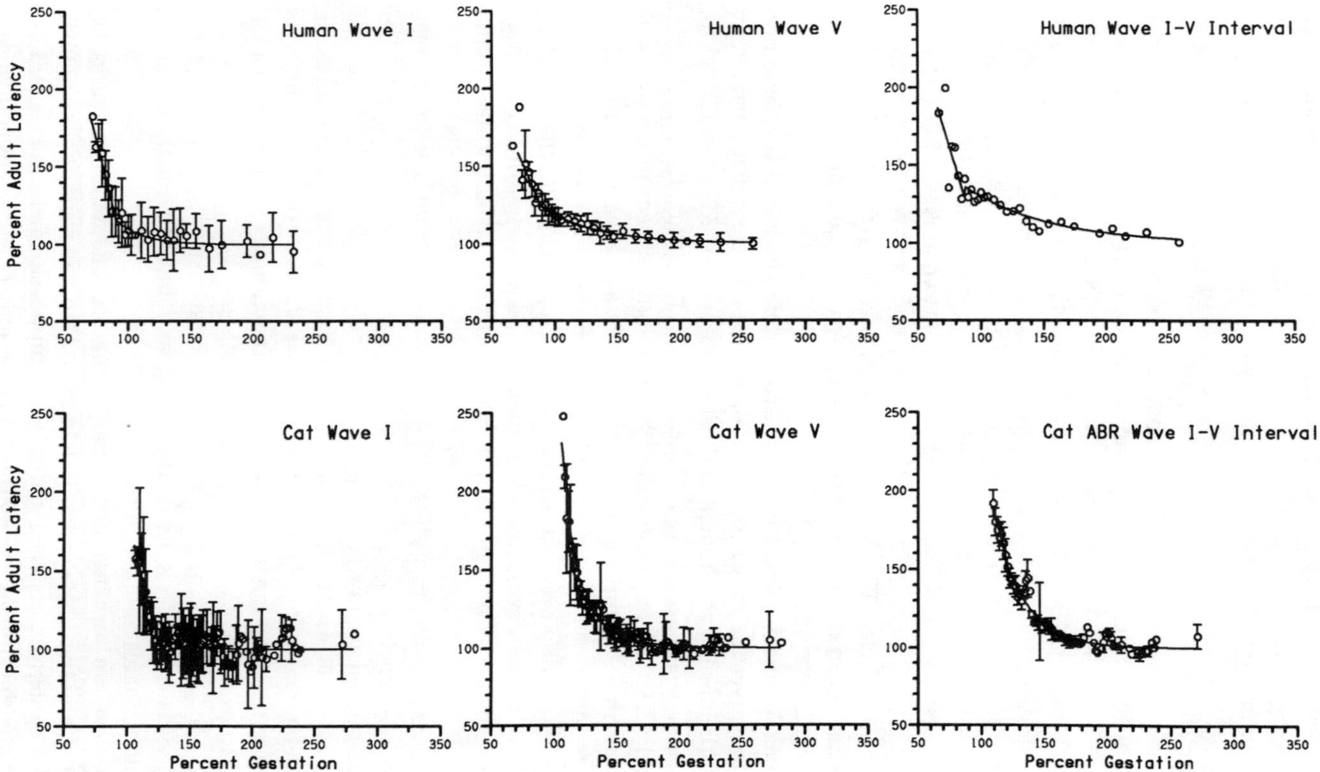

Figure 20. Maturation of ABR waves I and V and the wave I–V time interval in cats and humans. Age is expressed in terms of gestational duration, and latencies are expressed as percentages of adult values.

behave in very nearly the same way, we can accept the normalization procedure as being adequate, and we can make a preliminary statement that the relative maturation of human ABRs closely resembles the maturation of cat ABRs.

We are left with one minor problem, however,. The problem is that the breakpoints between the linear and exponential segments of the fitted curves occur at different times relative to birth. The final step, then, in completing this analysis is to introduce a correction factor that slides one set of data horizontally, bringing it into registration with the other. The easiest way to do this is simply to assume that the breakpoints between the linear and exponential segments represent functionally equivalent stages of development. Lining up the data this way produces the plots of normalized ABR wave I and wave V latency and the wave I–V time interval shown in Figure 21. The average human data are shown as filled circles, and the average cat data are shown as open circles. The x-axis annotations have been removed because the cat data have been shifted to the left; hence, there is no common set of annotations for the two species.

Product–moment correlation coefficients were computed for these normalizations over the range for which data were collected. The correlations between the normalized human and cat data were .998 for wave I, .973 for wave V, and .893 for the wave I–V time interval. It appears, then, that developmental ABR data from cats can be brought into excellent registraton with those from humans simply by normalizing the data relative to gestational duration, asymptotic latency, and the linear-exponential breakpoints. The acceptable correlation between the human and cat data implies that the auditory system of the developing cat is indeed a good model for the auditory system of the developing human, at least up to and including the inferior colliculus.

The preceding analysis allows us to construct a "map" or linear relationship between functionally equivalent stages in humans and cats. For postconceptional age in weeks, the equation is $C = 9/39\,H + 35/11.6$, or $C = 0.231\,H + 3.02$ where C represents the equivalent postconceptional age in cats for a human age of H postconceptional weeks. For example, a human at birth (39 postconceptional weeks) would be functionally equivalent to a kitten at 12 postconceptional (or 3 weeks postnatal) weeks. Notice that the slope, 9/39 or .231, is simply the ratio of the gestation periods and that the intercept, 35/11.6 or 3.02, is the ratio of the breakpoints between the linear and exponential phases of maturation.

Cats, then, are born in a functionally immature state, but they mature between four and five times faster than humans. More importantly, an equivalence can be derived between auditory system development in cats and humans at any time during the maturational period. Whether this equivalence extends to other sensory systems or even to higher levels of the auditory sys-

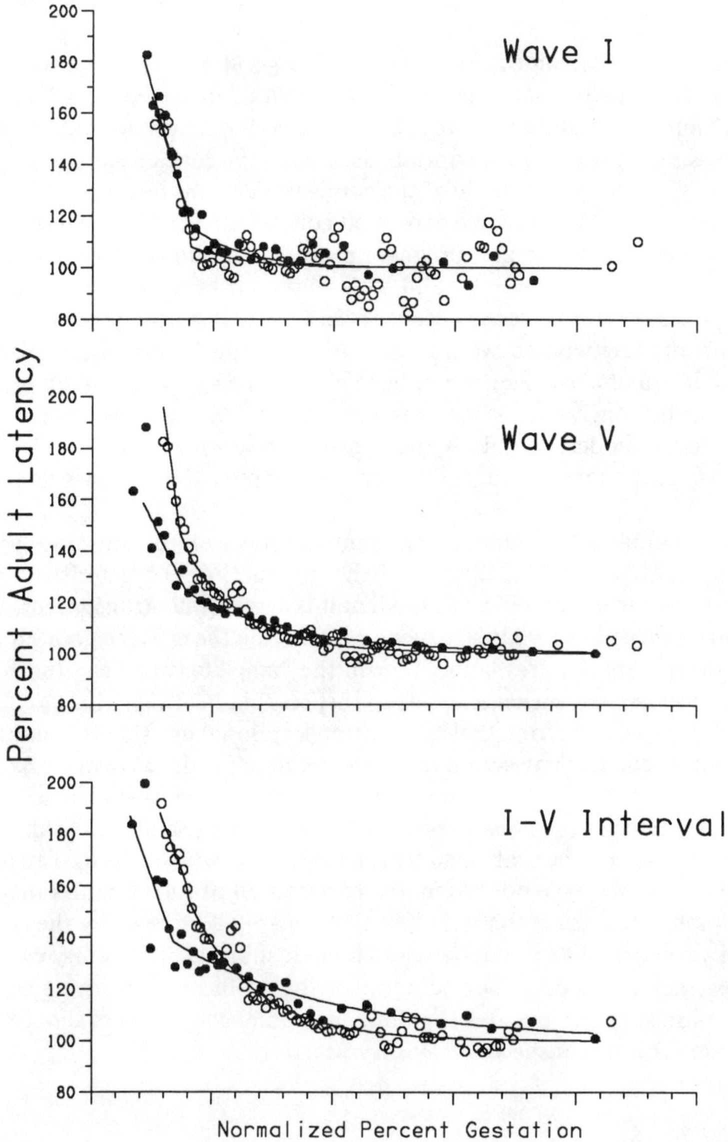

Figure 21. Fully normalized data for maturation of ABR wave I and V latency and ABR wave I–V time interval in cats and humans. Data from cats have been shifted to the left, with the data lining up at the breakpoints between the linear and exponential segments (see text).

tem cannot be determined, of course, but the good quality of the fit between cat and human ABR data suggests that certain unanswered questions about human auditory function during the early developmental period can be addressed simply by using appropriate data from the cat as a substitute.

Here is one simple example of the application of this technique: Recently, scientists and physicians have expressed concern that the hearing of unborn infants might be damaged if pregnant mothers are allowed to work in noisy environments. Is this concern valid, or is it unimportant? It is very difficult to address this question directly because even after disregarding the ethics of the experiment, few women would consent to having hydrophones placed in their uterus and allowing their unborn child to be exposed to high-intensity noise. In addition, acoustic measurements from other animals—and the classic obstetric model for this is the pregnant ewe—may not be relevant to humans, and the equipment needed to perform these measurements is expensive.

We can apply knowledge gained from kittens to address this question. To simplify matters, we will disregard the attenuation characteristics of the womb (itself an issue) and presume that it is acoustically transparent, which is probably true at very low frequencies. Merging the existing data on kitten ABR thresholds (Figures 4 and 5) with the "map" between cat and human maturation derived earlier leads us to suspect that hearing in human fetuses should be so poor before 35 weeks postconceptional age that it is unlikely a fetus will encounter any sound intense enough to produce cochlear damage. After this age, however, the unborn babies should be able to hear intense sounds, at which time noise exposure might be a hazard to be avoided.

We have been rather glib in addressing this issue, which is indeed an important one, and we have not attempted to assess all of the variables involved. The point, however, is that this question is easily addressed by the cat data and is very difficult to address using human subjects. The utility of simple models like the one described here for solving problems concerning auditory maturation supports the idea that human–animal equivalences should be investigated for other aspects of sensory function.

Summary

EPs in cats appear later in development than EPs in humans, but cat EPs mature faster. Linear–exponential fits to human EP data indicate that human EPs develop in much the same manner as cat EPs. EP data from cats can be compared directly with those from humans by performing a normalization that takes into account differences in gestation length and asymptotic wave latencies, and by lining up one set of curves with the other at the breakpoint between the early, fast-maturing segment and the late, slowly maturing segment. This process brings the data on the maturation of the cat wave I, wave V, and wave I–V time interval into excellent registration with those from the human. The normalized data indicate that the cat can be considered to be a good model for auditory EP development in man, at least to upper brainstem levels.

REFERENCES

Achor, L.J., & Starr, A. (1980) Auditory brain stem responses in the cat. II. Effects of lesion. *Electroencephalography and Clinical Neurophysiology, 48,* 174–190.

Black, R.C., Clark, G.M., O'Leary, S.J., & Walters, C. (1983). Intracochlear electrical stimulation of normal and deaf cats investigated using brainstem response audiometry. *Acta Otolaryngologica (Stockholm), Suppl., 399,* 5–17.

Bredberg, G. (1968). Cellular pattern and nerve supply of the human organ of Corti. *Acta Otolaryngologica (Stockholm), Suppl., 236,* 1–135.

Brugge, J.F., Javel, E., & Kitzes, L.M. (1978). Signs of functional maturation of peripheral auditory system in discharge patterns of neurons in anteroventral cochlear nucleus of kittens. *Journal of Neurophysiology, 41,* 1557–1579.

Brugge, J.F., Kitzes, L.M., & Javel, E. (1981). Postnatal development of frequency and intensity sensitivity of neurons in the anteroventral cochlear nucleus of kittens. *Hearing Research, 5,* 217–229.

Buchwald, J.S., & Huang, C.M. (1975). Far-field acoustic response: Origins in the cat. *Science, 189,* 382–384.

Carlier, E., Lenoir, M., & Pujol, R. (1979). Development of cochlear frequency selectivity tested by compound action potential tuning curve. *Hearing Research, 1,* 197–201.

Cox, L., Hack, M., & Metz, D. (1981). Brainstem-evoked response audiometry: Normative data from the preterm infant. *Audiology, 20,* 53–64.

Crowley, D.E., & Hepp-Reymond, M.-C. (1966). Development of cochlear function in the ear of the infant rat. *Journal of Comparative and Physiological Psychology, 62,* 427–432.

Davis, H., Davis, P.A., Loomis, A.L., Harvey, E.N., & Hobart, G. (1939). Electrical reactions of the human brain to auditory stimulation during sleep. *Journal of Neurophysiology, 2,* 500–514.

[1] It must be recalled that EP waveform structure depends on the placement of the active and reference electrodes. Most investigators put the active electrode on the midline vertex of the skull and the reference electrode on the ipsilateral mastoid. This is not the only montage that has been used, however, and ABRs obtained at other positions have been reported. In general, active electrode sites along the midline (relative to reference electrode sites that are truly indifferent) tend to emphasize the later EP waves, while positions near the ear tend to emphasize the earlier waves. Also, the position of the reference electrode influences EP waveforms. For example, an active electrode on the vertex usually produces six positive-going ABR waves when the reference electrode is at the mastoid, while a reference site at the nose produces seven waves with slightly different latencies. Furthermore, the numbering system used to describe ABR waves can vary from study to study, depending on an investigator's willingness to attach significance to certain waves. For example, Shipley, Buchwald, Normans, and Guthrie (1980) described one wave with two components (waves IIa and IIb) in young kittens, whereas our interpretation is that of two separate waves. Since the reference electrode sites were different in the two studies, we cannot compare the data reliably. The point to remember here is that different electrode positions may produce different ABR waveforms, which in turn can affect interpretations and comparisons of findings.

Eggermont, J.J. (1982). *Physiology of the development auditory system* Paper presented at the Symposium on Auditory Development in Infancy, University of Toronto, Canada.

Ehret, G. (1976). Development of absolute auditory thresholds in the house mouse (mus musculus). *Journal of the American Audiological Society, 1,* 173–184.

Ehret, G., & Romand, R. (1981). Postnatal development of absolute auditory thresholds in kittens. *Journal of Comparative and Physiological Psychology, 95,* 304–311.

Ellingson, R.J., & Wilcott, R.C. (1960). Development of evoked responses in visual and auditory cortices of kittens. *Journal of Neurophysiology, 23,* 363–375.

Fawer, C.-L., & Dubowitz, L.M.S. (1982). Auditory brain stem response in neurologically normal preterm and full-term newborn infants. *Neuropediatrics, 13,* 200–206.

Fernandez, C., & Hinojosa, R. (1974). Postnatal development of endocochlear potential and stria vascularis in the cat. *Acta Otolaryngologica (Stockholm), 78,* 173–186.

Galambos, R., & Hecox, K. (1978). Clinical applications of the auditory brain stem response. *Otolaryngology Clinics of North America, 11,* 708–722.

Gardi, J.N., & Schindler, R.A. (1983). Preoperative and intraoperative evaluation of nerve status. In *Proceedings of the 10th Anniversary Conference on Cochlear Implants: An International Symposium.*

Goldstein, P., Krumholz, A., Felix, J., Shannon, D., & Carr, R. (1979). Brainstem evoked response in neonates. *American Journal of Obstetrics and Gynecology, 135,* 622–628.

Gray, L., & Rubel, E.W. (1981). Development of responsiveness to suprathreshold acoustic stimulation in chickens. *Journal of Comparative and Physiological Psychology, 95,* 188–198.

Grossman, C. (1955). Electro-ontogenesis of cerebral activity. *A.M.A. Archives of Neurology and Psychiatry,* 186–202.

Harris, D.M., & Dallos, P. (1984). Ontogenetic changes in frequency mapping of the mammalian ear. *Science, 225,* 741–743.

Harris, S., Mollerstrom, B., Reimer, A., & Grennert, L. (1981). Auditory brainstem response and gestational age in the newborn. *Scandinavian Audiology Suppl., 13,* 147–148.

Hecox, K. (1975). Electrophysiological correlates of human auditory development. In L.B. Cohen & P. Salapatek (Eds.), *Infant perception: From sensation to cognition* (Vol. 2). New York: Academic Press.

Hecox, K., & Galambos, R. (1974). Brainstem auditory evoked response in human infants and adults. *Archives of Otolaryngology, 99,* 30–33.

Jacobson, J.T., Morehouse, C.R., & Johnson, M.J. (1982). Strategies for infant auditory brain stem response assessment. *Ear and Hearing, 3,* 263–270.

Jewett, D.L., & Romano, M.N. (1972). Neonatal development of auditory system potentials averaged from the scalp of rat and cat, *Brain Research, 36,* 101–115.

Jewett, D.L., & Williston, J.S. (1971). Auditory-evoked far fields averaged from the scalp of humans. *Brain, 94,* 681–696.

Kiang, N.Y.-S., & Moxon, E.C. (1972). Physiological considerations in artificial stimulation of the inner ear. *Annals of Otology, Rhinology and Laryngology, 81,* 714–730.

Larsell, O., McCrady, E., Jr., & Larsell, J.F. (1944). Development of the organ of Corti in relation to the inception of hearing. *Archives of Otolaryngology, 40,* 233–248.

Mair, I.W.S., Elverland, H.H., & Laukli, E. (1978). Development of early auditory evoked responses in the cat. *Audiology, 17,* 468–488.

Marty, R., & Thomas, J. (1963). Response electrocorticale a la stimulation du nerf cochleaire chez le chat nouveau-ne [Electrocortical response after stimulation of the cochlear nerve in the newborn cat]. *Journal de Physiologie (Paris), 55,* 165–166.

McGee, J., Walsh, E.J., & Javel, E. (1981). High-intensity "notches" in responses of auditory nerve fibers. *Journal of the Acoustical Society of America, 69,* S53.

Moller, A.R., Jannetta, P., & Moller, M.B. (1982). Intracranially recorded auditory nerve response in man: New interpretations of BSER. *Archives of Otolaryngology, 108,* 77–82.

Pujol, R. (1972). Development of tone-burst responses along the auditory pathway in the cat. *Acta Otolaryngologica, 74,* 383–391.

Pujol, R., & Hilding, D. (1973). Anatomy and physiology of the onset of auditory function. *Acta Otolaryngologica (Stockholm), 76,* 1–10.

Pujol, R., & Marty, R. (1970). Postnatal maturation in the cochlea of the cat. *Journal of Comparative Neurology, 139,* 115–126.

Relkin, E.M., & Saunders, J.D. (1980). Displacement of the malleus in neonatal golden hamster, *Acta Otolaryngologica (Stockholm), 90,* 6–15.

Retzius, G. (1884). *Das Gehörorgan der Wirbeltiere II: Das Gehörorgan der Reptilien, der Vögel und Säugetiere [The Hearing Organ of Vertebrates II: The Hearing Organ of Reptiles, Birds and Mammals].* Stockholm: Samson & Wallin.

Romand, R. (1971). Maturation des potentiels cochleaires dans la periode perinatale chez le chat et chez le cobaye [Maturation of cochlear potentials during the perinatal period in the cat and the guinea pig]. *Journal de Physiologie. (Paris), 63,* 763–782.

Romand, R. (1979). Development of auditory nerve activity in kittens. *Brain Research, 173,* 554–556.

Romand, R., & Romand, M.-R. (1982). Myelination kinetics of spiral ganglion cells. *Journal of Comparative Neurology, 204,* 1–5.

Romand, R., Sans, A., Romand, M.R., & Marty, R. (1976). The structural maturation of the stato-acoustic nerve in the cat. *Journal of Comparative Neurology, 170,* 1–16.

Rose, J.E., Adrian, H., & Santibanez, G. (1957). Electrical signs of maturation in the auditory system of the kitten. *Acta Neurologica Latinoamerica, 3,* 133–137.

Rubel, E.W. (1978). Ontogeny of structure and function in the vertebrate auditory system. In M. Jacobsen (Ed.), *Handbook of sensory physiology, Vol. IX: Development of sensory systems.* New York: Springer-Verlag.

Rubel, E.W. (1984). Ontogeny of auditory system function. *Annual Review of Physiology, 46,* 213–229.

Rubel, E.W., & Ryals, B. (1983). Development of the place principle: Acoustic trauma, *Science, 219,* 512–514.

Salamy, A., & McKean, C.M. (1976). Postnatal development of human brainstem potentials during the first year of life. *Electroencephalography and Clinical Neurophysiology, 40,* 418–426.

Schulman-Galambos, C., & Galambos, R. (1975). Brainstem auditory evoked responses in premature infants. *Journal of Speech and Hearing Research, 18,* 456–465.

Shipley, C., Buchwald, J.S., Norman, R., & Guthrie, D. (1980). Brain stem auditory evoked response development in the kitten. *Brain Research, 182,* 313–326.

Sohmer, H., & Feinmesser, M. (1967). Cochlear action potentials recorded from the external ear in man. *Annals of Otology, Rhinology and Laryngology, 76,* 427–436.

Starr, A. (1976). Auditory brainstem responses in brain death. *Brain, 99,* 543–554.

Starr, A., Amlie, R., Martin, W., & Sanders, S. (1977). Development of auditory function in newborn infants revealed by auditory brainstem potentials. *Pediatrics, 60,* 831–839.

Starr, A., & Farley, G.R. (1983). Middle- and long-latency auditory evoked potentials in cat. II. Component distribution and dependence on stimulus factors. *Hearing Research, 10,* 139–152.

Starr, A., & Hamilton, A. (1976). Correlation between confirmed sites of neurological lesions and far-field auditory brainstem responses. *Electroencephalography and Clinical Neurophysiology, 41,* 595–608.

Stockard, J.E., & Westmoreland, B.F. (1981). Technical considerations in the recording and interpretation of the brainstem auditory evoked potential for neonatal neurologic diagnosis. *American Journal of EEG Technology, 21,* 31–54.

Teas, D.C., Klein, A., & Kramer, S. (1982). An analysis of auditory brainstem responses in infants. *Hearing Research, 7,* 19–54.

Walsh, E.J. (1983). *Development of Auditory Evoked Potentials in Kittens: A Parametric Analysis.* Ph.D. dissertation, Creighton University, Omaha, Nebraska.

Walsh, E.J., McGee, J., & Javel, E. (1982). Development of auditory nerve fiber responses in kittens. *Neuroscience Abstracts, 8,* 94.

Walsh, E.J., McGee, J., & Javel, E. (1983). External ear effects during early development in the kitten. *Journal of the Acoustical Society of America, 73,* S61.

Walsh, E.J., McGee, J., & Javel, E. (1986a). Development of auditory evoked potentials in the cat. I. Onset of response and development of sensitivity. *Journal of the Acoustical Society of America, 79,* 712–724.

Walsh, E.J., McGee, J., & Javel, E. (1986b). Development of auditory evoked potentials in the cat. II. Wave latencies. *Journal of the Acoustical Society of America, 79,* 725–744.

Walsh, E.J., McGee, J., & Javel, E. (1986c). Development of auditory evoked potentials in the cat. III. Wave amplitudes. *Journal of the Acoustical Society of America, 79,* 745–754.

Walsh, E.J., McGee, J., Wagahoff, D., & Scott, V. (1985). Myelination of auditory nerve, trapezoidal, and brachium of the inferior colliculus axons in the cat. *Abstracts of the Association for Research in Otolaryngology, 8,* 28–29.

Waring, M.D., Don, M., & Brimacombe, J.A. (1983). ABR assessment of stimulation in induction coil implant patients. In *Proceedings of the 10th Anniversary Conference on Cochlear Implants: An International Symposium.*

Yakovlev, P.I., & Lecours, A.R. (1967). The myelogenetic cycles of regional maturation of the brain. In A. Minkowski (Ed.), *Regional development of the brain in early life.* Oxford, England: Blackwell.

7 Development of the Place Principle*

William R. Lippe
Department of Otorhinolaryngology
University of Oklahoma Health Sciences Center

Brenda M. Ryals
Audiology and Speech Pathology Service
Veterans Administration Medical Center
Richmond, Virginia

Edwin W Rubel
Departments of Otolaryngology and Physiology
University of Virginia Medical Center

> Another way of dealing with errors is to have friends who are willing to spend the time necessary to carry out a critical examination of the experimental design beforehand and the results after the experiments have been completed. An even better way is to have an enemy. An enemy is willing to devote a vast amount of time and brain power to ferreting out errors both large and small, and this without any compensation. The trouble is that really capable enemies are scarce; most of them are only ordinary. Another trouble with enemies is that they sometimes develop into friends and lose a good deal of their zeal. It was in this way that the writer lost his three best enemies. (Georg von Békésy, 1960, pp. 8–9)

INTRODUCTION

The place principle is one of the cornerstones of modern auditory science. This principle, first demonstrated in the classic studies of Georg von Békésy, states that each position along the basilar membrane is most sensitive to a particular frequency of sound. von Békésy showed that sound stimulation causes a traveling wave of motion along the basilar membrane and that the location of maximum vibration varies systematically as a function of sound frequency. High-frequency sounds cause a maximum deflection at the base, while lower frequencies are represented progressively toward the apex (von

* We express our appreciation to Bill Engling and Joan Schnute for assistance in the preparation of the figures and to Lore Steury for typing the manuscript. The preparation of this manuscript was supported by NIH grant NS20724 to W.R. Lippe.

Send correspondence to: Dr. William Lippe, Department of Otorhinolaryngology, University of Oklahoma Health Sciences Center, P.O. Box 26307, Oklahoma City, OK 73126.

Békésy, 1960).[1] The functional importance of the cochlear frequency map is seen best in pathologies and experimental studies where damage at a particular location along the cochlear partition results in a hearing loss that is selective for the frequencies normally represented at the damaged region (Schuknecht, 1953, 1974).

The spatial representation of frequency which originates at the cochlea is preserved within the central nervous system. Electrophysiological studies have shown that each auditory neuron is most sensitive to a particular tone, its best or characteristic frequency. At each level of the auditory pathway, from the cochlear nucleus to the auditory cortex, neurons are arranged into orderly tonotopic maps according to their characteristic frequencies (Rose, Galambos, & Hughes, 1959; Rose, Greenwood, Goldberg, & Hind, 1963; Tsuchitani & Boudreau, 1966; Goldberg & Brown, 1968; Aitkin, Anderson, & Brugge, 1970; Aitkin & Webster, 1971; Reale & Imig, 1980).

Ever since the pioneering observations of von Békésy, it has been implicitly assumed that the relationship between sound frequency and position along the cochlear partition is fixed and immutable. Although it has sometimes been suggested that this relationship might change or be altered (Ades, Trahiotis, Kokko-Cunningham, & Averbuch, 1974; Hecox, 1975), the concept of a fixed place code has never been seriously questioned. However, recent evidence that the relationship between frequency and place along the cochlea changes during the course of normal development now appears to challenge this assumption (Lippe & Rubel, 1983, 1985; Rubel & Ryals, 1983; Ryals & Rubel, 1985). In the present chapter we would like to describe the evidence for an ontogenetic shift in the place code. First, the history of the place principle will be summarized briefly. Then the observations which led to the idea of a shifting place code and the experimental studies that support this hypothesis will be described. The focus will be mainly on studies in the avian auditory system where this idea was first tested, although recent observations from mammals will be described as well. Finally, we will speculate about some of the implications which a changing place code might have for auditory system development and audition in general.

HISTORY OF THE PLACE PRINCIPLE[2]

The idea that sounds of different frequencies are separated and represented spatially in the ear can be traced back to the very early history of auditory sci-

[1] Recent studies suggest that hair cell stereocilia as well as basilar membrane mechanics may contribute to frequency representation along the cochlear partition (Holton & Hudspeth, 1983; Tilney, Saunders, Egelman, & De Rosier, 1982; Tilney, Egelman, De Rosier, & Saunders, 1983; Tilney & Saunders, 1983; Strelioff & Flock, 1984).

[2] The descriptions of the early history of auditory theory and Helmholtz's resonance theory of hearing have been summarized from the excellent reviews of Bast and Anson (1949), Wever (1949), Boring (1942), Carterette (1978), and Schubert (1978).

ence. Early theories of hearing proposed that a spatial analysis of sound frequency occurred by the mechanism of resonance, most likely because the phenomenon of resonance was well known from work with musical instruments and from observations of how sound behaves in auditoriums and closed cavities. However, these theories were largely speculative and had little basis in either anatomical or physiological fact. Although the gross anatomy of the external and middle ears and the existence of the cochlea and eighth nerve had been described by 1600, the detailed anatomy of the inner ear was not known. Progress was also hindered, because the Aristotelian concept of "aer implantus"—the idea that hearing results from the vibration of air permanently "implanted" or confined to the inner ear and other cavities of the temporal bone—dominated thinking until 1789, when the discovery that the inner ear is fluid filled was finally accepted.

Bauhin's (1605) resonance theory is typical of these early ideas. He proposed that the different air-filled cavities and passages of the ear resonate selectively to sounds of different frequency, the larger cavities vibrating to low frequencies and the smaller, narrower spaces and channels responding to higher frequencies. Du Verney's (1683) ideas are somewhat more modern in form. He believed that the cochlea, the vestibule, and the semicircular canals were the organs of hearing. His published drawings were the first that showed the cochlea being divided into two longitudinal channels by the bony spiral lamina and the basilar membrane (Fig. 1). Because he believed that the eighth nerve innervated the spiral lamina, he considered it, rather than the basilar membrane, to be the receptive structure. He noted that the width of the lamina decreased from its basal to apical ends and proposed that the wide basal end vibrates selectively to low-frequency sounds while the narrower, more

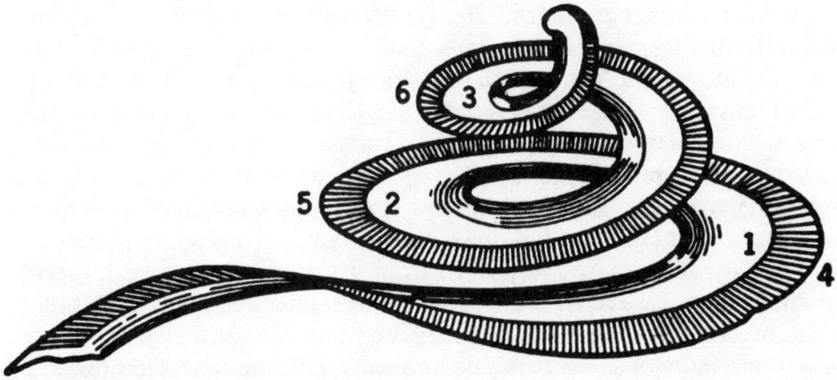

Figure 1. Du Verney's drawing of the spiral organ of Corti. The region of the spiral marked 1,2,3 is the bony lamina and the shaded region marked 4,5,6 is the membranous lamina (basilar membrane). This is the first published picture which showed the basilar membrane. (Reproduced from Wever, 1949, Fig. 1, by permission of the publisher.)

apical region responds to higher frequencies. In 1760 Cotugno reversed this order of frequency representation. He proposed that because of its greater elasticity, the basilar membrane, rather than the osseous lamina, responds to sound. Like many of his contemporaries, he pictured the membrane as composed of a series of parallel strings which were graded in length and under tension. Because Cotugno knew that the membranous lamina increases in width from base to apex, he located high frequency sounds at its basal end and low frequencies at the apex. This localization of frequencies agrees with modern theory. It is interesting that this early concept of the basilar membrane being composed of a series of tuned, vibrating strings anticipated Helmholtz's resonance theory by about a century.

Helmholtz first proposed his classic resonance theory of hearing in 1863. It was the first theory which was based upon anatomical and physiological fact and was widely accepted and dominated thinking for the next 80 years. Historians of science have emphasized that the success of the resonance theory is largely attributable to Helmholtz's genius in being able to draw together three bodies of previously unrelated information (Boring, 1942; Wever, 1949). First, the perfection of the compound microscope in 1830 led to a much greater understanding of the microscopic anatomy of the cochlea. Helmholtz was the beneficiary of Corti's (1851) classic studies which revealed the existence of the rods of Corti, the tectorial membrane, the tunnel of Corti, and the outer hair cells. Deiters (1860) described the inner hair cells and their supporting cells, and Reissner (1854), Claudius (1856), and Hensen (1863) identified the various structures and supporting cells of the cochlear partition which now bear their names. These studies provided Helmholtz with a much more modern picture of cochlear anatomy than had been available previously. Second, he drew upon Müller's law of specific nerve energies as a theoretical background. Müller (1838) had proposed that our qualitatively different sensations of vision, sound, etc., arise from excitation of different kinds of nerve fibers. Each nerve can give rise only to its own specific kind of sensation. Helmholtz extended Müller's theory to qualitative differences within a sensory dimension and proposed that each distinguishable pitch results from stimulation of a specific nerve fiber by an attached resonating structure. Third, Helmholtz drew upon Ohm's law of auditory analysis. Fourier (1829) had outlined the theorem that any complex function can be analyzed into, or constructed from, simple sine waves with specific amplitude and phase relationships. Ohm (1843) later applied Fourier's ideas to the functioning of the ear and suggested that the ear analyzes complex sounds into individual frequency components. Helmholtz was impressed by these ideas and believed that a series of mechanically tuned resonators was the only mechanism that could achieve such an analysis.

Helmholtz proposed that the ear consists of a graded series of tiny resonators, each tuned to a different frequency of sound. Corti had shown that the height of the pillar cells increases along the length of the cochlea, from about 0.06 mm at the base to 0.10 mm at the apex. Helmholtz believed that this slight variation in height was adequate for his theory and initially identified the pillars of Corti as the resonators. However, he later changed his thinking because of Hasse's (1867) finding that pillar cells are not present in birds and amphibians and the observation of Hensen (1863) that the basilar membrane increases in width by about twelvefold from base to apex. In later versions of the theory, Helmholtz identified the transverse fibers of the basilar membrane as the resonators.

Although Helmholtz's ideas were well received for about a decade, critics soon pointed out that many of the physical requirements of the resonance theory were inconsistent with the anatomy of the cochlea. It was noted that the transverse fibers could not vibrate as independent resonators, because they were embedded in a membranous structure. In addition, the damping of basilar membrane motion by the cochlear fluids would cause the resonating fibers to be very poorly tuned. Finally, some critics tried to show with physical models that stimulation of the basilar membrane would cause a standing wave pattern of vibration rather than a single point of resonance.

Several alternative theories of hearing were proposed between the late 1800s and the early 20th century (see Wever, 1949, for an excellent review of these theories). Some of these were only minor modifications of Helmholtz's resonance principle; they retained the notion of a place coding of sound frequency by resonance but differed in the identity of the resonators. Others retained the idea of place coding of frequency but proposed mechanisms other than resonance. The more extreme critics rejected the principle of place coding altogether and suggested that sound frequency is coded in the temporal discharge of the eighth nerve.

It is against this background that Georg von Békésy began his elegant and now-classic studies of hearing and basilar membrane mechanics. His studies were carried out between 1924 and 1958 and have been presented in collected form (von Békésy, 1960). It is a tribute to von Békésy's creative genius and insightful thinking that our present-day understanding of how the basilar membrane responds to sound is, in large part, based upon studies which were conducted by him without the aid of computers, laser interferometry, capacitive probes, Mössbauer analysis, and other modern techniques. He single-handedly invented techniques which ranged from procedures of anatomical dissection to the stroboscopic measurement of small-amplitude membrane vibrations. Von Békésy's achievements are all the more impressive when one realizes that throughout his life he worked alone, without students or collaborators (Davis, 1973).

Von Békésy used temporal bones from human and animal cadavers as well as physical models of the cochlear partition to study basilar membrane mechanics. Human temporal bones were typically prepared by drilling a hole in the apical end of the cochlear capsule under water and sealing the hole with a glass cover. Because the cochlear partition in fresh condition is an almost transparent, gelatinous mass, von Békésy replaced the lymph with a fluid containing finely ground particles of silver, carbon, or other metals. These particles adhered to the cochlear partition. By using a stereomicroscope and stroboscopic illumination, von Békésy was able to visualize the motion of the cochlear partition as well as the movements of the cochlear fluids themselves. In order to directly visualize the motion of the cochlear partition, vibrations must be in the order of magnitude of the wavelength of light. This required von Békésy to use very large amplitude stimuli in his experiments. To accomplish this, he replaced the delicate membranes of the oval and round window with rubber membranes. The vibrations of an electromechanical driver were transmitted to the cochlear fluids by a plunger attached to the artificial oval window membrane.

Von Békésy noted that all the major theories of hearing were consistent with the anatomy of the inner ear and differed only in the assumptions which they made about the mechanical characteristics of the basilar membrane. He demonstrated that the different patterns of vibrations predicted by these theories could all be obtained by simply varying the elastic properites and coupling between the adjacent parts of a rubber model of the basilar membrane (von Békésy, 1956). In order to decide between these alternative theories, von Békésy made measurements of fluid viscosity, cochlear partition stiffness, etc., from freshly preserved human cochleas. He approximated these natural conditions as best he could in a model cochlea and then observed the pattern of vibration that occurred when the model was stimulated with sound. Von Békésy first reported in 1928 that a traveling wave of motion propagated down the model basilar membrane. The traveling wave began at the stiffer end of the model membrane, gradually increased in amplitude as it traveled toward more elastic regions, reached a peak amplitude, and then quickly decreased in size. He then confirmed that a qualitatively similar type of traveling wave occurred along the cochlear partition in preserved human cochleas (Fig. 2).

In subsequent studies, von Békésy examined the properties of the traveling wave and obtained quantitative measures of basilar membrane motion and mechanics from preserved temporal bones. He showed that the position of maximum amplitude of the traveling wave along the cochlear partition varied systematically as a functon of sound frequency; high frequencies caused maximum deflections at the base, while low frequencies were represented progressively more apically (Fig. 3). In 1943–1944, von Békésy published the first quantitative maps of the relationship of sound frequency to place along the cochlea in humans, birds, and various animal species including the rat, mouse, guinea pig, cow, and elephant. Von Békésy also derived the first basilar membrane tuning curves by measuring the amplitude of

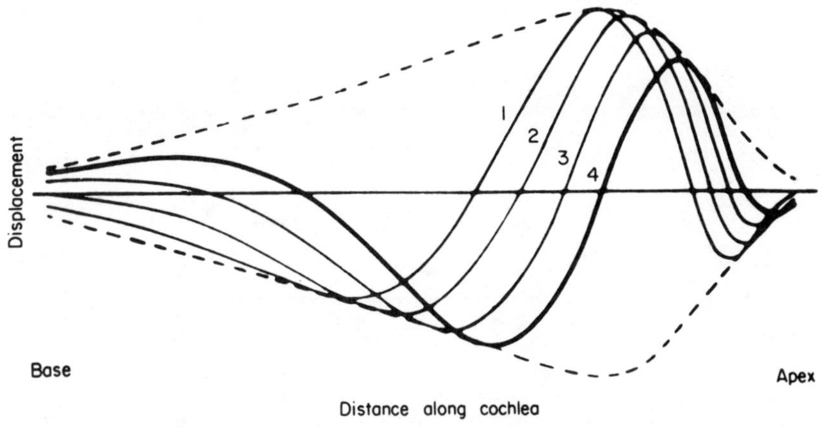

Figure 2. Traveling waves of motion along the human basilar membrane. Von Békésy first observed traveling waves in mechanical models and preserved human temporal bones in 1924. Solid lines show the displacement of the basilar membrane at four successive instants in time. The dashed line indicates the envelope of the traveling waves. 200-Hz stimulus. (Reproduced from Pickles, 1982, Fig. 3.7, based on von Békésy, 1960, Fig. 12–17, by permission of the publisher.)

deflection at the same position on the cochlear partition to different frequency sounds. With the use of fine hairs he measured the elasticity of the different structures of the cochlear partition: Reissner's membrane, the organ of Corti, the tectorial membrane, and the basilar membrane. He found that the elasticity of the basilar membrane decreased a hundredfold from base to apex, whereas the elasticity of the other structures remained relatively constant along the length of the cochlea (Fig. 4). Von Békésy concluded that the gradient of stiffness along the basilar membrane determines the movement of the cochlear partition and the location of maximum vibraton to different frequencies of sound. It is worth emphasizing that the elegance and aesthetic appeal of many of von Békésy's experiments lie in their pure simplicity. An excellent example, and one which von Békésy himself apparently regarded with great pride, was his demonstration that the basilar membrane is not under transverse tension (Davis, 1973). Von Békésy simply made a longitudinal cut along the basilar membrane and observed that the cut edges did not draw apart.

Von Békésy and subsequent investigators recognized several potential problems and limitations of his studies. He had to use nonphysiological levels of stimulation (140 dB SPL) to cause vibrations of the cochlear partition that were large enough to see, almost all his observations were restricted to the apical third or low-frequency end of the cochlea, and most of his studies were carried out on postmortem rather than live specimens. The subsequent development of more sensitive measuring techniques which can be used in live

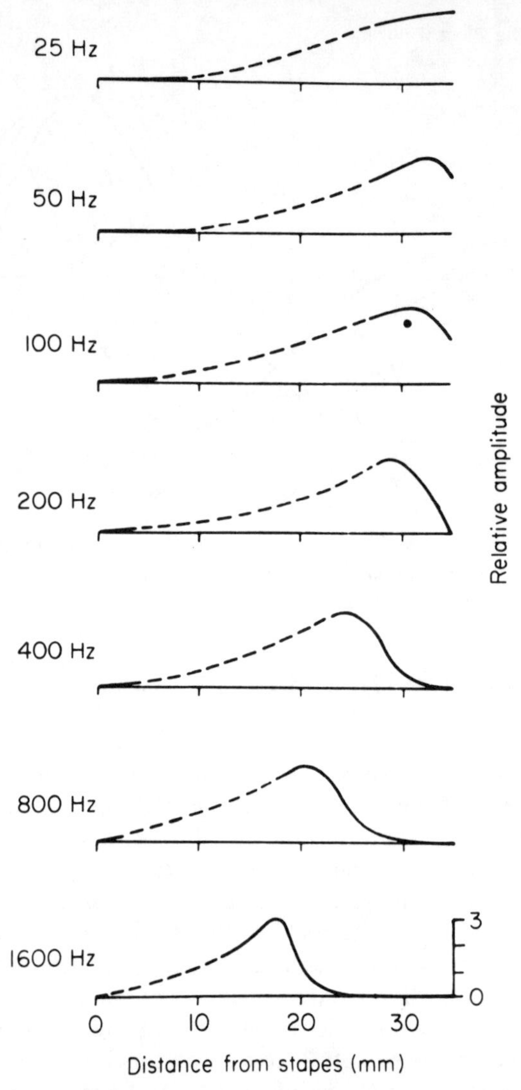

Figure 3. Displacement envelopes of the traveling wave along the cochlear partition to different frequencies. Von Békésy observed that the partition near the helicotrema vibrated with the same amplitude at all frequencies lower than approximately 30 Hz. At successively higher frequencies, the location of maximum deflection shifted progressively toward the base. Each plot was made by measuring the vibration amplitude of the cochlear partition at different distances from the stapes while stimulus frequency and peak stapes displacement were held constant. Different peak-stapes displacements were used for each frequency and therefore only relative amplitude is shown. Von Békésy was able to observe vibrations along the upper 8 mm of the cochlea by making a small hole in the apical end of the cochlear capsule. In order to measure vibrations at more basal locations, he had to cut away progressively more of the cochlea until the lowest turn was visible. The dashed lines indicate measurements which von Békésy considered to be inexact, because the upper end of the partition had been cut away. (Reproduced from von Békésy, 1960, Fig. 11–43, by permission of the publisher.)

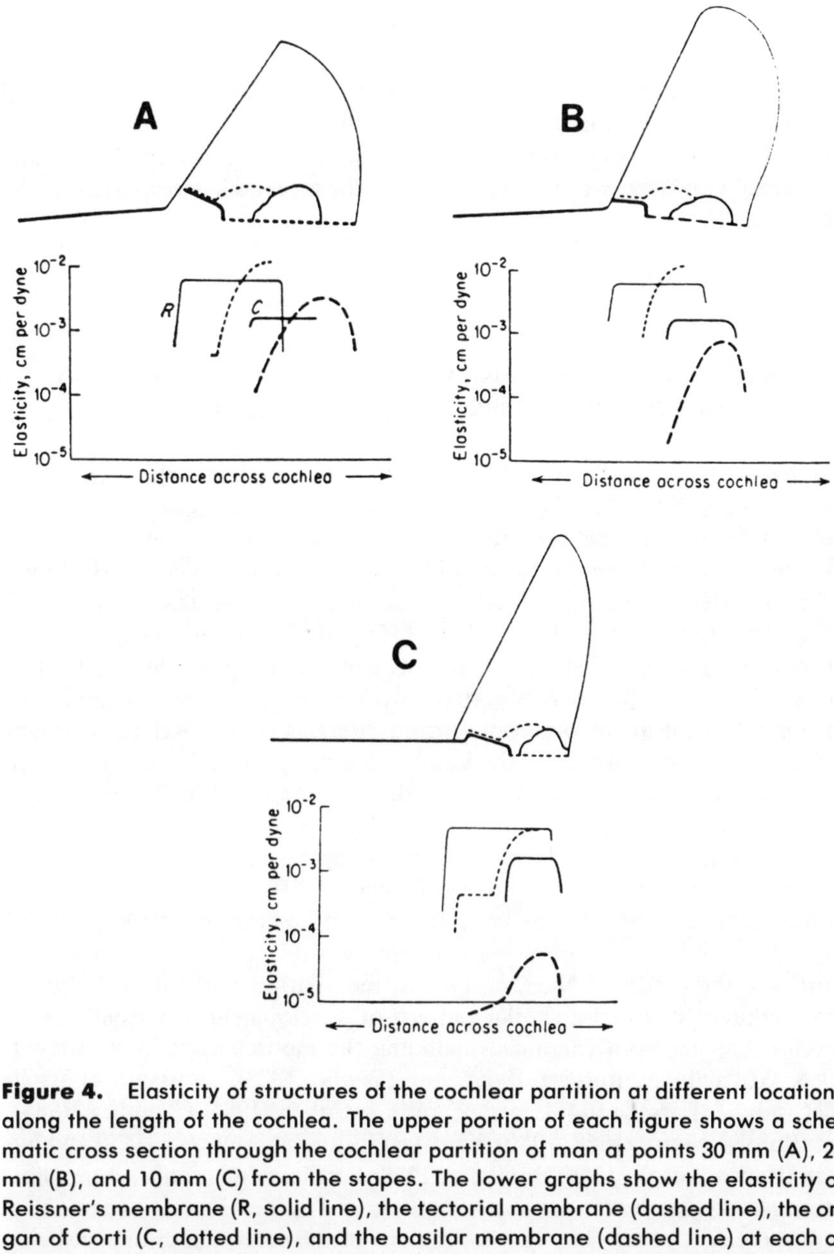

Figure 4. Elasticity of structures of the cochlear partition at different locations along the length of the cochlea. The upper portion of each figure shows a schematic cross section through the cochlear partition of man at points 30 mm (A), 20 mm (B), and 10 mm (C) from the stapes. The lower graphs show the elasticity of Reissner's membrane (R, solid line), the tectorial membrane (dashed line), the organ of Corti (C, dotted line), and the basilar membrane (dashed line) at each of these three locations plotted as a function of distance across the width of the cochlea. Von Békésy made these measurements under water using fine, calibrated hairs. The elasticity of Reissner's membrane, the tectorial membrane, and the organ of Corti changes very little as a function of distance along the cochlea. However, the elasticity of the basilar membrane increases progressively from base to apex. Von Békésy concluded that (a) the basilar membrane determines the elasticity of the cochlear partition, and that (b) the gradient of elasticity along the basilar membrane determines the relationship between frequency and the point of maximum amplitude of the traveling wave. (Reproduced from von Békésy, 1960, Figs. 11–64, 11–65, and 11–66, by permission of the publisher.)

specimens has allowed these and several other problems to be addressed (Johnstone, Taylor, & Boyle, 1970; Rhode, 1971; Wilson & Johnstone, 1975; Kohllöffel, 1972a). However, these more recent studies have, in large part, confirmed von Békésy's primary findings: The mechanical properties of the basilar membrane and its traveling wave vibrations to sound are mainly responsible for the spatial representation of frequency along the cochlea in mammalian vertebrates.

PARADOXICAL RELATIONSHIP BETWEEN THE STRUCTURAL AND FUNCTIONAL DEVELOPMENT OF THE AUDITORY SYSTEM

The hypothesis that the spatial coding of sound frequency along the cochlear partition changes during ontogeny was originally proposed to explain a peculiar discrepancy between the structural maturation of the cochlea and the onset of responsiveness to sound (Rubel, Smith, & Miller, 1976; Rubel, 1978). In brief, morphological differentiation does not take place simultaneously along the length of the cochlea. Differentiation occurs first at the base or midbasal region and spreads primarily toward the apex. This gradient of morphological development was first described in the very earliest studies of the development of the organ of Corti by Retzius (1884). Retzius's elegant drawings of sections through the basal, middle, and apical coils of the rabbit's organ of Corti at 2 days after birth are reproduced in Figure 5. They clearly show that differentiation is most advanced at the basal end, the middle coil is slightly less well developed, and the apical end is least mature. Subsequent studies using various indices of cochlear differentiation—the formation of afferent and efferent synapses, the differentiation of receptor and supporting cells, the formation of the internal spiral sulcus, the tunnel of Corti and the spaces of Nuel, and the differentiation of the tectorial membrane—have described a similar pattern of development in virtually every species that has been examined including the mouse (Kikuchi & Hilding, 1965; Mikaelin & Ruben, 1965), rat (Wada, 1923), opossum (Larsell, McCrady, & Larsell, 1944), bird (Fermin & Cohen, 1984; Chandler, 1984), cat (Pujol & Marty, 1968, 1970), hamster (Pujol & Abonnenc, 1977) and human (Bast & Anson, 1949; Bredberg, 1968; see Fig. 6, this chap.). More limited data suggest that a corresponding pattern of development may occur within the central nervous system; regions of the central auditory pathway which receive input from the basal region of the cochlea appear to differentiate prior to more apical projection areas. This has been described for the processes of cell growth, myelination, lamina formation, and dendritic differentiation in brainstem auditory nuclei of birds (Rubel et al., 1976; Smith, 1981), the innervation of the dorsal cochlear nucleus in neonatal hamsters (Schweitzer & Cant, 1984), and the myelination of spiral ganglion cells and the

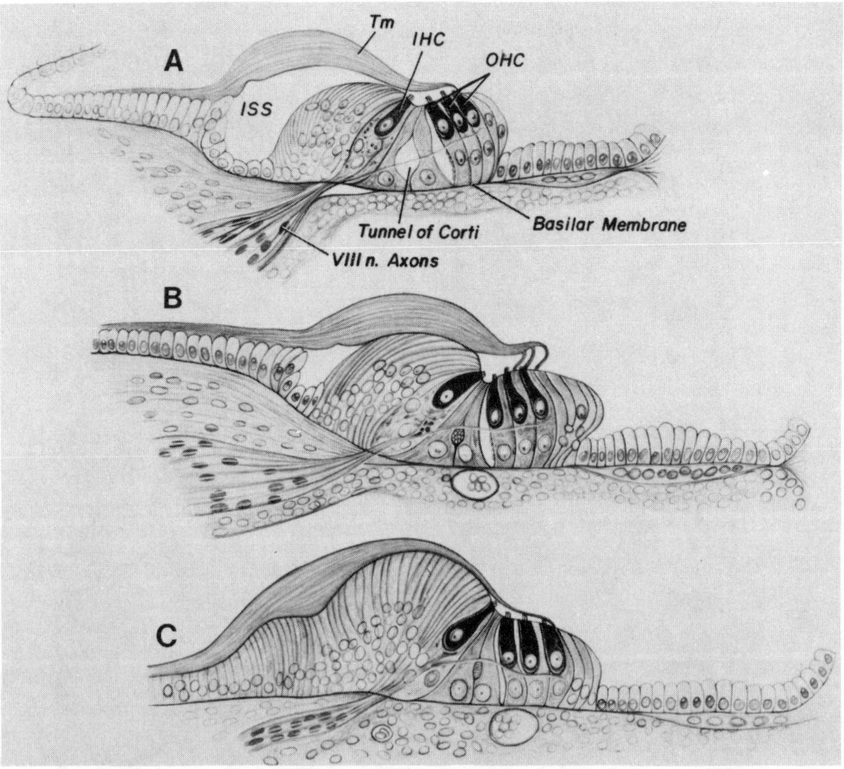

Figure 5. Retzius's drawings of cross sections through the basal (A), middle (B), and apical (C) coils of the rabbit cochlea at 2 days after birth. These have been redrawn from Retzius's original engravings. Note that the basal coil is most differentiated, the apical coil is least mature, and the middle coil is intermediate. This gradient of differentiation is seen in the relative size of the internal spiral sulcus and tunnel of Corti, the freeing of the tectorial membrane from its attachment to underlying structures, the thinning of the epithelial layer underlying the basilar membrane, and the separation of the inner from the outer hair cells. This illustrates the general finding that the morphological development of the cochlea generally occurs in a basal-to-apical direction. ISS, internal spiral sulcus; Tm, tectorial membrane; IHC, inner hair cells; OHC, outer hair cells; VIII n., eighth nerve. (Redrawn from Retzius, 1884.)

eighth nerve in mice and cats (Romand, Sans, Romand, & Marty, 1976; Romand & Romand, 1982; Anniko, 1983).

The base-to-apex sequence of morphological development along the cochlea predicts that animals should respond first to high frequency sounds and progressively later in development to lower frequencies. Paradoxically, electrophysiological and behavioral studies of functional development have consistently reported that responses occur first to low or midrange frequency

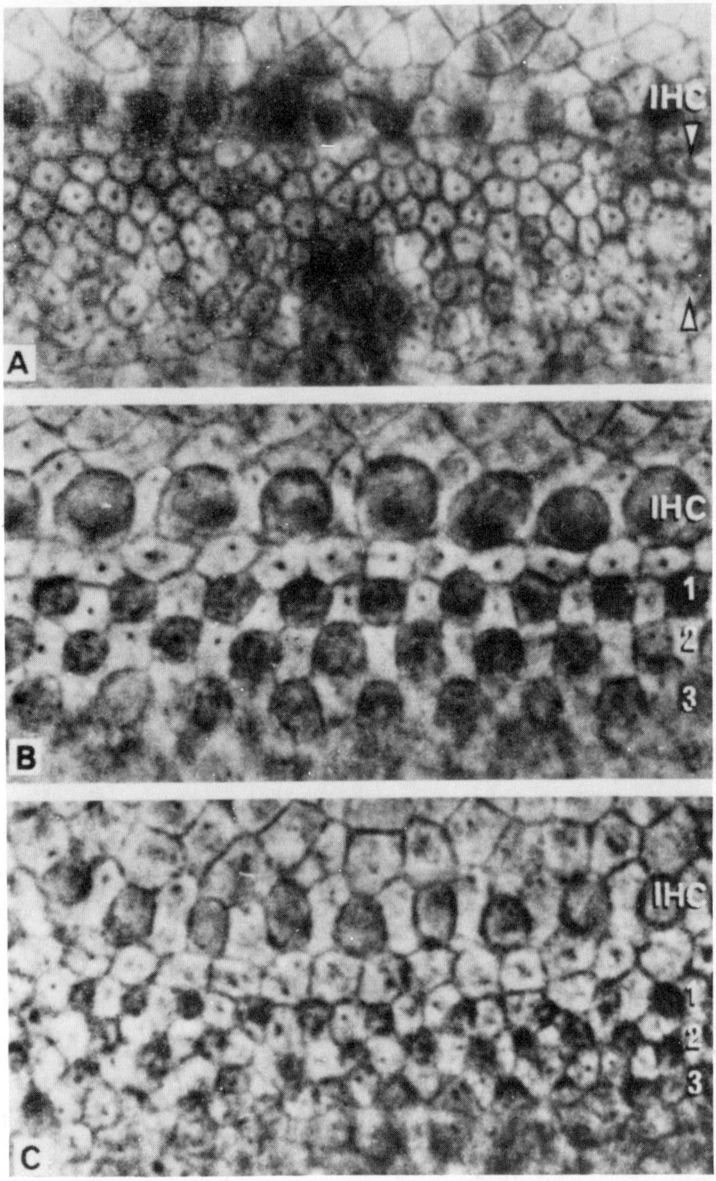

Figure 6. Surface preparations of the organ of Corti from a 3-month-old human fetus illustrating different stages of differentiation at positions 11 mm (A), 3–4 mm (B), and 1 mm (C) from the basal end of the cochlea. Inner hair cells (IHC) and three rows of outer hair cells (1,2,3) are clearly distinguishable at the midbasal location shown in B. At the extreme basal location (C), inner hair cells are well developed, but is is difficult to distinguish some of the outer hair cells from the supporting cells. The most apical region (A) is least mature. Here inner hair cells are not well differentiated, and it is not possible to distinguish either sensory or supporting cells in the region of the future outer hair cells (between arrows). (Reproduced from Bredberg, 1968, Fig. 11, by permission of the publisher.)

sounds, while responses to high frequencies are the last to mature (for reviews of this literature, see Gottlieb, 1971; Rubel, 1978; Ehret, 1983; Romand, 1983). A representative example of this finding for the development of the cochlear microphonic in rats is shown in Figure 7. Electrophysiological evidence for a progressive increase of high frequency sensitivity in infants is shown in Figure 8.

The literature on the low to high frequency order of functional development is summarized in Figure 9. It compares the adult hearing range of various species with the range of frequencies which first evoke behavioral or physiological responses. There are a number of interesting species differences. First, the particular range of low frequency sounds to which an animal responds initially is *relative* to its adult hearing range. For example, the "low" frequency sounds to which bats respond first are beyond the high-frequency hearing range of adult chickens and ducks. Second, in some species (e.g.,

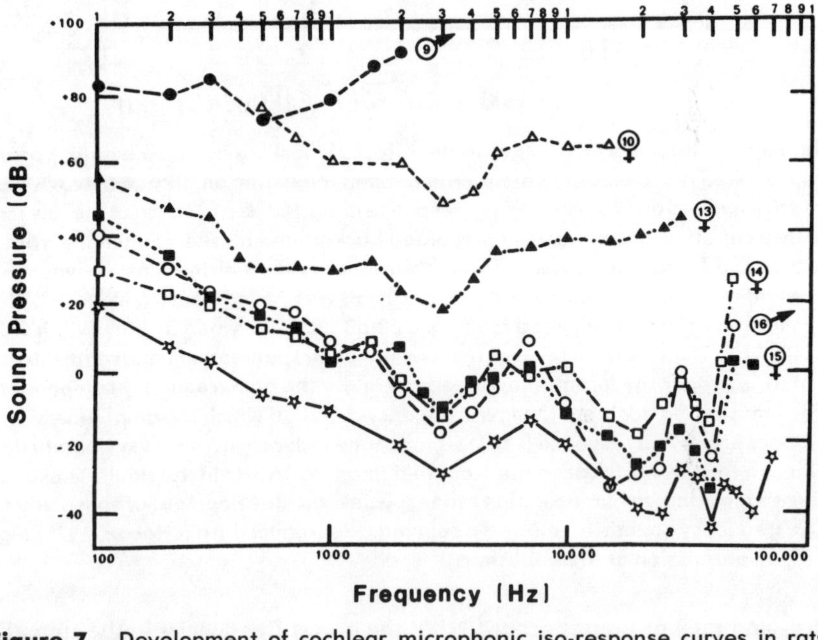

Figure 7. Development of cochlear microphonic iso-response curves in rats. Each curve was obtained from a single rat in the same litter. The symbols show the sex and age (days after birth) of each animal. The adult function is shown by the stars, and it represents the average of 12 animals. Each data point indicates the sound pressure (re. 1 dyne/cm^2) necessary to evoke a cochlear microphonic of 1 μv. Two trends can be seen: (a) Responses are initially elicited by relatively low frequency sounds and progressively change to include higher frequencies. (b) The point of maximum sensitivity shifts to higher frequencies during development. (Reproduced from Romand, 1983, Fig. 4, based on Crowley & Hepp-Reymond, 1966, Fig. 2, by permission of the publisher, © 1966 by the American Psychological Association.)

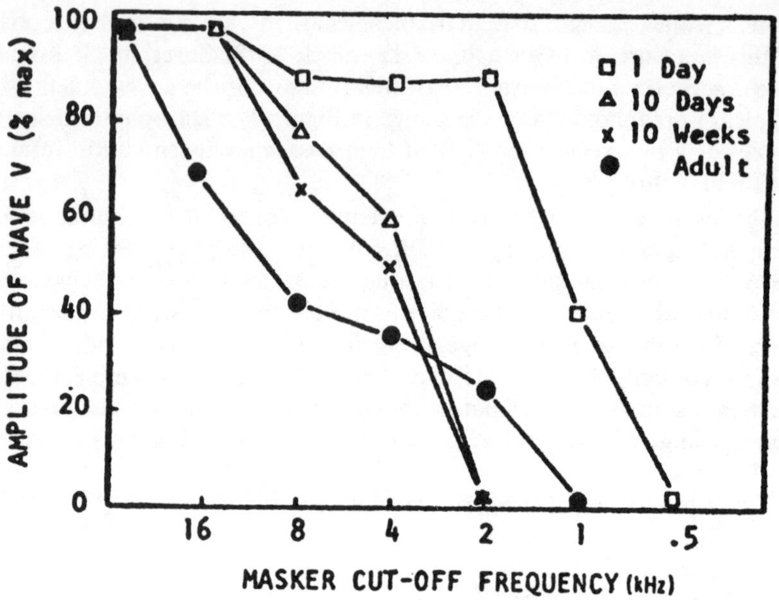

Figure 8. Ontogenetic changes in the effect of masking noise on auditory brain stem evoked responses in humans. The percent maximum amplitude of wave V of the click evoked auditory brainstem response is plotted as a function of the low frequency cut-off of a continuously presented background masker. Functions from 3 infants and 1 adult are shown. The high-frequency limit of the masker was held constant at 20 kHz, and its low-frequency cut-off was varied from 0.5 to 16 kHz. The masker intensity was adjusted to mask a 60-dB (SL) click when its bandwidth was 0.2–20 kHz. The spectrum level of the masker is the same for all bandwidths. Note that the younger the infant, the less effective are the high frequency components of the masker. In addition, the low-frequency cut-off at which the amplitude of the auditory brainstem response is first significantly reduced increases systematically with age from 1.0–2.0 kHz in the 1-day-old infant to 16 kHz in the adult. These results suggest that in humans, as in other species, the development of sensitivity to high frequency sounds is relatively delayed. (Reproduced from Hecox, 1975, Fig. 5.12, by permission of the publisher.)

birds and rats) responses occur first to the lowest frequencies in the animal's hearing range and change to include progressively higher frequencies. In other species (e.g., humans and cats), responses occur first to low-midrange frequency sounds and then gradually change to include responses to both lower and higher frequencies with responses to higher frequencies being the last to mature. Finally, a progressive increase in sensitivity to higher frequency sounds occurs at different times of development in different species. For example, this takes place during embryonic development (*in ovo*) in birds but not until after birth in such altricial species as mice and rats. However, despite these various differences, it appears to be a general characteristic of both mammalian and avian species that responses occur initially to relatively low frequency sounds and last to high frequencies (see Woolf & Ryan, 1984, for a possible exception). A low-to-high frequency sequence of functional development may also occur in the later maturation of physiological and behavioral thresholds and single neuron response properties. For example, the sounds to which an animal is most sensitive shift toward progressively higher frequencies during development (Ehret & Romand, 1981; Rebillard & Rubel, 1981; also see Fig. 7, this chap.), adult thresholds are reached first for low frequencies (Moore & Irvine, 1979; Gray & Rubel, 1981, 1985), and phase locking and adultlike tuning curves occur first in units that are tuned to low frequency sounds (Brugge, Javel, & Kitzes, 1978; Aitkin & Moore, 1975).

Two main types of explanations have been proposed to account for this apparent discrepancy between structural and functional development. The first attributes it to the transfer characteristics of the developing middle ear. According to this idea, such properties of the immature middle ear as the presence of mesenchymal fluids, a flaccid tympanic membrane, and carti-

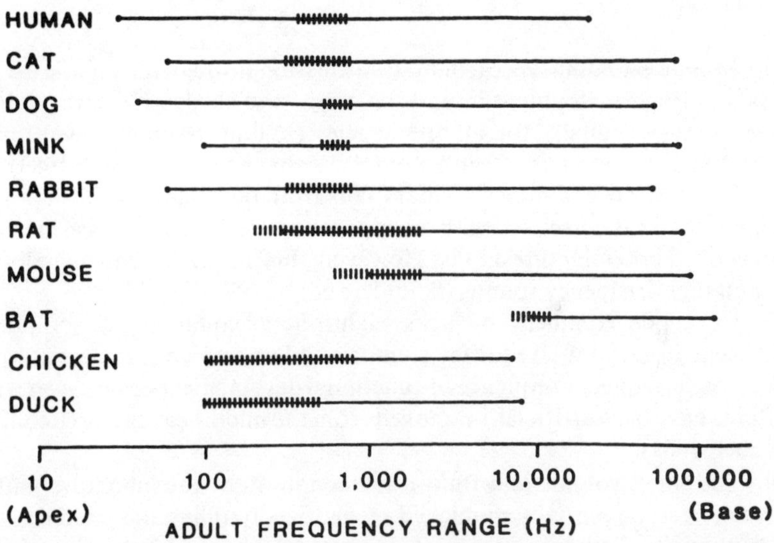

Figure 9. Frequency range at the onset of hearing for different mammalian and avian species. The adult frequency range of hearing (at approximately 70 dB SPL) is shown by the solid lines. The range of frequencies to which animals are sensitive at the youngest age that responses to sound first occur is shown by the vertical lines. Estimates have been made from both the behavioral and electrophysiological literature (see Rubel, 1978). Note that all animals respond initially to relatively low-frequency sounds. (Reproduced from Rubel, Lippe, & Ryals, 1984, Fig. 6, by permission of the publisher.)

lagenous ossicles which are incompletely coupled to each other, will selectively attenuate the transmission of high frequency energy to the cochlea (Finck, Schneck, & Hartman, 1972; Saunders, Coles, & Gates, 1973). The one experiment that is sometimes cited as evidence for this hypothesis is Ånggard's (1965) study of the development of the cochlear microphonic in neonatal rabbits. Ånggard eliminated the contribution of the developing middle ear to his recordings of the cochlear microphonic by removing the tympanic membrane and middle ear ossicles and directly stimulating the oval window with sound. He found that the threshold of the cochlear microphonic decreased uniformly across the frequency range during development. There was no evidence that responses to low frequency sounds either occurred earlier or matured at a faster rate than responses to high frequencies. However, the interpretation of this failure to observe a low-to-high frequency order of development is not clear, since comparable data on the development of the cochlear microphonic in rabbits with an intact middle ear system are not available.

Most other evidence indicates that the discrepancy between structural and functional development cannot be explained by differential middle ear attenuation:

1. Middle ear admittance (sound transmission through the middle ear) increases during development in both hamsters and chicks. However, admittance increases equally for all frequencies (Relkin, Saunders, & Konkle, 1979; Relkin & Saunders, 1980; Saunders, Kaltenbach, & Relkin, 1983).
2. The clearance of mesenchymal fluids from the middle ear cavity of developing chicks is correlated with an approximately 30-dB decrease in brainstem evoked potential thresholds. However, thresholds decrease equally for low and high frequency sounds (Saunders et al., 1973).
3. During development in chicks, eighth-nerve compound action potentials occur first to low frequency sounds and last to high frequencies. This low-to-high frequency sequence of functional development occurs even when all fluids have been artificially removed from the middle ear cavity (Rebillard & Rubel, 1981).
4. The small volume and fluid-filled condition of the immature middle ear cavity can be partially mimicked by artificially filling the middle ear of adult animals. This increases both behavioral and cochlear microphonic thresholds. However, thresholds are increased more for low rather than for high frequency sounds (Webster & Webster, 1972).
5. When chicks are exposed to high-intensity, broad-band, white noise during late embryonic development, hair cell damage is confined to the basal (high-frequency) half of the cochlea. In contrast, damage occurs along the entire length of the cochlea in birds which are exposed after hatching. The finding that damage is restricted to *high* frequency regions in the younger

birds is inconsistent with the idea that the immature middle ear primarily transmits *low* frequency sounds (Ryals & Rubel, 1985; also see Fig. 19, this chap.).

The second type of hypothesis suggests that the mechanics of the inner ear change during development (Larsell et al., 1944; Vanzulli & Garcia-Austt, 1963; Pujol & Marty, 1968, 1970). The possibility that this might explain the dissociation between structural and functional development was originally suggested to us by an observation that was made by Pujol and Marty (1968). They found that cortical auditory evoked potentials in the immature kitten were elicited only by relatively low frequency tones (0.5–2.5 kHz) and that the potentials were confined to the upper part of the anterior and central ectosylvian gyrus. Their original figure which shows the location of these potentials is reproduced in the upper part of Figure 10 (dotted region). However, when we compared the location of these early evoked potentials with the tonotopic map of auditory cortex from adult cats (lower portion of Figure 10), a curious finding emerged. It appeared that the low frequency responses which Pujol and Marty observed in young kittens were recorded from the region of primary auditory cortex which receives input from the basal part of the cochlea and responds to *high* frequency sounds in the adult. This suggested to us that the basal end of the cochlea in kittens responds to low rather than to high frequency sounds and that during development the representation of frequency along the cochlea changes.

The specific hypothesis we proposed and the predictions it makes are shown in Figure 11. The upper portion of each diagram schematically shows the basilar membrane, from base to apex, and the relative positions of the traveling waves to several pure tones, in kHz. The lower part of each diagram indicates the orderly projection of the eighth nerve into the central nervous system and the characteristic frequency (in kHz) of individual neurons. As depicted by the two left diagrams, we hypothesized that sound is first transduced by the early developing basal region of the cochlea. However, the basal end of the immature cochlea, unlike that in the adult, is maximally responsive to low rather than to high frequency sounds. During development the point of maximum sensitivity to low and midrange frequency sounds gradually shifts apically as the basal end becomes responsive to higher frequencies.

This hypothesis makes two testable predictions. The first is based on the finding that the frequency organization of the cochlea can be demonstrated by measuring the location of hair cell damage from exposure to high-intensity pure tones. In mature animals, high frequency sounds cause maximum damage at the base while lower frequencies result in damage at more apical locations (Stockwell, Ades, & Engstrom, 1969). Thus, if the frequency organization of the cochlea is changing during development, there should be

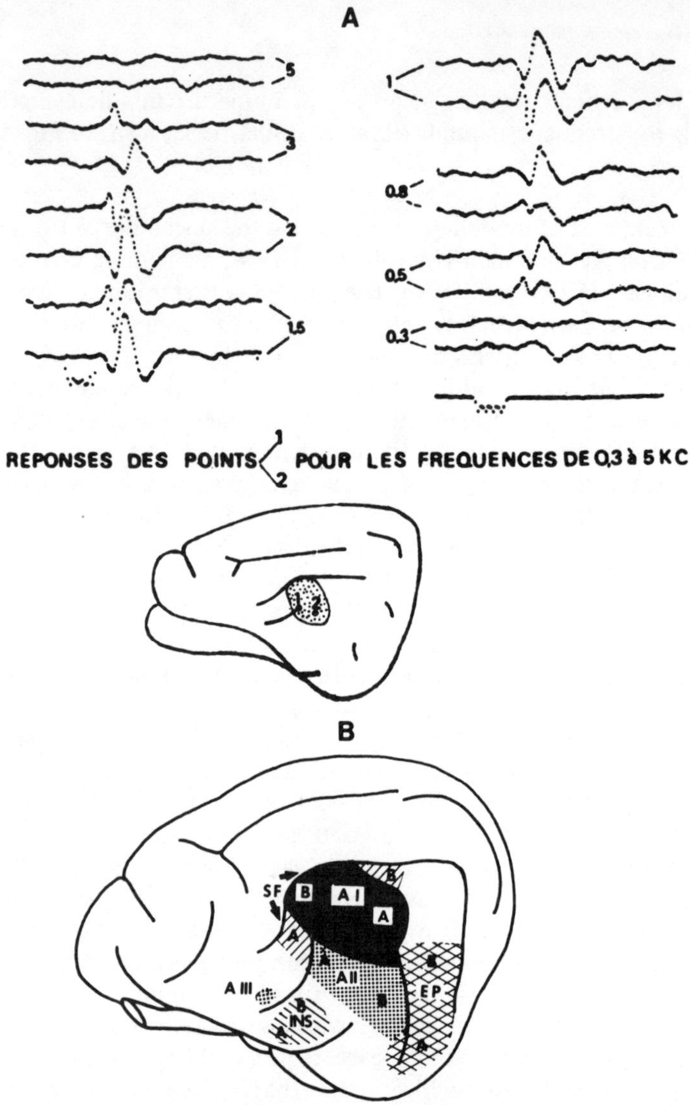

Figure 10. Comparison of the localization of auditory cortical evoked potentials in kittens and adult cats. (A) Outline drawing of the cerebral cortex of the kitten (brain facing left) showing the region (dotted) from which the first responses to sound were recorded in 2-day-old kittens. Initial responses were evoked only by relatively low frequency sounds. Responses recorded from points 1 and 2 to these low frequency sounds (0.5–3.0 kHz) are shown in the top tracings. (Reproduced from Pujol & Marty, 1968, Fig. 2, by permission of the publisher.) (B) Auditory areas of the cerebral cortex of the adult cat. Letters A and B indicate regions which receive input from the apical (low-frequency) and basal (high-frequency) regions of the cochlea. Note that the region of auditory cortex from which Pujol and Marty recorded low frequency responses in the kitten corresponds to the basal or high frequency projection region of AI in adults. AI, primary auditory field; AII, secondary auditory field; AIII, Tunturi's third auditory region; INS, insular region; SF, suprasylvian fringe sector; EP, posterior ectosylvian field. (Redrawn from Woolsey, 1959, Fig. 128, by permission of the publisher.)

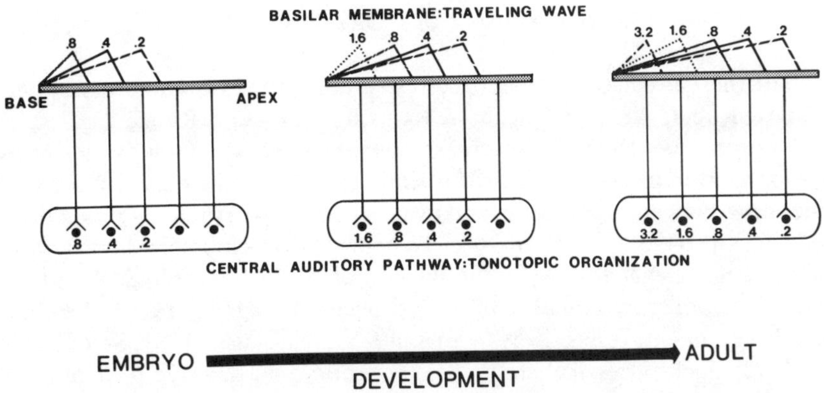

Figure 11. Model of the developmental shift in the place code described in text. The basilar membrane and the position of the traveling wave to several different frequencies are shown at the top. The tonotopic organization of an auditory region within the central nervous system is illustrated at the bottom. At the onset of auditory function (left) the basal portion of the basilar membrane responds to low and midrange frequency sounds. Regions of the central auditory pathway receiving projections from the basal part of the cochlea also respond to low frequencies. During the course of development (middle and right), the representation of low and midrange frequencies shifts apically along the cochlea, and the base responds to progressively higher frequency sounds. Within the central nervous system there is a corresponding shift in tonotopic organization; each neuron responds to progressively higher-frequency sounds during development. (Reproduced from Rubel, 1984, Fig. 1, with permission from the *Annual Review of Physiology*, Vol. 46, © 1984 by Annual Reviews Inc.)

a systematic ontogenetic shift in the position of hair cell damage produced by exposure to pure tone, high-intensity sounds. In particular, the position of maximum damage resulting from exposure to a particular low or midrange frequency tone should occur more apically in animals exposed at later times during development.

The second prediction is based on the assumption that any change in the spatial representation of frequency along the cochlea will be mirrored as a corresponding change of tonotopic organization within the central auditory system. During the period that the representation of low and midrange frequencies is shifting apically along the cochlea, the tonotopic organization of any neuronal region within the central auditory system should be (a) orderly and qualitatively similar to that in the adult, but (b) shifted to lower frequencies. Early in development, neurons should be tuned to lower frequency sounds than in the adult. As development proceeds, the characteristic frequency of an individual neuron should increase progressively towards its adult value.

THE AVIAN AUDITORY SYSTEM

Both of these predictions have been tested using the avian auditory system (Lippe & Rubel, 1983, 1985; Rubel & Ryals, 1983; Ryals & Rubel, 1985). This preparation was selected for several reasons. First, the chronology of hearing development in humans and birds is similar. In both, the onset of auditory function occurs embryonically, and by the time of birth (hatching) hearing is well developed but not fully mature. To provide a developmental framework for the studies that follow, it should be noted that physiological and behavioral responses to sound in birds first occur on days 11 and 14 of embryonic development, respectively (Vanzulli & Garcia-Austt, 1963; Saunders et al., 1973; Jackson & Rubel, 1978). By embryonic day 17, physiological thresholds have decreased to within 30 dB of mature levels, and the basilar papilla (avian cochlea) and its afferent innervation are well developed (Saunders et al., 1973; Hirokawa, 1978; Cohen & Fermin, 1978; Rebillard & Rubel, 1981; Fermin & Cohen, 1984). On day 19, the embryo enters the airspace and begins pulmonary respiration in preparation for hatching. Its external and middle ears are clear of embryonic fluids and physiological thresholds are near adultlike levels (Saunders et al., 1973). One day after hatching, behavioral and physiological thresholds have reached mature levels for all but the highest frequencies (Saunders et al., 1973; Kerr, Ostapoff, & Rubel, 1979; Rebillard & Rubel, 1981; Gray & Rubel, 1981, 1985). Cochlear growth (Tilney, 1984; Ryals, Creech, & Rubel, 1984), and increases in middle ear admittance (Saunders et al., 1983) continue for several months after hatching. However, by one week, posthatch thresholds have reached mature levels for all frequencies (Saunders et al., 1973; Rebillard & Rubel, 1981; Gray & Rubel, 1981, 1985).

Second, the basilar papilla has a short, uncoiled structure which allows the number of hair cells to be easily counted and quantified using standard methods of serial reconstruction. In addition, the relationship between frequency and place along the basilar papilla has been qualitatively described in adult birds (von Békésy, 1960; Ryals & Rubel, 1982). This provides a basis for studying changes in the place code during development. Third, nucleus magnocellularis and nucleus laminaris, first and second order auditory nuclei in the bird, have a relatively simple geometry and pattern of afferent innervation which makes them especially well suited for studying the development of tonotopicity. This stereotyped organization makes it possible to use quantitative methods to describe and compare tonotopic organization at different times during development (Rubel & Parks, 1975; Lippe & Rubel, 1983, 1985).

The brainstem auditory system in the adult bird is shown schematically in Figure 12. The basilar papilla sends a topographically organized projection to nucleus magnocellularis, the homologue of the "bushy cell" region of the mammalian anteroventral cochlear nucleus (Boord & Rasmussen, 1963;

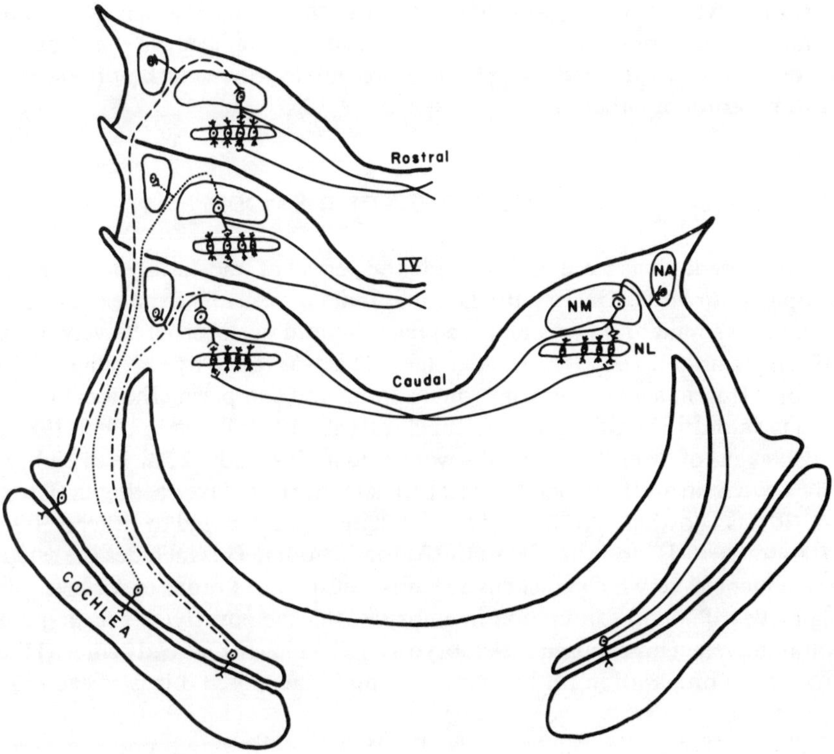

Figure 12. Schematic drawing showing the topographically organized projections from the uncoiled avian cochlea (basilar papilla) via the cochlear nerve to nucleus magnocellularis (NM) and nucleus angularis (NA); and the topographically organized, spatially segregated bilateral projections from nucleus magnocellularis to nucleus laminaris (NL). See text for details. IV, fourth ventricle. (Reproduced from Rubel et al., 1976, Fig. 1, by permission of the publisher.)

Jhaveri & Morest, 1982). Neurons at the anteromedial pole of nucleus magnocellularis receive projections from the proximal (basal) end of the papilla and respond to high frequency sounds; neurons at progressively posterolateral locations in nucleus magnocellularis are innervated by more distal (apical) points along the papilla and respond to progressively lower frequencies (Boord & Rasmussen, 1963; Rubel & Parks, 1975). Nucleus magnocellularis, in turn, sends a bilateral projection to nucleus laminaris, the avian homolog of the mammalian medial superior olivary nucleus (Boord & Rasmussen, 1963; Parks & Rubel, 1975; Rubel & Parks, 1975). Nucleus laminaris consists of a monolayer of neurons whose bipolar dendrites extend dorsally and ventrally into distinctive neuropil regions. The dorsal dendrites are innervated by the ipsilateral magnocellular nucleus, while the ventral dendrites receive a crossed projection from the contralateral nucleus magnocellularis. These bilateral projections are frequency matched, so that individual neurons in nucleus laminaris have approximately the same best frequency to stimulation of either ear.

EXPERIMENTAL TESTS OF THE MODEL

The two predictions were tested during the period of mid-to-late hearing development in birds. The first prediction is that hair cell loss from exposure to an intense sound of a particular frequency should occur progressively more apically in animals exposed at older ages. This was tested by exposing chickens of different ages to the same tonal stimuli and comparing the location of damage along the basilar papilla (Rubel & Ryals, 1983; Ryals & Rubel, 1985).

Chickens of three different ages were used in this study: 20 days of embryonic development (E20; one day prior to hatching), 10 days posthatch (P10), and 30 days posthatch (P30). Birds at each age were exposed to either a 500-, 1500-, or 3000-Hz tone at 125 dB (SPL) for 12 hours. This includes the range of frequencies to which chickens are most sensitive. In order to achieve this high level of sound stimulation in embryos, the shell overlying the airspace was removed. This exposed the embryo's head which had already entered the airspace in preparation for hatching. Normal (unexposed) birds of each age served as controls.

The birds were allowed to survive for 10 days following sound exposure. The basilar papillae were then fixed, embedded in Epon, and sectioned transversely to the longitudinal axis. A group of 3–4, 3μ thick sections was collected every 100μ along the length of the papilla and stained. The number of hair cells in each section was counted under the light microscope and plotted as a function of percent distance from the proximal (base) to the distal (apex) end of the papilla.

Initial studies examined the extent and location of hair cell loss in 10-day-old hatchlings which had been exposed to 500-, 1500-, and 3000-Hz tones. We observed that the effects of overstimulation in birds are similar to what has been described in mammals. Hair cells are lost, and many of the remaining hair cells in the damaged region have distorted cell bodies and clumped or missing cilia. In addition, the location of hair cell damage varies systematically as a function of sound frequency. This finding is illustrated in Figure 13. The mean total number of hair cells is plotted as a function of percent distance along the papilla for each exposure condition. The location of maximum hair cell loss along the papilla is indicated by the arrows. The mean number of hair cells ($\pm$ 1 S.E.M.) in control birds is shown by the shaded area. Exposure to the 500-Hz tone caused a broad area of damage with the location of maximum damage occurring about midway along the length of the

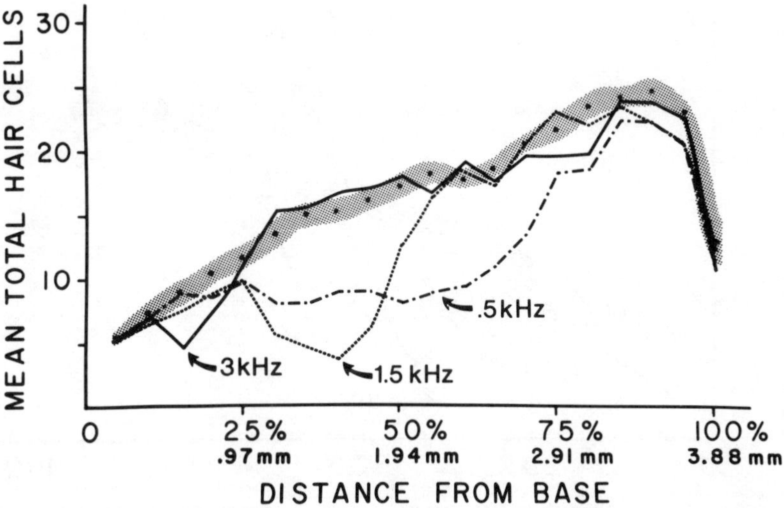

Figure 13. Location of hair cell loss varies as a function of sound frequency. Mean total number of hair cells is plotted as a function of distance along the papilla in 10-day-old chicks exposed to 500-Hz, 1500-Hz, or 3000-Hz tones at 125 dB SPL for 12 hours. The location of maximum percentage cell loss for each condition is indicated by the arrows. Survival time was 10 days. Shaded areas show mean total number of hair cells (± 1 S.E.M.) in control chicks. Note that the position of maximum percentage cell loss occurs progressively towards the base for higher frequencies of exposure. (Reproduced from Ryals & Rubel, 1982, Fig. 1, by permission of the publisher.)

papilla. The region of damage from exposure to the higher frequencies became narrower and more discrete and was localized progressively toward the base.

This same experiment was then performed in embryos one day before hatching (E20) and in 30-day posthatch birds. The same trend observed in 10-day hatchlings was found: higher frequency tones resulted in damage which was localized progressively toward the base. Most notably, however, the position of hair cell loss from exposure to the same frequency sound differed between ages. Both the overall region of hair cell loss and the position of maximum damage shifted systematically toward the apex in older birds. Figure 14 shows this finding for exposure to the 1500-Hz tone in the three age groups. In 20-day embryos the position of maximum loss is located about 30% of the distance from the base toward the apex. At 10-days posthatch, the location of maximum damage has shifted to 39% of length, and by 30 days posthatch it has moved even further apically to 49% of length.

The findings of this study are summarized in Figure 15. The position of maximum damage to each frequency is plotted as a function of age. No ap-

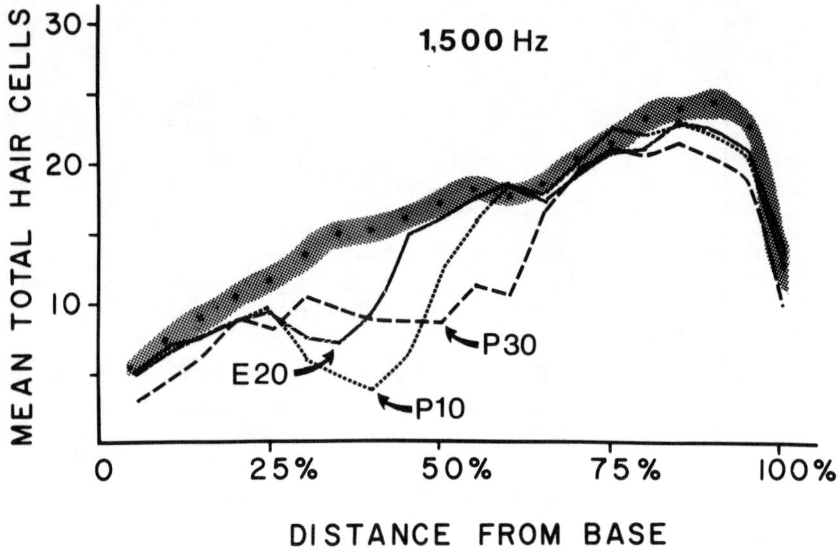

Figure 14. Location of hair cell loss varies as a function of age. Mean total number of hair cells is plotted as a function of percent distance along the papilla in 20 day embryos (E20), 10-day posthatch chicks (P10), and 30-day posthatch chicks (P30) exposed to a 1500-Hz tone at 125 dB SPL for 12 hours. The standard errors for the experimental groups have been omitted but are comparable to those in control birds. Shaded area shows mean total number of hair cells (± 1 S.E.M.) in control birds (the number of cells in normal birds is similar at these three ages). Arrows indicate locations of maximum percentage hair cell loss. Note that the location of maximum damage occurs more apically in older birds. (Reproduced from Rubel & Ryals, 1983, Fig. 1B, by permission of the publisher, © 1983 by the AAAS.)

preciable hair cell loss occurred in the 20-day embryos exposed to 3000 Hz, most likely because thresholds for high frequency sounds are still elevated at this age. Thus, no data point is shown for this condition. Aside from this one exception, the location of maximum damage to each frequency shifted progressively toward the apex in older birds. This finding confirms the first prediction.

The second prediction is that the tonotopic organization of any nucleus in the auditory system should change during development. Neurons at a given location within an auditory neuronal region should become maximally responsive to progressively higher frequency sounds during development. This prediction was tested by electrophysiologically mapping the tonotopic organization of nucleus magnocellularis and nucleus laminaris in chicks at different ages. The characteristic frequencies of neurons having the same relative location in each nucleus were then compared at different times during development (Lippe & Rubel, 1983, 1985).

Seventeen-day embryos (E17; 4 days before hatching), 12–24 hour posthatch chicks (PO), and 2–4 week posthatch chicks ("adults") were used in this experiment. The posthatch birds were anesthetized and prepared for electrophysiological recording according to methods which are used routinely in our labs (Rubel & Parks, 1975; Lippe & Rubel, 1985). In order to record from embryos, it was necessary to expose their head through a hole in the shell. The head was supported with a head holder, and the egg and embryo were po-

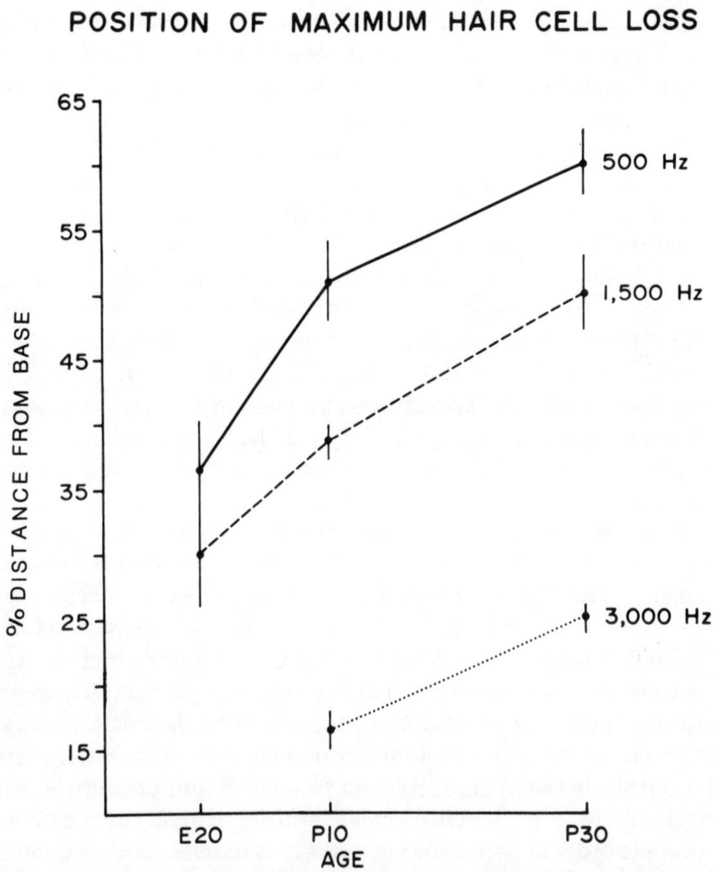

Figure 15. Summary of the effects of age and exposure frequency on location of hair cell loss. The mean percentage position along the papilla (± 1 S.E.M.) at which the maximum hair cell loss occurred is plotted for each frequency of exposure at each age. No significant cell loss occurred in embryos exposed to 3000 Hz, so a data point is not shown for this condition. These functions show that at each exposure frequency the location of maximum damage shifted progressively toward the apex in older birds. (Reproduced from Rubel & Ryals, 1983, Fig. 2, by permission of the publisher.)

sitioned inside a temperature-and-humidity-controlled chamber. Sound stimuli were delivered to embryos and hatchlings through a calibrated closed system sealed to the external auditory meatus. The characteristic frequency of single units and unit clusters was determined at several locations in nucleus magnocellularis and nucleus laminaris as a microelectrode was advanced through the brainstem. After several electrode penetrations had been completed, the brain was fixed *in situ,* embedded in paraffin, sectioned, and stained. The locations of all recorded units were determined and projected onto outline drawings of nucleus magnocellularis and nucleus laminaris as they would appear from the dorsal surface of the brain. The total posterior-anterior and lateral-medial extents of the outline drawings were set equal to 100%, and each unit cluster and its characteristic frequency were then specified in terms of its percentile posterior-anterior and lateral-medial positions. This method of normalization allowed us to combine data from birds of the same age and make comparisons between birds of different ages despite variations in the absolute size of the nuclei.

The tonotopic organization that was found in adult birds is shown in Figure 16. The scatter plots show the relationship between characteristic frequency and the percentile posterior-to-anterior (A,C) and lateral-to-medial (B,D) position of each unit and cluster of units which were recorded in nucleus magnocellularis (A,B) and nucleus laminaris (C,D). The solid and dashed lines are the best-fitting linear regression lines ± 1 standard error of estimate, respectively. These data show that nucleus magnocellularis and nucleus laminaris both have an orderly and highly predictable tonotopic organization. Progressively higher characteristic frequencies are recorded as an electrode is moved from posterior to anterior or from lateral to medial in either nucleus. The highest characteristic frequencies are located anteromedially and lower frequencies are recorded progressively posterolaterally.

In Figure 17, the tonotopic organization of adult birds is compared with the organization that was observed at the two younger ages. The regression lines and standard error of estimates which describe the tonotopic organization in adult birds have been replotted from Figure 16. The scatter plots show the relationship between characteristic frequency and position in embryos (top panel) and in newly hatched chicks (bottom panel). These data indicate that tonotopic order in both embryos and newly hatched birds is qualitatively similar to that in adults. Progressively higher characteristic frequencies were recorded at successively more medial and anterior positions in each nucleus in both embryos and 1-day-old birds, as in adults. However, the quantitative relationship between position and characteristic frequency is not the same. In embryos, each location in both nucleus magnocellularis and nucleus laminaris responded to lower frequencies than in adults. The characteristic frequencies in embryos averaged one octave below what would be predicted from the relationship between position and characteristic frequency in adult

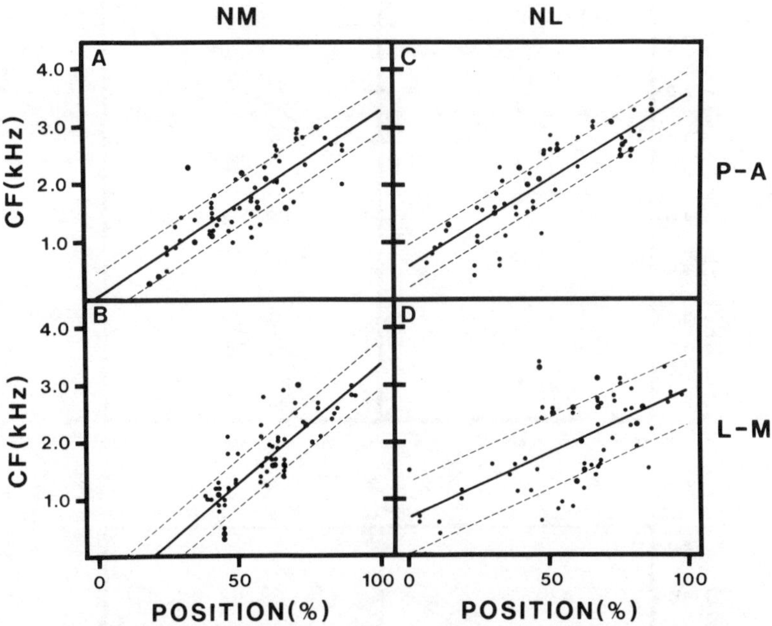

Figure 16. Tonotopic organization in "adult" birds. The scatter plots show the relationship between characteristic frequency (CF) and percentile distance along the posterior-to-anterior (A, C) and lateral-to-medial (B, D) dimensions of nucleus magnocellularis (NM; left-hand panels) and nucleus laminaris (NL; right-hand panels) in 2–4-week posthatch birds. Each point represents a recording from a single neuron or a cluster of neurons. The solid and dashed lines are the best fitting linear regression functions ± 1 standard error of estimate, respectively. Progressively higher characteristic frequencies are recorded at successively more medial and anterior locations in both nuclei. (Reproduced from Lippe & Rubel, 1985, Fig. 5, by permission of the publisher.)

birds. In newly hatched birds the characteristic frequencies were intermediate between those in adults and embryos and averaged one-third octave lower than their predicted values. Thus, each region of nucleus magnocellularis and nucleus laminaris becomes maximally responsive to progressively higher frequencies during development.

This systematic shift in tonotopic organization is shown more clearly in Figure 18. The top portion of the figure shows outline drawings or horizontal projections of both nuclei as they would be seen from the dorsal surface of the brain. The arrows which are superimposed on the projections indicate the tonotopic gradients or direction of increasing frequency. The outline drawings of nucleus laminaris and nucleus magnocellularis have been divided into four and five sectors, respectively, perpendicular to their tonotopic gradi-

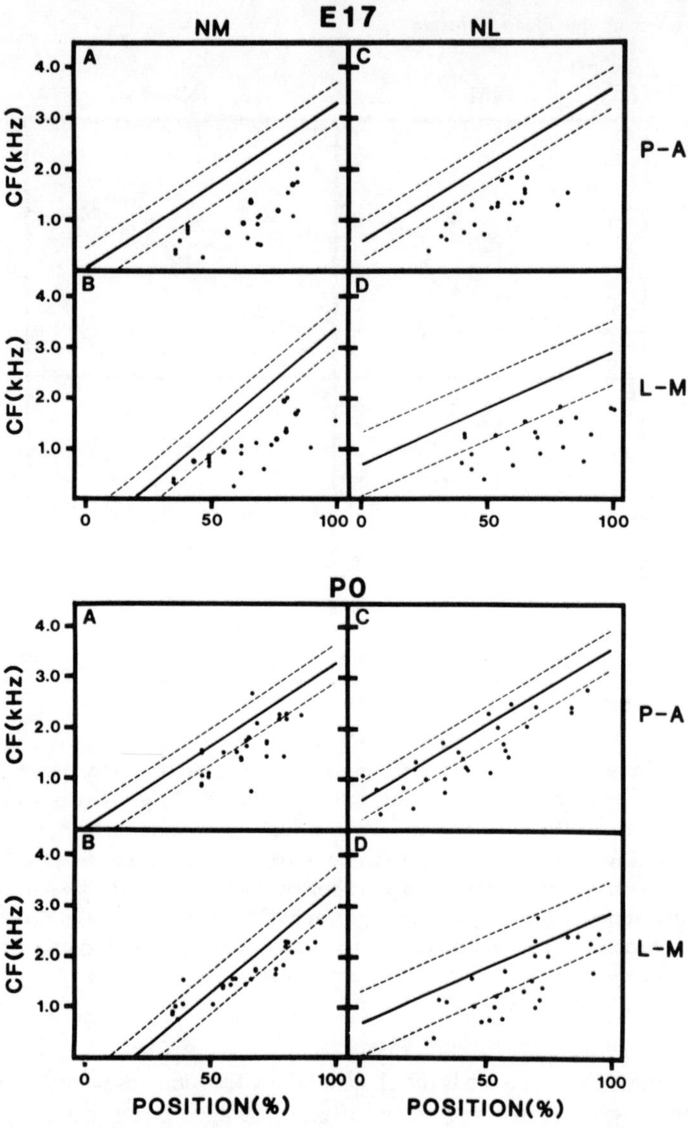

Figure 17. Comparison of tonotopic organization in nucleus magnocellularis and nucleus laminaris at different ages. The linear regressions that predict best frequency as a function of position in nucleus magnocellularis (NM) and nucleus laminaris (NL) in adult birds are shown by the solid lines; the dashed lines represent ± 1 standard error of estimate. They have been replotted from Figure 16. The relationship between best frequency and position that was actually observed in 17-day-old embryos (E17) and newly hatched birds (P0) is shown by the scatter plots. The order of tonotopic organization is similar at all ages, but a given position in either nuclei responds to lower frequencies sounds in embryos and newly hatched chicks than in adults. (Reproduced from Lippe & Rubel, 1985, Fig. 8, by permission of the publisher.)

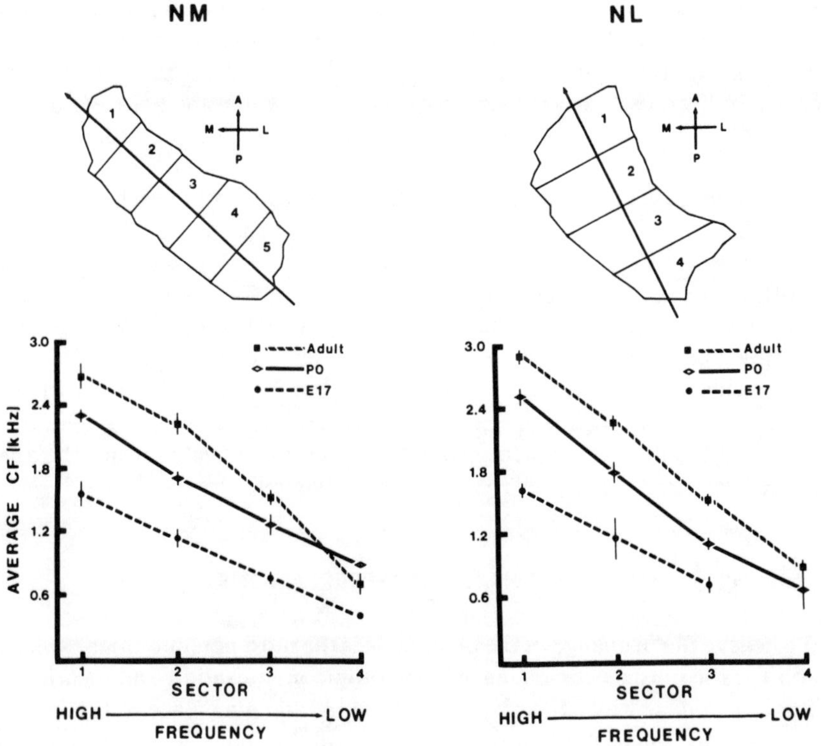

Figure 18. Summary of the developmental changes in tonotopic organization in nucleus magnocellularis and nucleus laminaris. Outline drawings of nucleus magnocellularis (NM) and nucleus laminaris (NL) are divided into equal sectors perpendicular to their tonotopic axes (indicated by arrow). The posterior-anterior and lateral-medial dimensions of the brain are indicated. The average characteristic frequency (± 1 S.E.M.) which was recorded in each sector at every age is plotted in the lower graphs. No data points are plotted for sector 5 of nucleus magnocellularis, because this region does not receive auditory input. The average characteristic frequency within each sector increased progressively during development. See text for details. (Reproduced from Lippe & Rubel, 1985, Fig. 10, by permission of the publisher.)

ents. The most caudolateral sector in nucleus magnocellularis (sector 5) does not receive auditory input. The remaining four sectors in each nucleus comprise regions that receive input from progressively more apical regions along the basilar papilla as one moves from sector 1 (anteromedial) to sector 4 (posterolateral). The average characteristic frequency (± 1 S.E.M.) that was observed in each of the four sectors at the different ages is plotted in the bottom graphs.

The data points for embryos and newly hatched chicks in the most posterolateral or low-frequency sector (sector 4) are based upon very few recordings and cannot be meaningfully compared between groups. The data points in the remaining sectors show two clear trends. The systematic decrease in average characteristic frequency from anteromedial (sector 1) to posterolateral (sector 3) at all ages indicates that tonotopic order remains similar during development. However, the progressive and statistically significant increase of frequency that occurs across ages within each sector indicates that each region becomes most sensitive to or is maximally stimulated by progressively higher frequency sounds during development. This finding confirms the second prediction.

The converging results of these two studies strongly support the model of a shifting place code. According to this model, only the basal end of the cochlea transduces sound early in development, but it is maximally sensitive to low rather than to high frequencies. During development the representation of low and midrange frequency sounds shifts progressively toward the apex as the base becomes responsive to successively higher frequencies.

ALTERNATIVE INTERPRETATIONS

We believe that a change in the place code is the most parsimonious explanation for the ontogenetic changes in tonotopic organization and location of hair cell damage which have been observed. A changing place code is probably the only *single* mechanism that can easily account for *both* findings. However, there are alternative mechanisms which might explain either finding alone, and it would be worthwhile to briefly consider these.

Ontogenetic Shifts in Position of Hair Cell Damage

Cochlear Growth. The basilar papilla continues to increase in length until at least 3 months after hatching (Tilney, 1984; Ryals et al., 1984). Between 20 days of embryonic development and 30 days posthatch the average length of the papilla increases approximately 30%, from 4.6 mm to 6 mm. New sensory cells are not being added during this time, so this growth reflects the addition of new supporting cells and/or the growth of existing structures. The position of hair cell loss would not be affected by this growth, if the papilla grows equally along its length. However, if growth occurs primarily at the basal end, then the position of damage would shift systematically during development, even if the place code remains fixed. In this case, exposure to a given tone will damage the same population of hair cells (i.e., the same absolute position along the papilla) at different ages. However, the relative location of damage will shift progressively toward the apex in birds exposed at later times during development.

Two observations make it unlikely that this accounts for the systematic change in the location of damage which occurred. First, the location of maximum damage does not differ significantly between birds which are exposed to the same frequency sound but allowed to survive for different periods of time (Rubel & Ryals, 1982). This is inconsistent with the idea that the papilla grows primarily at its basal end. Second, we have calculated the change in location of damage that would occur under the assumption that the basilar papilla grows only at its basal end. Table 1 shows that even under this unlikely condition, cochlear growth cannot account fully for the ontogenetic shift in the position of hair cell loss that occurred.

Developmental Changes in Sound Stimulating the Inner Ear. The study of high-intensity sound exposure is based on the assumption that the spectrum and intensity of sound stimuli reaching the inner ear do not change

Table 1. Comparison of the Observed and Predicted Locations of Maximum Hair Cell Loss Along the Basilar Papilla Following Pure Tone Overstimulation

	Position of Maximum Hair Cell Loss		
Frequency	**Observed**		**Predicted**
	E20	*P10*	*P10*
500	37%	52%	42%
1500	30%	38%	35%
	P10	*P30*	*P30*
500	52%	60%	55%
1500	38%	50%	41%
3000	17%	25%	22%

Notes:

1. E20—embryonic day 20; P10—posthatch day 10; P30—posthatch day 30.
2. Position is expressed as percent distance from the proximal (basal) to the distal (apical) end of the basilar papilla.
3. The observed locations of maximum hair cell loss following pure tone overstimulation are from the data of Rubel and Ryals (1983). The predicted locations of hair cell loss were calculated by assuming that a given frequency stimulates the same hair cells at different times during development and that the basilar papilla grows only at its basal end. The calculations are based on the data of Rubel and Ryals (1983) and Ryals et al. (1984). The first entry in the table (predicted location of hair cell loss at P10 following exposure to 500 Hz at E20) will serve as an example of how the predicted location of damage was calculated: Predicted percent location of damage at P10 = [(Observed % location of damage at E20 for 500Hz) × (Average length of papilla at E20) + (Increase in length of papilla between E20 and P10)]/Average length of papilla at P10.

systematically during the ages that were studied. There is little reason to suspect that spectral differences occurred. The acoustic fields were similar at all ages, harmonics were well attenuated, and the resonant frequencies associated with the growth of the ear canal are higher than the sounds to which the birds were exposed (Ryals, 1981). Distortion products are likely reflected in the pattern of hair cell loss. However, there is no reason to believe that the spectral characteristics of these distortion products would change systematically during development. The possibility that the effective sound intensity which reached the middle ear might have changed systematically across ages is more likely, especially because middle ear admittance continues to increase during the ages which were studied (Saunders et al., 1983). Intensity differences were of concern because of findings in mammals that the position of both hair cell loss and the peak of the traveling wave along the basilar membrane vary with sound intensity (von Békésy, 1960; Rhode, 1971; Stockwell et al., 1969). However, as already noted, the experiments on high-intensity sound exposure were conducted during the period of late hearing development and mature function when the sensitivity of the auditory system is changing very little. By embryonic day 20, the youngest age which was tested, the middle ear is fluid-free and in its last stages of development (Saunders et al., 1973; Jaskoll & Maderson, 1978). Electrophysiological thresholds to low frequencies have reached mature levels but are still somewhat elevated for frequencies above 800 Hz (Saunders et al., 1973). However, by 10 days after hatching, electrophysiological and behavioral thresholds have reached adult levels for all frequencies (Saunders et al., 1973; Rebillard & Rubel, 1981; Gray & Rubel, 1981, 1985). Thus, with the exception of the embryos exposed to the highest frequency sounds, the changes in position of damage took place when normal or near normal thresholds had been established. This makes it highly unlikely that the shifts in location of damage reflected age-related differences in the effective intensity of sound at the inner ear.

Developmental Changes in Tonotopic Organization

Changes in Middle Ear Transmission Properties. The most likely alternative explanation for the change in tonotopic organization is that the immature middle ear cannot effectively transmit high-frequency energy to the cochlea (Finck et al., 1972; Saunders et al., 1973, 1983; Brugge et al., 1978). In the section on "Paradoxical Relationship Between the Structural and Functional Development of the Auditory System" it was noted that this same mechanism has also been proposed to explain the discrepancy between structural and functional development. According to this proposal, neurons in the developing and mature auditory systems might be tuned alike. However, because the middle ear acts as a low pass filter, some point on the low frequency slope of a neuron's tuning curve would appear to be its best frequency. There are several findings which are not consistent with this explanation. First, this predicts that the relative amount of shift to lower best frequencies would be greatest for high-frequency neurons (those located in the anteromedial regions of nucleus magnocellularis and nucleus laminaris) and progressively less for lower-frequency units (those located more posterolaterally). However, the percent change in characteristic frequency was comparable, regardless of position within either nucleus (see Fig. 18). Second, tonotopic organization is still shifting one day after hatching, although by this time the middle ear is cleared of mesenchyme and thresholds to all but the highest-frequency sounds are no longer changing (Saunders et al., 1973; Rebillard & Rubel, 1981; Gray & Rubel, 1985). Third, the increase in middle ear admittance which occurs during development in both hamsters and chicks is not greater for high- versus low-frequency sounds (Relkin et al., 1979; Relkin & Saunders, 1980; Saunders et al, 1983). Finally, if the immature middle ear is functioning as a low pass filter, one would predict that hair cell damage resulting from exposure to white noise would extend more toward the apex in older animals. This was tested by exposing 20-day-old embryos and 10-day posthatch chicks to high-intensity, white noise (Ryals & Rubel, 1985). The results of this study are shown in Figure 19. The mean numbers of hair cells in exposed and normal birds are plotted as a function of percent distance along the basilar papilla for both ages. The results show that hair cell loss in embryos was restricted to the basal half of the papilla and spread to include more apical regions in older birds. This finding is inconsistent with the idea that the immature middle ear selectively transmits low frequency sounds.

Structural Changes. Two types of structural changes could account for the changes in tonotopic organization. First, the relative positions of neurons in nucleus magnocellularis and nucleus laminaris might shift during development. This is unlikely, because cell migration, cell death, and other morphogenetic processes which could result in such a shift have ended by embryonic day 17 (Rubel et al., 1976). Second, a systematic remapping of connections, similar to that which occurs during the development of retinotectal connections in both fish and amphibians (Gaze, Chung, & Keating, 1972; Gaze, Keating, & Chung, 1974; Longley, 1978; Reh & Constantine-Paton, 1984; Easter & Stuermer, 1984), might occur between nucleus magnocellularis and the basilar papilla. Although we consider this unlikely, none of the results from the mapping study exclude this possibility. However, a change in connections does not explain the ontogenetic shift in position of hair cell loss. Neither can it account for the progressive increase in the cut-off frequency of the cochlear microphonic which has been found in the developing gerbil (Harris & Dallos, 1984; see Fig. 21, this chap.).

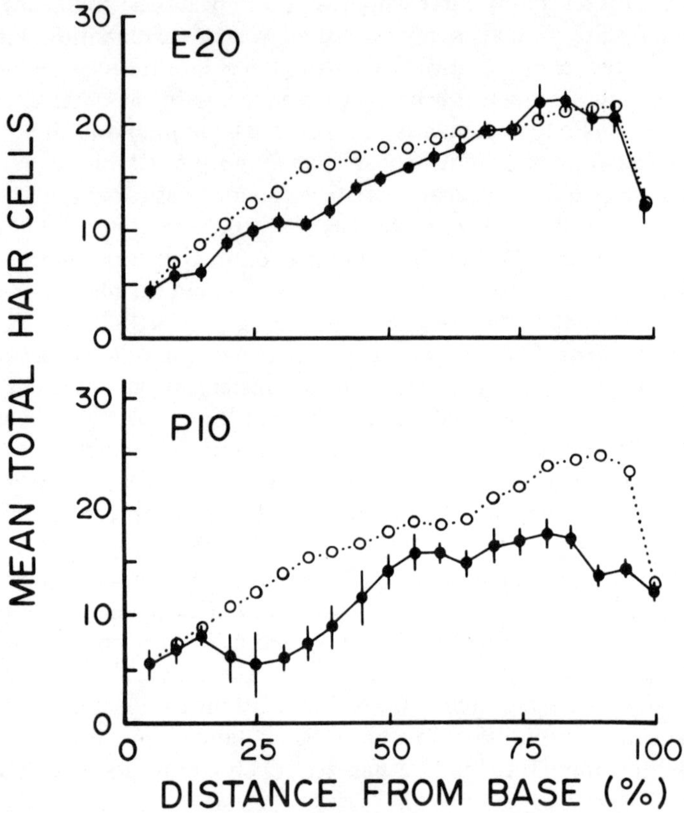

Figure 19. Mean total number of hair cells (± 1 S.E.M.) is plotted as a function of percent distance along the papilla in chicks exposed at either 20 days of embryonic development (E20) or 10 days after hatching (P10) to broad-band white noise at 125 dB SPL for 12 hours. Open circles show the average number of hair cells in control birds. Damage is confined to approximately the basal half of the papilla in embryos but extends to include more apical locations in the posthatch birds. (Reproduced from Ryals & Rubel, 1985, Fig. 8, by permission of the publisher.)

SPECIES GENERALITY

The model of a changing place code has been tested mainly in chickens. Is this process specific to birds? Several lines of evidence indicate that it is not. An ontogenetic shift in the cochlear frequency map appears to be general across vertebrate species.

First, the paradoxical dissociation between cochlear development and functional ontogeny described earlier is universal across species. Second, results suggesting that the tonotopic organization within the central auditory system changes during development have also been reported for cats and gerbils. The findings of Pujol and Marty, described previously, indicate that regions of auditory cortex which respond to high frequency sounds in adult cats are activated by relatively low frequencies in kittens (Pujol & Marty, 1968). Ryan and Woolf (1985) have reported similar findings in their 2-deoxy-glucose studies of the development of tonotopic organization in the gerbil. Figure 20 shows representative radiographs through the cochlear nuclei of adult and 12 day-old gerbils that were exposed to either a 0.75-kHz, 3.0-kHz,

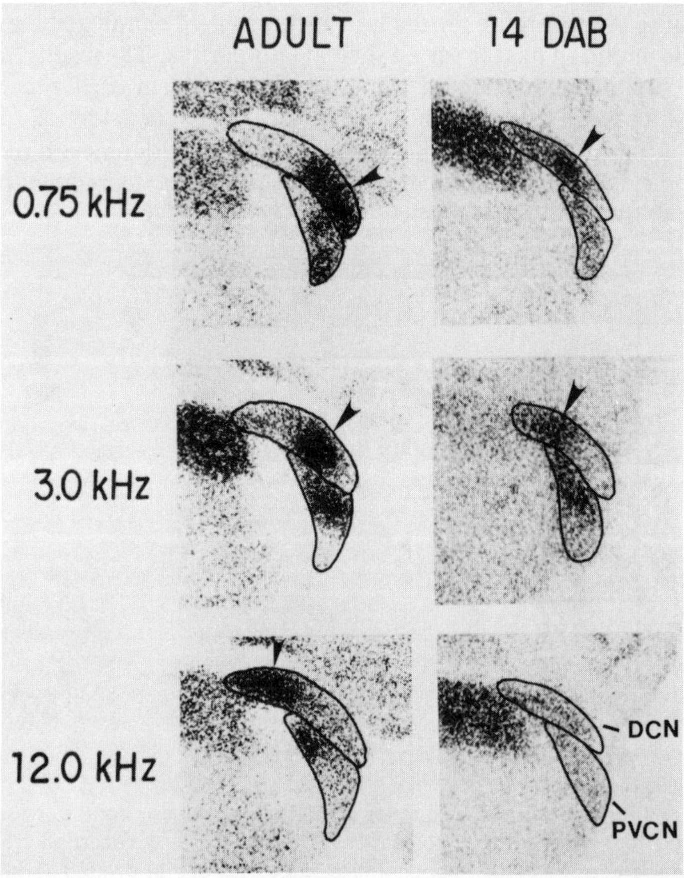

Figure 20. Radiographs showing the distribution of 2-deoxy-glucose uptake (dark areas) in the posterior ventral (PVCN) and dorsal (DCN) cochlear nuclei of adult and 14-day-old gerbils after exposure to 0.75-kHz, 3.0-kHz, or 12.0-kHz tones. The arrows indicate the region of maximum uptake in the DCN for each exposure condition. Note that the same region of the DCN is "marked" by lower-frequency sounds in the 14-day-old gerbils than in the adults. (Reproduced from Ryan & Woolf, 1985, by permission of the publisher.)

or 12.0-kHz tone. Comparison of the radiographs between the two ages shows that the region of the dorsal cochlear nucleus which increases its metabolic activity (glucose uptake) in response to a given frequency of stimulation changes during development. The regions that are "marked" by the 0.75-kHz and 3.0-kHz tones in the immature gerbil respond to higher-frequency sounds in the adult. Third, Harris and Dallos (1984) have recently examined the development of place coding in the gerbil cochlea. They compared the best frequency of the cochlear microphonic recorded from the midbasal turn of the cochlea in animals at different ages. This study is particularly important, because the recording procedure which was used eliminated the influence of the maturing middle ear on their measurements. The results of their study are summarized in Figure 21. It shows that the cut-off frequency or most sensitive frequency at their recording location in the midbasal turn increased during development. This finding is probably the most direct and convincing evidence to date that changes in frequency representation are occurring at the level of the cochlea.

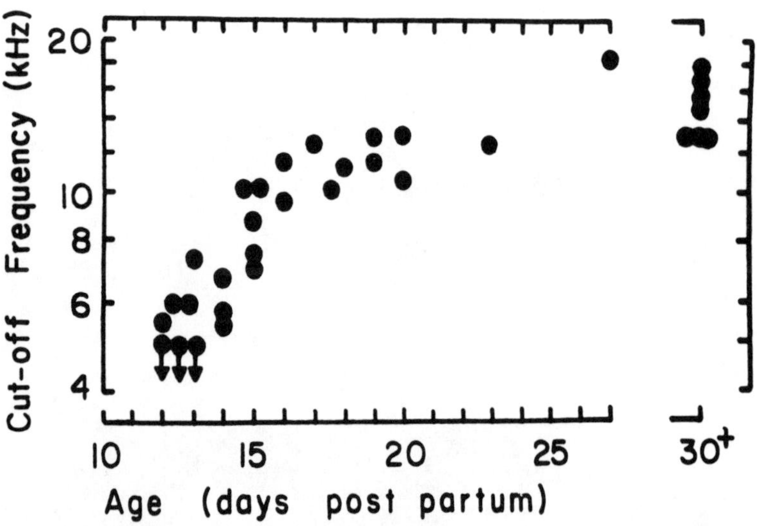

Figure 21. Change in cut-off frequency of the cochlear microphonic as a function of age. Cochlear microphonic iso-response functions were recorded from an intracochlear electrode in the midbasal turn of a series of age-graded gerbils and subtracted from similar functions recorded from the round window. The difference between these two functions provides a measure of the frequency sensitivity at the intracochlear recording site, which is independent of the frequency characteristics of the developing middle ear. The results show that the cut-off frequency increases systematically during development. (Reproduced from Harris & Dallos, 1984, Fig. 2, by permission of the publisher.)

MECHANISMS UNDERLYING A SHIFT IN THE PLACE CODE

The mechanism or mechanisms which underlie the ontogenetic change in frequency representation along the cochlea are presently unknown and a matter of speculation. Future studies which correlate quantitative measurements of the morphological development of the cochlear partition with functional measures of shifts in the cochlear place code will provide important insights. However, on the basis of what is presently known about frequency representation in the adult, we can speculate about the processes which might be involved.

The spatial coding of sound frequency along the cochlear partition has classically been attributed to the graded elasticity of the basilar membrane and its traveling wave vibration to sound (von Békésy, 1960; Dallos, 1981). Thus, maturational changes in the mechanical properties of the basilar membrane would seem to be the most likely explanation for a shifting place code. Several investigators have described developmental changes in cellular structure which would likely affect the response of the basilar membrane to sound (Kraus & Aulbach-Kraus, 1981; Pujol & Marty, 1970; see Romand, 1983, for a recent review of this literature). There is a progressive thinning of the basilar membrane and its associated epithelial layer. The loss of internal spiral sulcus cells results in the formation of the internal spiral sulcus and the freeing of the tectorial membrane. At the same time, the tunnel of Corti gradually enlarges, and the pillar cells move apart and change their orientation. Concommitant with this loss of cellular structure, filaments form and gather into bundles in both the basilar membrane and pillar cells. The effect of these structural changes on the transduction properties of the cochlear partition and tuning is not known. However, it seems reasonable that the increase in stiffness and decrease in mass which are implied by several of these changes might shift the resonance at any point along the cochlear partition to progressively higher-frequency sounds during development (Kraus & Aulbach-Kraus, 1981; Harris & Dallos, 1984).

Age-related changes in the mechanical properties of sensory hair cell bundles might also contribute to an ontogenetic shift in the cochlear place code. In several nonmammalian vertebrates which lack a traveling wave of basilar membrane motion, tonotopic organization and frequency tuning likely result from the tuned mechanical resonance of sensory hair cells whose cilia are graded in length (Holton & Hudspeth, 1983; Peake & Ling, 1980; Weiss, Peake, Ling, & Holton, 1978; Turner, Muraski, & Nielson, 1981). Sensory hair cell mechanical tuning has not yet been demonstrated in either the mammalian or avian cochlea. However, several lines of evidence make it likely that stereocilia contribute to frequency selectivity and representation in these species as well: (a) a progressive gradation in stereocilia height, similar to that which underlies tuned mechanical resonance in nonmammalian vertebrates, also occurs along the length of the cochlea in the chinchilla (Lim, 1980), mouse (Garfinkle & Saunders, 1983), bird (Tilney & Saunders, 1983), human (Wright, 1981), and guinea pig (Strelioff & Flock, 1984); (b) in guinea pigs, the stiffness of sensory hair cell bundles decreases progressively from base to apex (Strelioff & Flock, 1984), and (c) various manipulations which alter neural tuning also affect the rigidity of stereocilia (Hunter-Duvar, & Mount, 1977; Tilney et al., 1982). In view of these observatons, future studies of the developmental relationships between the structure and physical properties of stereocilia and frequency tuning will be important.

Finally, the possible contribution of active or energy dependent processes needs to be considered (Gold, 1948; Davis, 1983). Several findings indicate that the vibration of the basilar membrane is affected by physiological processes in the organ of Corti, possibly mediated via the efferent innervation of the outer hair cells (Mountain, 1980; Siegel & Kim, 1982; Brownell, Bader, Bertrand, & de Ribaupierre, 1985). Two findings should be noted in this context. First, the efferent innervation and synaptology of the outer hair cells are still changing well after the onset of hearing (Pujol, Carlier, & Devigne, 1978; Pujol, Carlier, & Lenoir, 1980). Second, the location of maximum vibration of the traveling wave along the basilar membrane to a given frequency is "physiologically vulnerable," i.e., it is altered by conditions which would likely affect physiological processes (Rhode, 1973; Khanna & Leonard, 1982; Kelly & Khanna, 1984; Kohllöffel, 1972b, 1972c). Thus, it is tempting to speculate that physiological processes mediated via the efferent outer-hair-cell system might systematically alter basilar membrane mechanics during development. Whether active processes affect the cochlear place code in this manner or by some other mechanism remains an important question for future studies.

IMPLICATIONS

What are the implications of an ontogenetic shift in frequency representation along the cochlear partition? First, it helps explain the curious incongruity between the basal-to-apical gradient or morphological development along the cochlea and the low-to-high frequency order of physiological and behavioral maturation. Second, it implies that neurons within the central auditory system will be maximally stimulated by different frequency sounds at different times during development. Looked at slightly differently, each cochleotopic region within the nervous system will be maximally stimulated by low frequency sounds at some stage during ontogeny. In this context it is interesting to note that the early acoustic environment of young organisms, whether it be in an egg or *in utero,* is dominated by relatively low-frequency sounds (Walker, Grimwade, & Wood, 1971; Armitage, Baldwin, & Vince, 1980; Grimwade, Walker, Bartlett, Gordon, & Wood, 1971). Figure 22 illustrates this finding for the human fetus. The ambient *in utero* sound pressure level (dashed line; left vertical axis) and the amount of attenuation of sound by the maternal body wall (solid line; right vertical axis) are plotted as a function of sound frequency. These functions indicate that both the spectrum of internally generated sounds (heart beat, fetal movement, etc.) as well as the attenuation of sounds from outside the mother to the uterus favor low frequencies. The consequence is that between the time that the human is first capable of hearing at approximately 26 weeks of gestation until birth at 40 weeks, it is exposed to predominantly low frequency sounds. Several studies have now demonstrated that in the auditory system the normal development of physiological response properties (Clopton & Winfield, 1976; Clopton & Silverman, 1977, 1978; Silverman & Clopton, 1977), neural structure (Webster & Webster, 1979; Coleman & O'Connor, 1979; Feng & Rogowski, 1980;

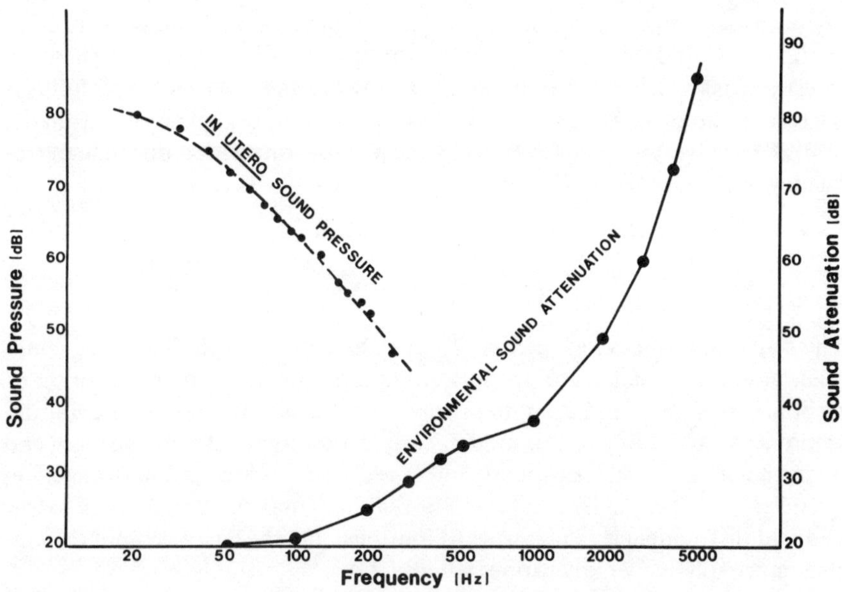

Figure 22. Intrauterine acoustic environment of the human fetus. The curve to the left shows the ambient level of intrauterine noise and the right-hand curve shows the attenuation of externally produced sound by the maternal tissues. Both sets of measurements were obtained from condenser microphones that were placed within the uterine cavity of 16 pregnant and 7 nonpregnant women. The functions indicate that predominantly low frequency sounds are available to the fetus. Similar findings have been reported from hydrophones implanted inside the intact amniotic sac of fetal sheep (Armitage et al., 1980). (Adapted from Walker et al., 1971, Figs. 2 and 3, by permission of the publisher.)

Conlee & Parks, 1981; Gray, Smith, & Rubel, 1982) and perceptual behavior (Tees, 1967; Gottlieb, 1976; Clements & Kelly, 1978; Kerr et al., 1979; Knudsen, Knudsen, & Esterly, 1982) depend upon early sensory stimulation. Thus, it is tempting to speculate that a change in spatial coding along the cochlear partition may be a mechanism to ensure that normally occurring low frequency sounds provide stimulation necessary for normal development to *all* tonotopic regions in central auditory nuclei and not only to those regions which are maximally sensitive to low frequencies in the adult.

Third, and probably most notably, a change in the spatial coding of frequency during development indicates that the values assigned to the place code are not necessarily fixed and immutable. This raises the possibility that the place code may change or be altered under other conditions as well as during normal development. For example, there is circumstantial evidence that the representation of frequency along the cochlea may be altered by trauma resulting from exposure to aminoglycoside antibiotics (Robertson & Johnstone, 1979) and high-intensity sound (Ades et al., 1974). The possibility that the place code may shift during the normal process of aging is even more intriguing. Could this account, in part, for the loss of high-frequency hearing (presbycusis) which commonly occurs during old age? Consistent with this is the recent finding of Willott (1982) that the tonotopic organization within the central nervous system appears to change in aging rats with reduced high frequency sensitivity.

CONCLUSIONS

The discrepancy between the base-to-apex order of morphological development along the cochlea and the low-to-high frequency sequence of onset of responsiveness to sound led us to propose that the place code shifts during development. According to this model, early in development only the basal end of the cochlea transduces sound, but it responds to low and midrange frequencies. As the organism matures, the region of maximum sensitivity to low and middle frequencies shifts toward the apex, and the base becomes responsive to progressively higher tones (Figure 23).

Various experimental approaches, including acoustic overstimulation, mapping of tonotopic organization within the central auditory pathway, and measurement of the cut-off frequency of the cochlear microphonic have been used in both birds and mammals to test this model. The results of all these studies have strongly supported the conclusion that the spatial coding of sound frequency along the cochlea changes during development in a manner that is predicted by the model. On the other hand, that part of the model which hypothesizes that the apical region of the cochlea does not respond to

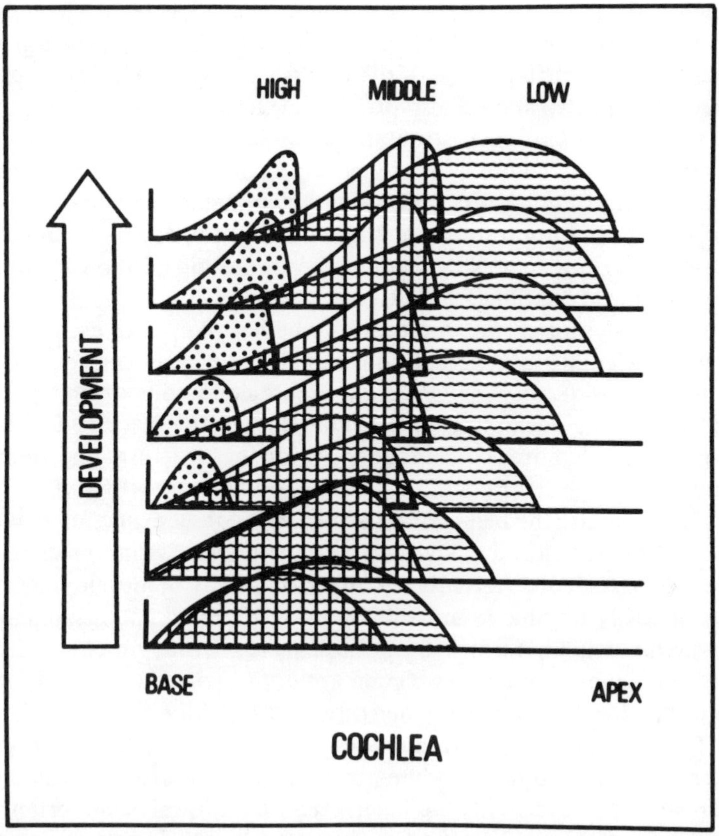

Figure 23. Schematic representation of the hypothesized shift in the position of the traveling wave during development for high, middle, and low frequency sounds. See text for details. (Adapted from Rubel et al., 1984, Fig. 6, by permission of the publisher.)

sound during the early development of hearing has not yet been addressed and needs to be examined.

The mechanism(s) which underlie the shift in the place code will be an important question for future studies. Our ideas and experimental approaches will change as new mechanisms for the spatial coding of sound frequency along the mature cochlea are uncovered (Weiss et al., 1978; Crawford & Fettiplace, 1980). Developmental studies which correlate changes in the structure and dimensional characteristics (e.g., mass and stiffness) of the cochlear partition with shifts in frequency representation should provide important insights. The recent development of *in vitro* techniques for studying hair cell mechanics will be especially valuable (Strelioff & Flock, 1984;

Brownell et al., 1985). Comparative studies between species in which the spatial coding of frequency undergoes a shift during development but whose cochlear structure differs (e.g., birds lack a true organ of Corti with inner and outer pillar cells) should also provide suggestions as to possible mechanisms and rule out particular structures as being essential for a change in the place code. In this context, it will be especially interesting to determine whether the place code shifts in those nonmammalian vertebrates in which tonotopic organization results from the resonant properties of hair cells and not from a traveling wave of basilar membrane motion (Holton & Hudspeth, 1983; Crawford & Fettiplace, 1980).

As previously noted, the question of whether the values assigned to the place code shift under other conditions as well as during normal development needs to be considered. Conversely, are there conditions or manipulations which prevent the normal developmental shift in the place code from occurring? If so, what are the consequences for the structural and functional development of the central auditory pathway and for hearing?

Finally, what are the behavioral (perceptual) consequences of a changing place code? One obvious but "bothersome" prediction is that the same sound should be perceived differently at different stages of development. This should be easily testable in animals by using standard conditioning procedures. In this context, it is worth emphasizing again that present evidence indicates that changes in the place code are *not* restricted to the very earliest stages of hearing development, when thresholds are high and sound likely has little effect on the developing auditory system. In both birds and gerbils, changes continue into the very late period of hearing development and past the time that adult sensitivity has been established. It will be important to determine the generality of this finding in other species. However, on the basis of current data it seems likely that changes in the place code are still occurring after birth in humans (Hecox, 1975). This raises important questions about the role of a changing place code in hearing and language development in infants and children. This as well as the other implications already outlined, need to be examined critically in future studies.

REFERENCES

Ades, H.W., Trahiotis, C., Kokko-Cunningham, A., & Averbuch, A. (1974). Comparison of hearing thresholds and morphological changes in the chinchilla after exposure to 4kHz tones. *Acta Otolaryngologica (Stockholm), 78,* 192–206.

Aitkin, L.M., Anderson, D.J., & Brugge, J.F. (1970). Tonotopic organization and discharge characteristics of single neurons in nuclei of the lateral lemniscus of the cat. *Journal of Neurophysiology, 33,* 421–440.

Aitkin, L.M., & Moore, D.R. (1975). Inferior colliculus. II. Development of tuning characteristics and tonotopic organization in the central nucleus of the neonatal cat. *Journal of Neurophysiology, 38,* 1208–1216.

Aitkin, L.M., & Webster, W.R. (1971). Tonotopic organization in the medial geniculate body of the cat. *Brain Research, 26,* 402–405.

Ånggard, L. (1965). An electrophysiological study of the development of cochlear function in the rabbit. *Acta Otolaryngologica (Stockholm), Supplement, 203,* 1–64.

Anniko, M. (1983). Early development and maturation of the spiral ganglion. *Acta Otolaryngologica (Stockholm), 95,* 263–276.

Armitage, S.E., Baldwin, B.A., & Vince, M.A. (1980). The fetal sound environment of sheep. *Science, 208,* 1173–1174.

Bast, T.H., & Anson, B.J. (1949). *The temporal bone and the ear.* Springfield, IL: Thomas.

Bauhin, Casper (1605). *Theatrum anatomicum [The Anatomical Theater].* Frauncofurti at Moenum.

Boord, R.L., & Rasmussen, G.L. (1963). Projection of the cochlear and lagenar nerves on the cochlear nuclei of the pigeon. *Journal of Comparative Neurology, 120,* 463–475.

Boring, E.G. (1942). *Sensation and perception in the history of experimental psychology.* New York: Appleton-Century-Crofts.

Bredberg, G. (1968). Cellular pattern and nerve supply of the human organ of Corti. *Acta Otolaryngologica (Stockholm), Supplement, 236,* 1–135.

Brownell, W.E., Bader, C.R., Bertrand, D., & de Ribaupierre, Y. (1985). Evoked mechanical responses of isolated cochlear outer hair cells. *Science,* 227, 194–196.

Brugge, J.F., Javel, E., & Kitzes, L.M. (1978). Signs of functional maturation of peripheral auditory system in discharge patterns of neurons in anteroventral cochlear nucleus of kittens. *Journal of Neurophysiology, 41,* 1557–1579.

Carterette, E.C. (1978). Some historical notes on research in hearing. In C. Carterette & M.P. Friedman (Eds.), *Handbook of perception. Volume 4.* (pp. 3–39). *Hearing.* New York: Academic.

Chandler, J.P. (1984). Light and electron microscopic studies of the basilar papilla in the duck, *Anas platyrhynchos.* II. Embryonic development. *Journal of Comparative Neurology, 222,* 523–542.

Claudius, M. (1856). Bemerkungen über den Bau der häutigen Spiralleiste der Schnecke [Remarks on the structure of the cutaneous spiral moulding of the snail], *Zeitschrift für wissenschaftliche Zooligie, 7,* 154–161.

Clements, C., & Kelly, J.B. (1978). Auditory spatial responses of young guinea pigs (*Cavia porcellus*) during and after ear blocking. *Journal of Comparative Physiology, 92,* 34–44.

Clopton, B.M., & Silverman, M.S. (1977). Plasticity of binaural interaction. II. Critical period and changes in midline response. *Journal of Neurophysiology, 40,* 1275–1280.

Clopton, B.M., & Silverman, M.S. (1978). Changes in latency and duration of neural responding following developmental auditory deprivation. *Experimental Brain Research, 32,* 39–47.

Clopton, B.M., & Winfield, J.A. (1976). Effect of early exposure to patterned sound on unit activity in rat inferior colliculus. *Journal of Neurophysiology, 39,* 1081–1089.

Cohen, G.M., & Fermin, C.D. (1978). The development of hair cells in the embryonic chick's basilar papilla. *Acta Otolaryngologica (Stockholm), 86,* 342–358.

Coleman, J.R., & O'Connor, P. (1979). Effects of monaural and binaural sound deprivation on cell development in the anteroventral cochlear nucleus of rats. *Experimental Neurology, 64,* 553–566.

Conlee, J.W., & Parks, T.N. (1981). Age- and position-dependent effects of monaural acoustic deprivation in nucleus magnocellularis of the chicken. *Journal of Comparative Neurology,* 202, 373–384.

Corti, Alphonse (1851). Recherches sur l'organe de l'ouïe des mammifères [Research on the gill organ of mammals]. *Zeitschrift für wissenschaftliche Zooligie, 3,* 109–169.

Crawford, A.C., & Fettiplace, R. (1980). The frequency selectivity of auditory nerve fibres and hair cells in the cochlea of the turtle. *Journal of Physiology,* 306, 79–125.

Crowley, D.E., & Hepp-Reymond, M.C. (1966). Development of cochlea function in the ear of the infant rat. *Journal of Comparative and Physiological Psychology, 62,* 427–432.

Dallos, P. (1981). Cochlear physiology. *Annual Review of Psychology, 32,* 153–190.

Davis, H. (1973). Introduction: v. Békésy. In R. Moller (Ed.), *Basic mechanisms in hearing* (pp. 1–7). New York: Academic.

Davis, H. (1983). An active process in cochlear mechanics. *Hearing Research, 9,* 79–90.

Deiters, Otto (1860). Untersuchungen über die Lamina spirals membranacea [Investigations on the lamina of the spiral membrane]. Bonn.

Du Verney, Joseph, G. (1683). *Traité de l'organe de l'ouie [Treatis on the gill].* Paris.

Easter, S.S., Jr., & Stuermer, C.A.O. (1984). An evaluation of the hypothesis of shifting terminals in goldfish optic tectum. *Journal of Neuroscience, 4,* 1052–1063.

Ehret, G. (1983). Development of hearing and response behavior to sound stimuli: Behavioral studies. In R. Romand (Ed.), *Development of auditory and vestibular systems* (pp. 211–237). New York: Academic.

Ehret, G., & Romand, R. (1981). Postnatal development of absolute auditory thresholds in kittens. *Journal of Comparative and Physiolgoical Psychology, 95,* 304–311.

Feng, A.S., & Rogowski, B.A. (1980). Effects of monaural and binaural occlusion on the morphology of neurons in the medial superior olivary nucleus of the rat. *Brain Research, 189,* 530–534.

Fermin, C.D., & Cohen, G.M. (1984). Developmental gradients in the embryonic chick's basilar papilla. *Acta Otolaryngologica (Stockholm), 97,* 39–51.

Finck, A., Schneck, C.D., & Hartman, A.F. (1972). Development of cochlear function in the neonate Mongolian gerbil (*Merinoes unguiculatis*). *Journal of Comparative and Physiological Psychology, 78,* 375–380.

Fourier, J.B.J. (1982a). La théorie analytique de la chaleur [Analytic theory of heat]. *Academei des sciences, Paris, Member of the Royal Academy of Science, 8,* 581–622.

Garfinkle, T.J., & Saunders, J.C. (1983). Morphology of inner hair cell stereocilia in C57BL/6J mice as studied by scanning electron microscopy. *Otolaryngology—Head and Neck surgery, 91,* 421–426.

Gaze, R.M., Chung, S.H., & Keating, M.J. (1972). Development of the retinotectal projection in *Xenopus. Nature (New Biology.), 236,* 133–135.

Gaze, R.M., Keating, M.J., & Chung, S.H. (1974). The evolution of the retinotectal map during development in *Xenopus. Proceedings of the Royal Society of London (Biology), 185,* 301–330.

Gold, T. (1948). The physical basis of the action of the cochlea. *Proceedings of the Royal Society of London (Series B.), 135,* 492–498.

Goldberg, J.M., & Brown, P.B. (1968). Functional organization of the dog superior olivary complex: An anatomical and electrophysiological study. *Journal of Neurophysiology, 31,* 639–656.

Gottlieb, G. (1971). Ontogenesis of sensory function in birds and mammals. In E. Tobach, L.A. Aronson, & E. Shaw (Eds.), *The biopsychology of development* (pp. 67–128). New York: Academic.

Gottlieb, G. (1976). Early development of species-specific auditory perception in birds. In G. Gottlieb (Ed.), *Neural and behavioral specificity. Studies on development of behavior and the nervous system (Vol. 3) (pp. 237–280).* New York: Academic.

Gray, L.C., & Rubel, E.W. (1981). Development of responsiveness to suprathreshold acoustic stimulation in chickens. *Journal of Comparative and Phsyiological Psychology, 95,* 188–198.

Gray, L.C., & Rubel, E.W. (1985). Development of absolute thresholds in chickens. *Journal of the Acoustical Society of America, 77,* 1162–1172.

Gray, L., Smith, Z., & Rubel, E.W. (1982). Developmental and experiential changes in dendritic symmetry in n. laminaris of the chick. *Brain Research, 244,* 360–364.

Grimwade, J.C., Walker, D.W., Bartlett, M., Gordon., S., & Wood, C. (1971). Human fetal heart rate change and movement in response to sound and vibration. *American Journal of Obstetrics and Gynecology, 109,* 86–90.

Harris, D.M., & Dallos, P. (1984). Ontogenetic changes in frequency mapping in a mammalian ear. *Science, 225,* 741–743.

Hasse, Carl (1867). Die Schnecke der Vögel (Cochlea of birds). *Zeitschrift für wissenschaftliche Zooligie, 17,* 56–104.

Hecox, K. (1975). Electrophysiological correlates of human auditory development. In L.B. Cohen & C.P. Salaptek (Eds.), *Infant perception: From sensation to cognition. (Vol. 2)* (pp. 151–191). New York: Academic.

Hensen, V. (1863). Zur Morphologie der Schnecke des Menschen und der Säugethiere [Concerning the morphology of the human and mammalian cochlea]. *Zeitschrift für wissenschaftliche Zooligie, 13,* 481–512.

Hirokawa, N. (1978). Synaptogenesis in the basilar papilla of the chick. *Journal of Neurocytology, 1,* 283–300.

Holton, T., & Hudspeth, A.J. (1983). A micromechanical contribution to cochlear tuning and tonotopic organization. *Science, 222,* 508–510.

Hunter-Duvar, I.M., & Mount, R.J. (1977). Morphology of the normal and the acoustically damaged cochlea. *SEM/1977/II* (pp. 421–428). Chicago, IL: IIT Research Institute.

Jaskson, H., & Rubel, E.W. (1978). Ontogeny of behavioral responsiveness to sound in the chick embryo as indicated by electrical recordings of motility. *Journal of Comparative and Physiological Psychology, 92,* 680–694.

Jackoll, T.F., & Maderson, P.A. (1978). A histological study of the development of the avian middle ear and tympanum. *Anatomical Record, 190,* 17–199.

Jhaveri, S.R. & Morest, D.K. (1982). Neuronal architecture in nucleus magnocellularis of the chicken with observations on nucleus laminaris: A light and electron microscope study. *Neuroscience, 7,* 809–835.

Johnstone, B.M., Taylor, K.J., & Boyle, A.J. (1970). Mechanics of the guinea pig cochlea. *Journal of the Acoustical Society of America, 47,* 504–509.

Kelly, J.P., & Khanna, S.M. (1984). Ultrastructural damage in cochleas used for studies of basilar membrane mechanics. *Hearing Research, 14,* 59–78.

Kerr, L.M., Ostapoff, M., & Rubel, E.W. (1979). Influence of acoustic experience on the ontogeny of frequency generalization gradients in the chicken. *Journal of Experimental Psychology, 5,* 97–115.

Khanna, S.M., & Leonard, D.G.B. (1982). Basilar membrane tuning in the cat cochlea. *Science, 215,* 305–306.

Kikuchi, K., & Hilding, D. (1965). The development of the organ of Corti in the mouse. *Acta Otolaryngologica (Stockholm), 60,* 207–222.

Knudsen, E.I., Knudsen, P.F., & Esterly, S.D. (1982). Early auditory experience modifies sound localization in barn owls. *Nature, 295,* 238–240.

Kohllöffel, L.U.E. (1972a). A study of basilar membrane vibrations I. Fuzziness-detection: A new method for the analysis of microvibrations with laser light. *Acustica, 27,* 49–65.

Kohllöffel, L.U.E. (1972b). A study of basilar membrane vibrations II. The vibratory amplitude and phase pattern along the basilar membrane (postmortem). *Acustica, 27,* 66–81.

Kohllöffel, L.U.E. (1972c). A study of basilar membrane vibrations III. The basilar-membrane frequency response curve in the living guinea pig. *Acustica, 27,* 82–89.

Kraus, H.J., & Aulbach-Kraus, K. (1981). Morphological changes in the cochlea of the mouse after the onset of hearing. *Hearing Research, 4,* 89–102.

Larsell, O., McCrady, E., & Larsell, J.F. (1944). Development of the organ of Corti in relation to the inception of hearing. *Archives of Otolaryngology, 40,* 233–248.

Lim, D.J. (1980). Cochlear anatomy related to cochlear micromechanics: A review. *Journal of the Acoustical Society of America, 67,* 1686–1695.

Lippe W.R., & Rubel, E.W. (1983). Development of the place principle: Tonotopic organization. *Science, 219,* 514–516.

Lippe, W.R., & Rubel, E.W. (1985). Ontogeny of tonotopic organization of brain stem auditory nuclei in the chicken: Implications for development of the place principle. *Journal of Comparative Neurology, 237,* 273–289.

Longley, A. (1978). Anatomical mapping of retino-tectal connections in developing and metamorphosed *Xenopus*: Evidence for changing connections. *Journal of Embryology and Experimental Morphology, 45,* 249–270.

Mikaelin, D., & Ruben, R.J. (1965). Development of hearing in the normal CBA-J mouse: Correlation of physiological observations with behavioral responses and with cochlear anatomy. *Acta Otolaryngologica (Stockholm), 59,* 451–461.

Moore, D.R., & Irvine, D.R.F. (1979). The development of some peripheral and central auditory responses in the neonatal cat. *Brain Research, 163,* 49–59.

Mountain, D.C. (1980). Changes in endolymphatic potential and crossed olivocochlear bundle stimulation alter cochlear mechanics. *Science, 210,* 71–71.

Müller, Johannes (1838). *Handbook der Physiologie des Menschen* [Handbook of the physiology of humans], II, book 5.

Ohm, G.S. (1843). Ueber die Definition des Tones, nebst daran geknüpfter Theorie der Sirene und ähnlicher tonbildener Vorrichtungen [On the definition of sound, in addition to related theories on the siren and similar sound producing mechanisms]. *Annalen des Physik, 59,* 497–565.

Parks, T.N., & Rubel, E.W. (1975). Organization and development of the brain stem auditory nuclei of the chicken: Organization of projections from n. magnocellularis to n. laminaris. *Journal of Comparative Neurology, 164,* 435–448.

Peake, W.T., & Ling, A., Jr. (1980). Basilar membrane motion in the alligator lizard: Its relation to tonotopic organization and frequency selectivity. *Journal of the Acoustical Society of America, 67,* 1736–1745.

Pickles, J.O. (1982). *An introduction to the physiology of hearing.* New York: Academic.

Pujol, R., & Abonnenc, M. (1977). Receptor naturationa and synaptogenesis in the golden hamster cochlea. *Archives of Oto-Rhino-Laryngology, 217,* 1–12.

Pujol, R., Carlier, E., & Devigne, C. (1978). Different patterns of cochlea innervation during the development of the kitten. *Journal of Comparative Neurology, 177,* 529–535.

Pujol, R., Carlier, E., & Lenoir, M. (1980). Ontogenetic approach to inner and outer hair cell function. *Hearing Research, 2,* 423–430.

Pujol, R., & Marty, R. (1968). Structural and physiological relationships of the maturing auditory system. In L. Vilek & S. Trojan (Eds.), *Ontogenesis of the brain.* Prague, Czechoslovakia: Charles University Press.

Pujol, R., & Marty, R. (1970). Postnatal maturation in the cochlea of the cat. *Journal of Comparative Neurology, 139,* 115–126.

Reale, R.A., & Imig, T.J. (1980). Tonotopic organization in auditory cortex of the cat. *Journal of Comparative Neurology, 192,* 265–291.

Rebillard, G., & Rubel, E.W. (1981). Electrophysiological study of the maturation of auditory responses from the inner ear of the chick. *Brain Research, 229,* 15–23.

Reh, T.A., & Constantine-Paton, M. (1984). Retinal ganglion cell terminals change their projection sites during laural development of *Rana pipiens. Journal of Neuroscience, 4,* 442–457.

Reissner, Ernest (1854). Zur Kenntniss der Schnecke im Gehörogan der Säugethiere und des Menschen [Concerning knowledge of the cochlea in the hearing organ of mammals and the human]. *Archi für anatomische Physiologie und wissenschaftliche Medizin,* 420–427.

Relkin, E.M., & Saunders, J.C. (1980). Displacement of the malleus in neonatal golden hamster. *Acta Otolaryngologica (Stockholm), 90,* 6–15.

Relkin, E.M., Saunders, J.C., & Konkle, D.F. (1979). The development of middle ear admittance in the hamster. *Journal of the Acoustical Society of America, 66,* 133–139.

Retzius, G. (1884). *Das gehororgan der wirbeltiere. II. Das gehorogan der reptillien, der vogel und saugetiere* [The hearing organ of vertebrates. II. The hearing organ of reptiles, birds and mammals]. Stockholm, Sweden: Samson & Wallin.

Rhode, W.S. (1971). Observations of the vibration of the basilar membrane in squirrel monkeys using the Mössbauer technique. *Journal of the Acoustical Society of America, 49,* 1218–1231.

Rhode, W.S. (1973). An investigation of post-mortem cochlear mechanisms using the Mössbauer effect. In A. Moller (Ed.), *Basic mechanisms in hearing* (pp. 49–67). New York: Academic.

Robertson, D., & Johnstone, B.M. (1979). Aberrant tonotopic organization in the inner ear damaged by Kanamycin. *Journal of the Acoustical Society of America, 66,* 466–469.

Romand, R. (1983). Development of the cochlea. In R. Romand (Ed.), *Development of auditory and vestibular systems* (pp. 47–88). New York: Academic.

Romand, R., & Romand, M.R. (1982). Myelination kinetics of spiral ganglion cells in kittens. *Journal of Comparative Neurology, 204,* 1–5.

Romand, R.A., Sans, M.R., & Marty, R. (1976). The structural maturation of the stato-acoustic nerve in the cat. *Journal of Comparative Neurology, 170,* 1–16.

Rose, J.E., Galambos, R., & Hughes, J.R. (1959). Microelectrode studies of the cochlear nuclei of the cat. *Bulletin of Johns Hopkins Hospital, 104,* 211–251.

Rose, J.E., Greenwood, D.D., Goldberg, J. M., & Hind, J.E. (1963). Some discharge characteristics of single neurons in the inferior celliculus of the cat. I. Tonotopical organization, relation of spike counts to tone intensity and firing patterns of single elements *Journal of Neurophysiology, 26,* 294–320.

Rubel, E.W. (1978). Ontogeny of structure and function in the vertebrate auditory system. In M. Jacobsen (Ed.), *Handbook of sensory physiology, Volume 9. Development of sensory systems.* (pp. 135–237). New York: Springer-Verlag.

Rubel, E.W. (1984). Ontogeny of auditory system function. *Annual Review of Physiology, 46,* 213–229.

Rubel, E.W., Lippe, W.R., & Ryals, B.M. (1984). Development of the place principle. *Annals of Otology, Rhinology and Laryngology, 93,* 609–615.

Rubel, E.W., & Parks, T.N. (1975). Organization and development of the brain stem auditory nuclei of the chicken: Tonotopic organization of N. magnocellularis and N. laminaris. *Journal of Comparative Neurology, 164,* 411–434.

Rubel, E.W., & Ryals, B.M. (1982). Patterns of hair cell loss in chick basilar papilla after intense auditory stimulation. Exposure duration and survival time. *Acta Otolaryngologica (Stockholm), 93,* 31–41.

Rubel, E.W., & Ryals, B.M. (1983). Development of the place principle: Acoustic trauma. *Science, 219,* 512–514.

Rubel, E.W., Smith, D.J., & Miller, L.C. (1976). Organization and development of the brain stem auditory nuclei of the chicken: Ontogeny of N. magnocellularis and N. laminaris *Journal of Comparative Neurology, 166,* 469–490.

Ryals, B.M. (1981). *Ontogenetic effects of acoustic trauma in chick basilar papilla,* Unpublished doctoral dissertation, University of Virginia, Charlottesville.

Ryals, B.M., Creech, H.B., & Rubel, E.W. (1984). Postnatal changes in the size of the avian cochlear duct. *Acta Otolaryngologica (Stockholm), 98,* 93–97.

Ryals, B.M., & Rubel, E.W. (1982). Patterns of hair cell loss in chick basilar papilla after intense auditory stimulation. Frequency organization. *Acta Otolaryngologica (Stockholm), 93,* 205–210.

Ryals, B.M., & Rubel, E.W. (1985). Ontogenetic changes in the position of hair cell loss after acoustic overstimulation in avian basilar papilla. *Hearing Research, 19,* 135–142.

Ryan, A.F., & Woolf, N.K. (in press). Development of tonotopic organization in the mongolian gerbil: A 2-deoxyglucose study. *Experimental Brain Research.*

Saunders, J.C., Coles, R.B., & Gates, G.R. (1973). The development of auditory evoked responses in the cochlea and cochlear nuclei of the chick. *Brain Research, 63,* 59–74.

Saunders, J.C., Kaltenbach, J.A., & Relkin, E.M. (1983). The structural and functional development of the outer and middle ear. In R. Romand (Ed.), *Development of auditory and vestibular systems* (pp. 3–25). New York: Academic.

Schubert, E.D. (1978). History of research on hearing. In C. Carterette & M.P. Friedman (Eds.), *Handbook of perception. Vol. IV. Hearing* (pp. 41–80). New York: Academic.

Schuknecht, J.F. (1953). Techniques for study of cochlear function and pathology in experimental animals. *Acta Otolaryngologica (Stockholm), 58,* 377.

Schuknecht, J.F. (1974). *Pathology of the ear.* Cambridge, MA: Harvard University Press.

Schweitzer, L., & Cant, N.B. (1984). Development of the cochlear innervation of the dorsal cochlear nucleus of the hamster. *Journal of Comparative Neurology, 225,* 228–243.

Siegel, J.H., & Kim, D.O. (1982). Efferent neural control of cochlear mechanics? Olivocochlear bundle stimulation affects cochlear biomechanical nonlinearity. *Hearing Research, 6,* 171–182.

Silverman, M.S., & Clopton, B.M. (1977). Plasticity of binaural interaction. I. Effect of early auditory deprivation. *Journal of Neurophysiology, 40,* 1266–1274.

Smith, Z.D.J. (1981). Organization and development of brain stem auditory nuclei of the chicken: Dendritic development of n. laminaris. *Journal of Comparative Neurology, 203,* 309–333.

Stockwell, W.W., Ades, H.W., & Engstrom, H. (1969). Patterns of hair cell damage after intense auditory stimulation. *Annals of Otology, Rhinology and Laryngology, 78,* 1144.

Strelioff, D., & Flock, Å. (1984). Stiffness of sensory-cell hair bundles in the isolated guinea pig cochlea. *Hearing Research, 151,* 19–28.

Tees, R.C. (1967). Effects of early auditory restriction in the rat on adult pattern discrimination. *Journal of Comparative and Physiological Psychology, 63,* 389–393.

Tilney, L.G. (1984). *The organization of actin filaments in stereocilia.* Paper presented at the Seventh Midwinter Research Meeting of the Association for Research in Otolaryngology, St. Petersburg, FL.

Tilney, L.G., Egelman, E., DeRosier, D.J., & Saunders, J.C. (1983). Actin filaments, stereocilia, and hair cells of the bird cochlea. II. Packing of actin filaments in the stereocilia and in the cuticular plate and what happens to the organization when the stereocilia are bent. *Journal of Cell Biology, 96,* 822–834.

Tilney, L.G., Saunders, J.C., Egelman, E., & DeRosier, D. J. (1982). Changes in the organization of actin filaments in the stereocilia of noise-damaged lizard cochleae. *Hearing Research, 7,* 181–197.

Tilney, L.G., & Saunders, J.C. (1983). Actin filaments, stereocilia, and hair cells of the bird cochlea I. Length, width, and distribution of stereocilia of each hair cell are related to the position of the hair cell on the cochlea. *Journal of Cell Biology, 96,* 807–821.

Tsuchitani, C., & Boudreau, J.C. (1966). Single unit analysis of cat superior olive S segment with tonal stimuli. *Journal of Neurophysiology, 29,* 684–697.

Turner, R.G., Muraski, A.A., & Nielson, D.W. (1981). Cilium length: Influence on neural tonotopic organization. *Science, 213,* 1519–1521.

Vanzulli, A., & Garcia-Austt, E. (1963). Development of cochlear microphonic potentials in the chick embryo. *Acta Neurophysiologica Latinoamerica, 9,* 19–23.

von Békésy, G. (1956). Current status of theories of hearing. *Science, 123,* 779–783.

von Békésy, G. (1960). *Experiments in hearing.* (E.G. Wever, Trans.). New York: McGraw Hill.

Wada, T., (1923). Anatomical and physiological studies on the growth of the inner ear of the albino rat. *American Anatomical Memoirs, 10,* 1–74.

Walker, D., Grimwade, J., & Wood, C. (1971). Intrauterine noise: A component of the fetal environment. *American Journal of Obstetrics and Gynecology, 109,* 91–95.

Webster, D.B., & Webster, M. (1972). Kangaroo rat auditory thresholds before and after middle ear reduction. *Brain, Behavior and Evolution, 5,* 41–53.

Webster, D.B., & Webster, M. (1979). Effects of neonatal conductive hearing loss on brainstem auditory nuclei. *Annals of Otology, Rhinology and Laryngology, 88,* 684–688.

Wever, E.G. (1949). *Theory of hearing.* New York: Wiley.

Weiss, T.F., Peake, W.T., Ling, A., Jr. & Holton, T. (1978). Which structures determine frequency selectivity and tonotopic organization of vertebrate cochlear nerve fibers? Evidence from the alligator lizard. In R. Naunton & C. Fernandez (Eds.), *Evoked electrical activity in the auditory nervous system* (pp. 91–112). New York: Academic.

Willott, J.F. (1982). Response changes of inferior colliculus neurons in aging C57BL/6 mice: Gains and losses. *Society for Neuroscience Abstracts, 8*(1), 443.

Wilson, J.P., & Johnstone, J.R. (1975). Basilar membrane and middle ear vibrations in guinea pig measured by capacitive probe. *Journal of the Acoustical Society of America,57,* 705;0723.

Woolf, N.K., & Ryan, A.F. (1984). The development of auditory function in the cochlea of the Mongolian gerbil. *Hearing Research, 13,* 277–283.

Woolsey, C.N. (1959). Organization of cortical auditory system: A review and a synthesis. In G.L. Rasmussen & W.F. Windle (Eds.), *Neural Mechanisms of the auditory and vestibular systems* (pp. 165–180). Springfield, IL: Thomas.

Wright, A. (1981). Scanning electron microscopy of the human cochlea-organ of Corti. *Archives of Otorhinolaryngology, 230,* 11–19.

8 The Development of Sound Localization and Auditory Processing in Mammals*

Jack B. Kelly
Department of Psychology
Carleton University
Ottawa, Canada, K1S 5B6

This chapter will review studies of the development of directional responses to sounds in mammals. Emphasis will be placed on investigations of the albino rat for which the most complete behavioral data are available. Where appropriate, comparisons among species will be made to illustrate the major dimensions of diversity among mammals or to establish the generality of observations and principles of development. The interpretation of directional responses depends upon what is known about the development of auditory sensitivity generally and structures involved in sound localization more specifically. The chapter will, therefore, provide a selective coverage of studies of the onset and development of cochlear and central nervous system function in the rat.

DEVELOPMENT OF COCHLEAR FUNCTION

In the rat the cochlear microphonic potential can be demonstrated first around 8–9 days after birth in response to intense acoustic stimuli of approximately 100–130 dB SPL (Crowley & Hepp-Raymond, 1966; Uziel, Romand, & Marot, 1981). At this age the range of sound frequencies capable of eliciting a response is limited, and the amplitude of the cochlear microphonic is quite small relative to adult values. Over the next few days the frequency range broadens, threshold sensitivity increases dramatically, and the amplitude of the microphonic response becomes greater. By 16 or 17 days of age this period of rapid change has begun to plateau. Under conditions of free-field stimulation, there is a particularly large shift in sensitivity of approximately 20–30 dB around days 12–13, which can be attributed to the opening of the external auditory meatus (see Fig. 1). Also, between days 9–17 there is

*The preparation of this chapter was supported by an operating grant from the Natural Sciences and Engineering Research Council of Canada (7654).

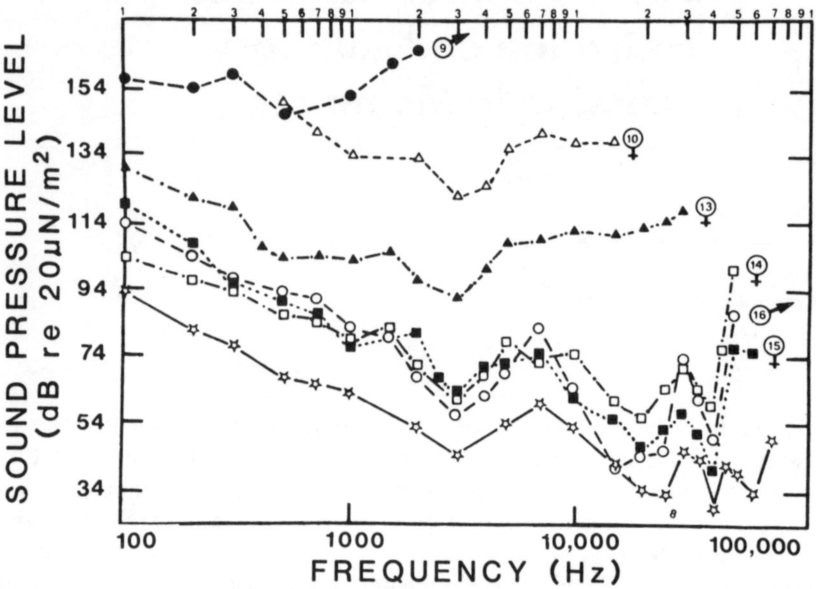

Figure 1. The development of cochlear microphonic responses is shown for albino rat pups from 9 to 16 days after birth. The sound pressure necessary to elicit a 1-mV microphonic response is indicated for a wide range of sound frequencies. An averaged adult curve (stars) is included for comparison with infant response data. Attention is drawn to the fact that sound pressure levels are expressed here with reference to $20\mu N/m^2$ (i.e., 0.0002 $dynes/cm^2$) rather than the 1 $dyne/cm^2$ used in the original study. (Adapted from Crowley & Hepp-Raymond, 1966, by permission of the publisher and authors; © 1966 by the American Psychological Association.)

a progressive shift in maximum sensitivity from low to high frequencies. For example, at postnatal days 9 to 13 the best frequencies for eliciting cochlear microphonic responses are less than 4 kHz, whereas at days 14 and 16 the best frequencies are closer to 20 kHz. There is clearly a tendency for low frequency responses to develop earlier in ontogeny than high frequency ones.

The low-to-high frequency sequence of functional development in the cochlea corresponds to a morphological development of the inner ear which proceeds from the basal turn of the cochlea toward the more apical turns (Wada, 1923). This correspondence of structure and function is paradoxical, because in the adult ear it is well established that the basal turns mediate responses to high frequency stimuli, whereas the apical turns are activated by low frequencies (see Rubel, 1978, pp. 174–178; Rubel, 1984; Lippe, Ryals, & Rubel, this volume, for further discussion). It seems likely that this discrepancy is related to mechanical differences between the infant and adult ears. Whatever the underlying basis for this phenomenon, however, it is clear that the earliest responses of infant rats are based upon low-frequency sensitivity mediated by the basal end of the cochlear partition.

The development of the summating and the endocochlear potentials closely parallels that of the cochlear microphonic (Romand, 1983). In the rat the endocochlear potential has been examined in detail by Schmidt and Fernández (1963) and Bosher and Warren (1971). As in the case of the cochlear microphonic, the magnitude of the potential is low during the period between 8 and 11 days and increases to near adult values between 11 and 16 days of age.

Also, the development of the eighth nerve action potential has been investigated in the rat by Carlier, Lenoir, and Pujol (1979) and Uziel et al. (1981). Recording the compound, or whole nerve, action potential from electrodes placed on the round window, these investigators have shown that the first responses to sounds occur around postnatal days 11–12 with sound pressure levels of approximately 100 dB. Over the next 10 days there is a rapid increase in the sensitivity of the response and a broadening of the range of effective stimuli for eliciting an action potential. There is also an increased sharpness of tuning for responses to specific frequencies as demonstrated by the effectiveness of a masking tone on action potentials elicited by a standard tone. The increase in tuning first appears around day 13 and achieves adult values around day 16 (Carlier et al., 1979). These studies support the generalization that the eighth-nerve action potential typically emerges one or two days after the cochlear microphonic response and thereafter follows a closely comparable rate of development (Romand, 1983).

Developmental changes are also seen in the wave form and latency of eighth-nerve action potentials. The earliest potentials are characterized by relatively slow wave forms and long latencies up to around day 13. Thereafter, both wave forms and latencies change progressively until they reach adult values around day 25 or 30. These changes occur independently of changes in threshold which are taking place at the same time (Uziel et al., 1981), and probably reflect a tendency toward greater synchrony of firing and faster conduction times in underlying neural elements. Such changes are highly significant for sound localization, which depends at least in part on the timing of physiological activity in the nervous system.

The general features of cochlear development in the rat are also found in other mammalian species. Opossum, guinea pig, gerbil, mouse, rabbit, cat, and dog all show a progressive increase in the sensitivity of the cochlear microphonic and a broadening of the effective frequency range as the animals grow older. Typically, sensitivity to a low- or low–middle range of frequencies appears first followed by an increased sensitivity to high frequencies, the gerbil being a possible exception to this pattern (Romand, 1983; Rubel, 1978). Pronounced differences among species are seen primarily in the age of onset and the rate of development of cochlear responses. For example, the age of initial appearance of the cochlear microphonic response ranges from before birth in highly precocial species such as the guinea pig or sheep to well after birth in altricial species such as the opossum, *Didelphis marsupialis,* with an onset as late as 59 days of age. Cochlear function in other species first appears at ages between these extremes. For example, cochlear microphonics have been recorded 2 days prior to birth in kittens, 4–5 days after birth in dogs and rabbits, 8–11 days after birth in various strains of mice, and around 12 days after birth in gerbils. In this context the rat can be considered a relatively altricial mammal.

Diversity is also found in the rate of functional development following initial responses. In this respect the rat shows an extremely rapid development of cochlear function reaching adult values in a period of approximately 1 week, compared, for example, to the much slower development found in the cat which requires approximately 3 weeks to obtain an equivalent degree of maturity (Bosher & Warren, 1971; Crowley & Hepp-Raymond, 1966; Fernández & Hinojosa, 1974; Pujol & Marty, 1970).

DEVELOPMENT OF CENTRAL AUDITORY FUNCTION

The development of the central auditory system has received considerable attention particularly in recent years. Studies of single neuronal responses in brainstem structures, primarily the cochlear nucleus and inferior colliculus, have been recently reviewed by Brugge (1983) and Moore (1983). Studies of the development of forebrain auditory responses, based largely on analysis of cortical evoked potentials, have also been recently reviewed by Mysliveĉek (1983). For the purpose of this chapter, it is important to point out that the rat has not been as thoroughly investigated as one might hope and that the experimental animal of preference has been the cat, probably because of the relatively enormous wealth of data on the physiological properties of the adult auditory system in that species. Nevertheless, it is possible to provide a general indication of the onset and development of central responses to sounds and to arrive at some general conclusions regarding the nature of changes which take place.

In the rat the ^{14}C-2-deoxyglucose method has been used to study the onset of auditory responses in the central nervous system. This method is based upon an autoradiographic analysis of the level of metabolic activity in central nervous system structures during sensory stimulation. Deoxyglucose, which is injected into the circulatory system just prior to stimulation, is distributed in the nervous system in proportion to the amount of local glucose utilization. Thus, comparison of the distribution of deoxyglucose in stimulated and unstimulated animals can provide an indication of the pattern of activity associated with sensory function (Plum, Gjedde, & Samson, 1976). Kelly and Skeen (1979; Kelly, 1981) have examined the metabolic response of 8-, 11-, 14-, 17-, 20-, and 30-day-old rat pups to 70-ms broadband noise bursts (2–32 kHz, 80 dB SPL) presented from an overhead loudspeaker at a rate of 5 to 10 per s. The animals were unanesthetized and were free to move about in a small cage located below the loudspeaker. For control purposes these animals were compared to animals which received no deliberate stimulation. In addition, for nonstimulated animals with open ear canals, the middle ear cavities were filled with an acrylic material to further reduce the possibility of auditory input. Following injections of deoxyglucose, animals were placed in a sound-attenuated chamber for 45 min during which they were exposed to either noise or silence. They were then removed and sacrificed under the influence of barbiturate anesthesia (Nembutal). Frontal sections of the brains of these animals were placed against the photographic emulsion of an x-ray film (SB-5), and the distribution of deoxyglucose was determined by the density of exposure of the film.

The differences between stimulated and nonstimulated animals were most pronounced in the cochlear nucleus and inferior colliculus. These structures typically showed high levels of metabolic activity in stimulated animals and provided a maximum contrast for evaluating developmental trends. Responses in forebrain auditory structures were less pronounced as can be seen in Figure 2.

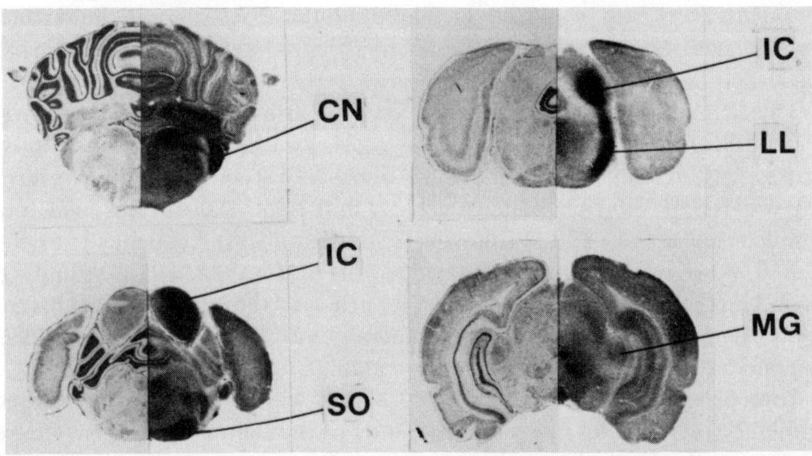

Figure 2. The pattern of deoxyglucose activity at different levels of the auditory system for a 17-day-old rat pup stimulated with broadband white noise pulses. The ^{14}C-deoxyglucose autoradiograph is shown on the right half of each of the four brain sections, and a cresyl violet stain of the corresponding neural tissue is shown on the left. The level of metabolic activity is reflected in the optical density of the autoradiograph. High levels of activity can be seen in the cochlear nucleus (CN), superior olivary complex (SO), lateral lemniscus (LL), and inferior colliculus (IC). In comparison, the level of activity in the medial geniculate (MG) was quite low. No consistent stimulus-induced response could be identified in the auditory cortex in our material.

Comparisons of stimulated and nonstimulated rat pups revealed no differences in the metabolic activity of auditory structures on days 8 or 11. The first evidence of stimulus-induced activity was seen in 14-day-old pups in both cochlear nucleus and inferior colliculus. At later ages, days 17, 20, 30, and 60, a more intense response was evident at both levels of the central auditory system.

These results have been confirmed by studies of rat pups between 11 and 16 days of age with one ear blocked using the previously described procedures (see Fig. 3). In these studies, direct comparison of deoxyglucose responses on the left and right sides of the brain permitted an assessment of the effect of stimulation on metabolic activity in the central auditory system. As in the previous study, no consistent left/right differences were seen in animals at 11 days of age. In older animals, increased metabolism was seen in the cochlear nucleus ipsilateral to the unblocked ear and in the inferior colliculus and medial geniculate nucleus contralateral to the unblocked ear. The exact age of onset of these stimulus-induced responses differed among individuals. The earliest response was found in a 12-day-old rat pup, but other animals failed to show definite responses by the twelfth or thirteenth days postpartum. By day 14, however, consistent stimulus-related metabolic differences were apparent. In every case, responses appeared simultaneously at each level of the auditory pathway with no indication of a sequential trend from caudal to rostral structures.

The first responses to appear in brainstem structures frequently showed some indication of being restricted in spatial location. For example, in the clearest case of limited responding, a binaurally stimulated 14-day-old rat pup was found to have a band of activity in the cochlear nucleus, which resembled that seen in adults following stimulation with frequency restricted stimuli. Also, on the contralateral side of the brain, there was a spatially localized increase in activity in the central nucleus of the inferior colliculus (see Fig. 4). The active area corresponds generally with regions in the adult which respond maximally to high frequency stimuli (Clopton & Winfield, 1973).

Comparing results of the deoxyglucose study with studies of cochlear function in the rat, it seems likely that the onset of the central nervous system response was determined largely by peripheral factors. Given that only moderate sound pressures were used in the deoxyglucose studies, the initiation of a central response around day 14 corresponds closely with the expected onset of cochlear potentials at the same sound pressure. Furthermore, the limited deoxyglucose response in the cochlear nucleus and inferior colliculus of day-14 animals might reflect a corresponding limitation in the response of the cochlea at this developmental period. It is difficult to infer from the central response exactly what the nature of the limitation at this age might be. Assuming that the topography of connections from the cochlea to brainstem is roughly comparable in infants and adults, one might speculate that the

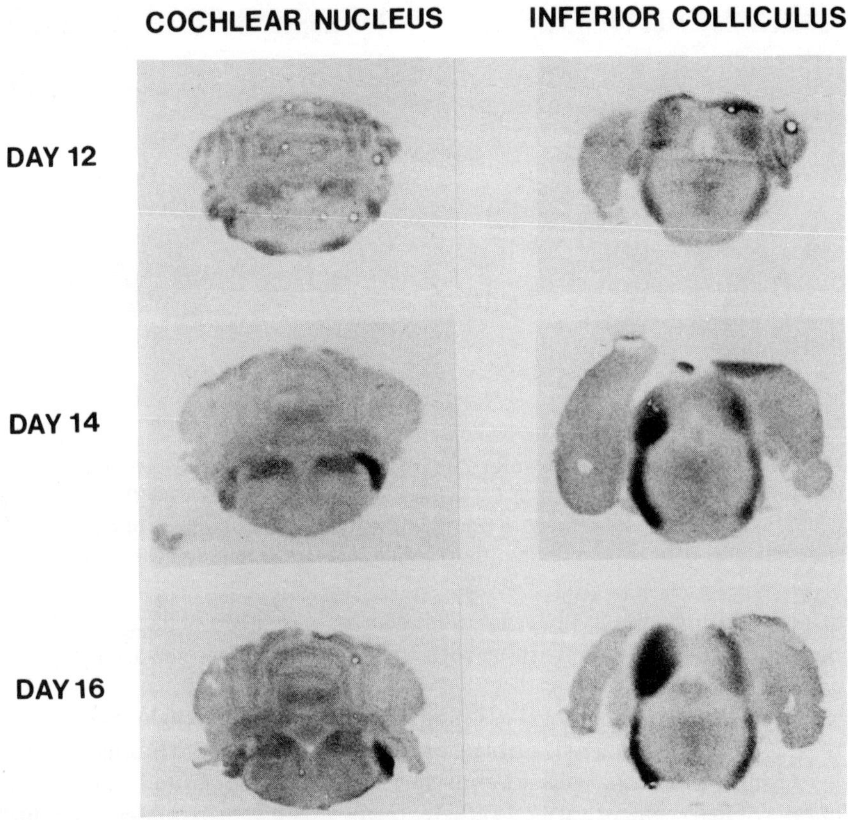

Figure 3. The level of metabolic activity revealed by the ^{14}C-deoxyglucose procedure is shown for 12-, 14-, and 16-day-old rat pups exposed to broadband noise pulses (80 dB SPL). The animals' ears were occluded on the left side only. Thus, comparisons of structures on the left and right side of the brain provide an indication of the effectiveness of auditory stimulation at different levels of the central pathway. At day 12 no substantial difference was found between left and right cochlear nuclei or inferior colliculi. By days 14 and 16 a clearly asymmetrical response was apparent in both structures. Increased metabolic activity was seen in the right cochlear nucleus and the left inferior colliculus at both ages.

deoxyglucose response reflects relatively higher levels of activity in basal than apical turns of the cochlea. This does not necessarily imply, however, that the central response is associated with preferential sensitivity to high frequencies. Because of the dynamic changes that are occurring in the frequency response of the auditory system during early development, it is equally likely that these restricted responses are associated with low-frequency sensitivity. Studies with pure tone stimulation would be necessary to determine the most

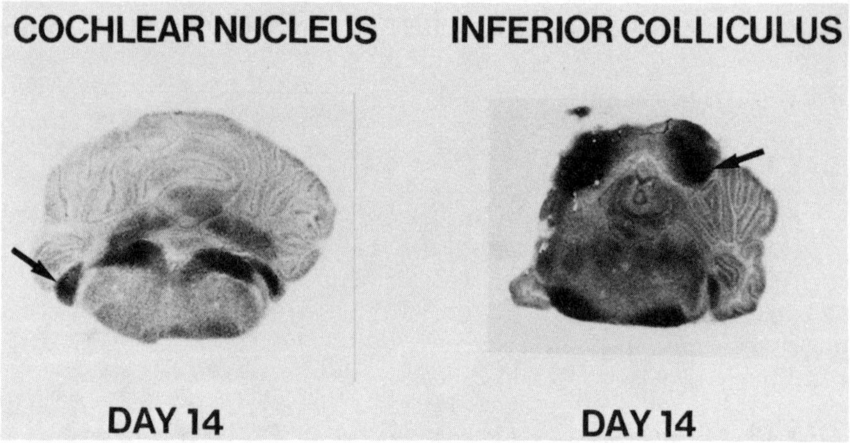

Figure 4. ^{14}C-deoxyglucose autoradiographs taken through the cochlear nucleus (A) and inferior colliculus (B) of a 14-day-old rat pup stimulated with broadband white noise pulses. Note the dark bands in the left cochlear nucleus and right inferior colliculus indicating a limited metabolic response within each region.

effective frequencies at different ages. The increased deoxyglucose response on days 17 and 20 is consistent with the development of sensitivity of the cochlea at these ages.

Ryan, Woolf, and Sharp (1982) have also used the deoxyglucose method to study the development of central auditory responses in the Mongolian gerbil. Using a wideband noise stimulus at 105 dB SPL, they found an increased uptake of deoxyglucose at 12 days after birth, which approximately coincides with the onset of the cochlear microphonic response in this species (Finck, Schneck, & Hartman, 1972). At this age only the ventral cochlear nucleus was affected, however. Increased activity in other lower brainstem auditory structures was not seen until day 14, and evidence of stimulus-induced increases in the dorsal nucleus of the lateral lemniscus, inferior colliculus, and medial geniculate was not found until day 16. Thus, in the gerbil there is a clear indication of a caudal-to-rostral sequence of development, which was not found in the albino rat.

The possibility of a similar caudal-to-rostral sequence of development cannot be completely ruled out for the albino rat. So far, studies of the rat have employed stimuli of 80 dB SPL, but with more intense stimulation equivalent to that used with gerbils, central responses might be induced at earlier developmental ages. A caudal-to-rostral sequence may emerge only during these very early periods of development. Also, because developmental changes are occurring very rapidly in the albino rat, it is possible that trends may be overlooked even when sampling on a daily basis.

Electrophysiological studies of the auditory pathway provide a further index of central auditory development in the rat. Jewett and Romano (1972) have recorded averaged click-evoked potentials from the scalps of developing rat pups and have reported on the short latency components. Responses from brainstem loci appeared first in 13-day-old animals and steadily decreased in latency and increased in reliability over the next week. Other investigators have shown that the first cortical responses appear at approximately the same time. Bures (1953) and Myslivec̆ek and Chaloupka (1959), as reported by Myslivec̆ek (1983), found cortical evoked potentials for the first time in day-14 rat pups. Recordings from older animals revealed a changing wave form with progressively decreasing latencies over a period of about two weeks. König and Marty (1974) recorded cortical slow potentials in the rat over the period of 11–15 days, and Mourek, Himwich, Myslivec̆ek, and Callison (1967) have reported cortical evoked potentials as early as 10–12 days of age, although the sound pressure level of the initiating stimulus was not given in these studies. Our own recordings of averaged evoked potentials from the primary auditory cortex of the rat indicate an early onset of activity with stimuli of moderate sound pressures. Responses to a broadband click (0.5–32 kHz) were first seen in day-14 animals at sound pressure levels between 60–70 dB SPL. No responses could be elicited in animals 11 days old or younger with clicks of 100 dB SPL (see Fig. 5).

The development of central auditory function has also been characterized by microelectrode recordings from central structures, although very few data are available for the albino rat. The majority of single unit studies have focused on the development of brainstem responses in the cat at the level of the cochlear nucleus, lateral superior olive, and inferior colliculus. As might be expected, the onset of single unit activity follows closely upon the development of input from the eighth nerve. Initially, one finds elevated thresholds and long latency responses followed by a gradual maturation over the first postnatal month (Pujol, 1972; Romand & Marty, 1975; Romand, Granier, & Marty, 1973; Moore & Irvine, 1979a). In addition, in the cochlear nucleus and the inferior colliculus there is an increase in the sharpness of frequency response curves of single neurons which may be related in part to synaptic changes among populations of central neurons as well as changes which are also occurring in the eighth nerve at about the same time (see Brugge, 1983, and Moore, 1983, for discussion of this effect). Of great interest for studies of sound localization and directional responding to sound is the further developmental change in the timing of action potentials in the cochlear nucleus which affects the temporal pattern of events in the auditory pathway. Brugge, Javel, and Kitzes (1978) report that the early responses of cells in the cochlear nucleus show less phase locking to low-frequency stimulation than at later stages of development and that the synchrony of neural discharges undergoes a dramatic change during the first weeks of development. One might expect that this trend would affect sound localization by disrupting the accuracy of binaural cues, particularly those associated with the utilization of small binaural time differences.

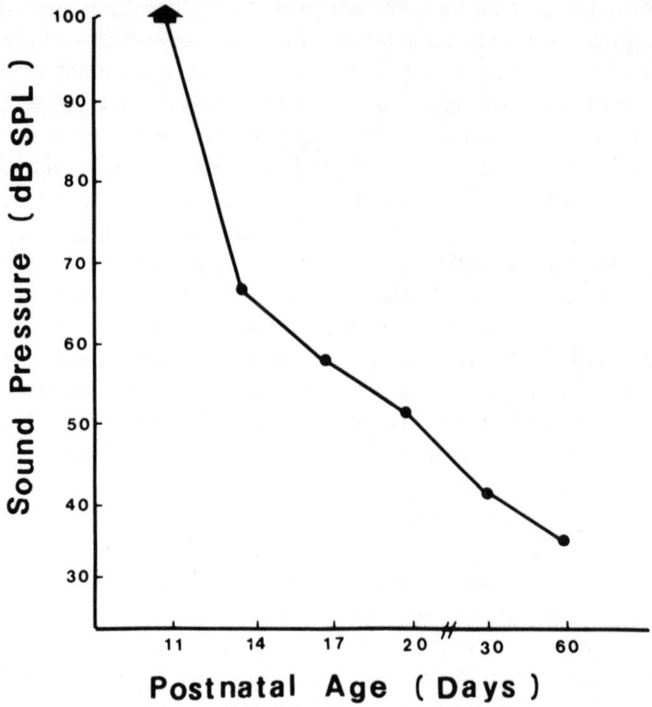

Figure 5. Threshold sound pressure levels needed to elicit cortical evoked potentials in rat pups of different ages. Stimuli were clicks presented to the left ear, and recordings were made from the contralateral auditory cortex with a silver ball electrode. Evoked potentials were averaged ($N = 50$), and thresholds were determined by reducing the sound pressure to produce a response of $10\mu V$ peak-to-peak amplitude.

DEVELOPMENT OF BINAURAL INTERACTIONS

The early development of binaural interactions has been demonstrated in both rat and cat (Clopton & Silverman, 1977; Aitkin & Reynolds, 1975; Moore & Irvine, 1981). In the rat, some evidence of binaural interaction can be seen in pups 14 to 17 days after birth. The interaction at this age is characterized by an ipsilateral inhibition of responses produced by a contralateral auditory stimulus under conditions of dichotic input. Variation of interaural intensity results in a pattern of response interactions which closely resembles that found in adults (Clopton & Silverman, 1977). So far there have been no reports on the development of responses to binaural *time* differences rather than interaural intensity differences, although it is possible that the two cues may change independently. Also, there have been no studies of the development of binaural interactions at levels other than the inferior colliculus.

In the cat, evidence of binaural interaction is found in cells of the inferior colliculus as early as 5 days after birth, which for stimuli of moderate intensity is quite soon after the onset of cochlear function (Aitkin & Reynolds, 1975). More recent studies of the nature of binaural interactions at these early stages of postnatal development have indicated that while early responses are certainly present, the sensitivity of cells to binaural intensity differences is not adultlike until approximately 1 month after birth. In very young animals, the responses of cells to changes in interaural intensity were variable and irregular at least for high-frequency stimuli (Moore & Irvine, 1981). These results suggest that the ability to localize sounds in space, a function which depends in part upon central processing of binaural intensity cues, may be delayed relative to the onset of peripheral sensitivity in the cat. The development of sensitivity to binaural time differences, which is also very important for sound localization in the cat, has not been investigated.

Directional sensitivity to free-field stimulation has been investigated in the bat, *Antrozous pallidus*. The responses of cells in the inferior colliculus of this species first appear around 6 days of age, but responses which depend upon the spatial position of sounds do not begin to achieve the precise spatial tuning seen in adults until around day 21 (Brown, Grinnell, & Harrison, 1978). Thus, in the bat there is a progressive development of physiological responses to the spatial locus of an auditory stimulus.

DIRECTIONAL RESPONSES TO SOUNDS

Behavioral studies of the development of directional sensitivity have emphasized two quite different unconditioned responses involving the localization of sounds in space. First, the tendency of infants to approach the source of auditory stimulation has been examined, and the incidence and accuracy of responses have been measured. Second, the occurrence of reflexive head movement toward a brief acoustic stimulus has been observed at various postnatal ages. Both responses permit an estimate of the onset of differential responding to the spatial locus of a sound source.

Approach Responses

Approach responses to sounds have been studied in rats, guinea pigs, and gerbils with the use of nearly identical procedures. In these studies infants were placed in the center of a circular maze as shown in Figure 6, and an auditory stimulus was presented from a loudspeaker located in one of eight possible positions around the perimeter of the maze. A start gate was then lifted, permitting an animal to execute a response toward any of the eight positions. The direction of an animal's response was observed through an overhead tele-

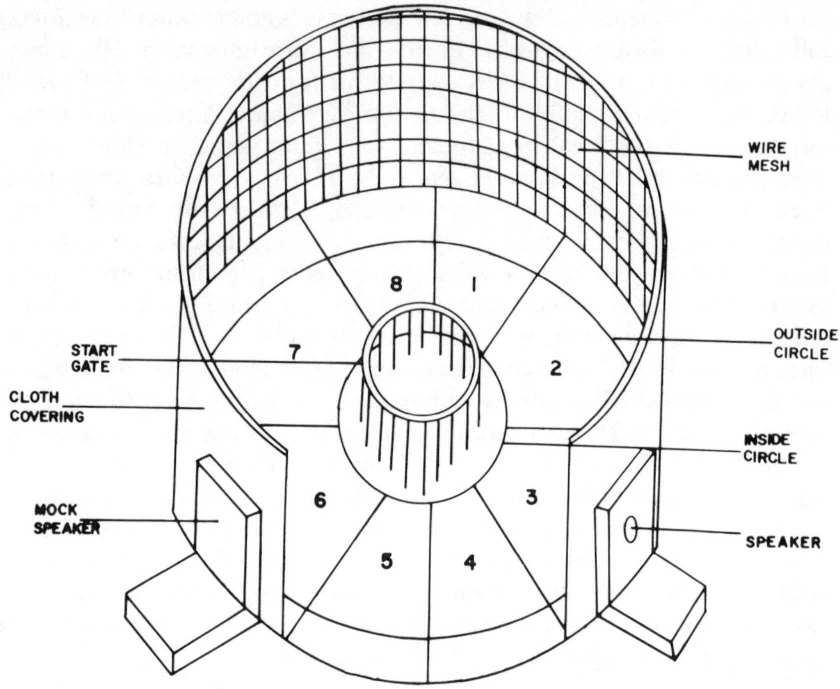

Figure 6. A cutaway view of the circular apparatus used to test auditory approach responses in rats. The maze was constructed of wire mesh covered with cotton cloth. Sounds were presented from a loudspeaker located out of view behind the maze wall. Animals were placed inside a start gate which was lifted by a pulley arrangement to initiate a trial. Responses could be executed toward any of the eight segments of the maze. The position of the loudspeaker was randomly distributed from trial to trial. (From Potash & Kelly, 1980, by permission of the publisher and authors; © 1980 by the American Psychological Association.)

vision camera. Measures of performance were based upon the percentage of trials on which an animal made a response toward the active loudspeaker. Two measures of approach have been employed in these studies. The first is based upon responses to the single segment of the maze containing the loudspeaker, and the second includes also indirect responses to the two segments on either side of the loudspeaker position. These measures will be referred to as direct and general approach responses. The direction of responses was determined by the animals' initial responses as they left the start area. Typically, the direction of response did not change as the animals approached the perimeter of the maze, and, for that reason, data regarding the animals' final responses at the edge of the maze will not be reported.

Potash and Kelly (1980) have examined directional approach responses in rat pups over the period from 13–20 days after birth. As discussed earlier, this period follows closely the onset of sensitivity to moderately intense auditory stimuli and is characterized by dynamic growth and development in the auditory system. Two qualitatively different acoustic stimuli were used in this study based upon tape-recordings of vocalizations from 8-day-old rat pups. One stimulus was referred to as a "distress" call and was elicited by pinching a rat pup's tail. The second stimulus was a "social" call and was obtained from a litter of rat pups huddled together in their nest after the mother had been removed. Tape loops were made of segments of these calls and were played back in a continuous fashion during test trials for directional responses. Sonagrams sampled from the stimuli are shown in Figure 7. As can be seen, both signals had complex temporal features and covered a broad frequency range. The frequency content of the two stimuli was quite similar, covering a range from 1–32 kHz with a peak around 4 kHz (see Fig. 8). Each stimulus was played back during testing at one of two intensity levels. In the high-intensity condition the peak sound pressure level for both stimuli was around 80 dB SPL. In the low-intensity condition the peak was around 45–50 dB SPL. In addition to the four stimulus conditions, there were two control conditions with blank tapes played back at low- and high-intensity levels. Six separate groups of animals were tested under each of these stimulus conditions.

Directional responses to sound were found only with the social call played back at low-intensity levels (see Fig. 9). Under this condition, 67% of responses led to a general approach toward the stimulus, whereas in all other conditions the level of approach was not different from the 37.5% expected by chance alone (i.e., three out of eight possible correct responses). The responses to the low-intensity social call were not precisely directed toward the active loudspeaker but rather included many indirect responses as well. The percentage of direct approach responses was 23.6% compared to 12.5% expected by chance (i.e., one out of eight possible correct responses). Thus, the level of approach responding to low-intensity social calls, while not high, was significantly above the level expected by chance.

One of the most remarkable aspects of this study is the fact that young rat pups will approach the source of a sound without the necessity of special training or reinforcement and that they will maintain this response over a period of about a week following the onset of hearing. Older animals, after about 21–23 days of age, do not maintain spontaneous approach responses. The existence of the response seems to be based on a specific motivation to approach auditory stimulation during a particular period of development. Similar observations have been made in avian and other mammalian species (Beer, 1970; Clements & Kelly, 1978a; Collias & Collias, 1956; Evans, 1970; Gottlieb, 1965; Potash & Kelly, 1978).

The motivation to approach an auditory stimulus is highly selective. In the first place, there is a greater tendency to approach a low-intensity than a

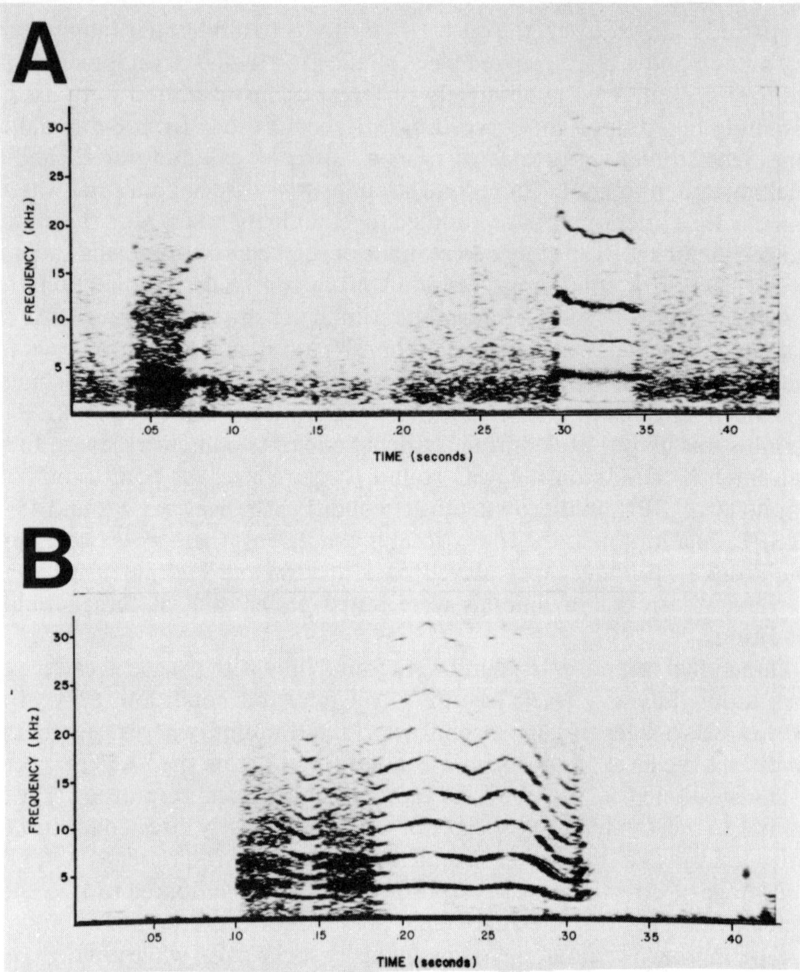

Figure 7. Sonagrams from the two vocalizations used to investigate approach responses in rat pups. Both social call (A) and distress call (B) were presented at low and high sound pressure levels. Frequency is shown on the *y*-axis in kilohertz. Time is indicated on the *x*-axis in seconds. The relative intensity of different components of the calls is indicated by the darkness of the print. (From Potash & Kelly, 1980, by permission of the publisher and authors; © by the American Psychological Association.)

high-intensity stimulus. Although this result seems unexpected from the perspective of psychophysics or perceptual saliency, it is consistent with Schneirla's (1965) theory of approach/withdrawal processes in the development of animal behavior. In addition, these data indicate selectivity based on stimulus quality. Infant rat pups will approach a social call but not a distress

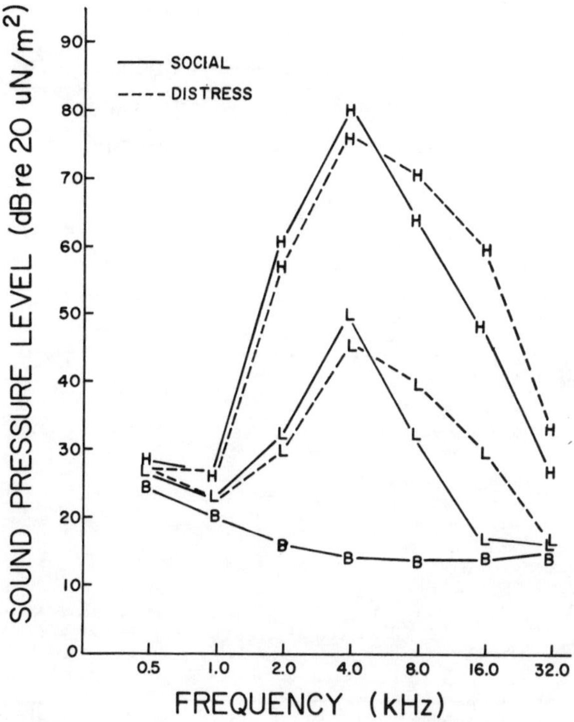

Figure 8. Frequency analysis of the low-intensity (L) and high-intensity (H) playback of the social (solid lines) and distress (dashed lines) calls used in studies of approach responding by rat pups. Measures are based on peak readings of sound pressure levels with a ½ inch microphone and ⅓ octave bandpass filters (Brüel & Kjaer Type 1613). Background noise levels are indicated as a solid line (B). (From Potash & Kelly, 1980, by permission of the publisher and authors; © 1980 by the American Psychological Association.)

call, even though the frequency content and the sound pressure levels of the two stimuli are closely matched. It seems unlikely that this differential response is based upon limits in the animals' sensory capacity. For example, there is no reason to believe that one stimulus was more readily heard than the other in this study. It is more likely that the difference between the two calls was based upon response preferences.

The occurrence of directional responses to sounds in early development implies the existence of basic mechanisms for the localization of sounds in space. Indeed, it is evident that rat pups are capable of sound localization during the first week following the onset of auditory sensitivity. Considering the complexity and duration of the signals employed, a variety of response strategies might have served to mediate sound localization in our study of rat

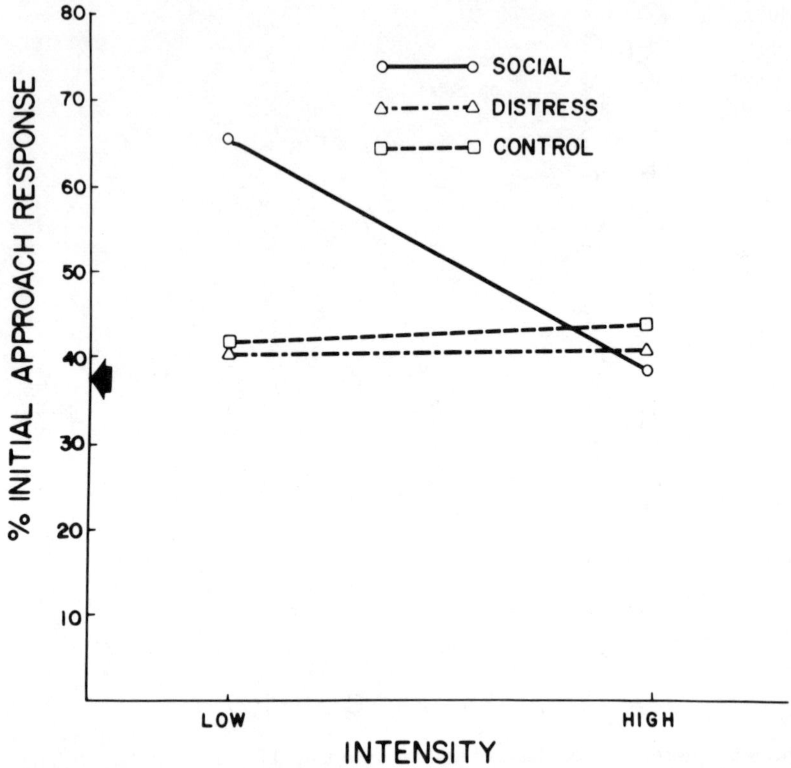

Figure 9. Average performance levels for executing a general approach response are shown for high- and low-intensity social calls, distress calls, and blank-tape control conditions. The performance level expected in this situation by chance alone (37.5%) is indicated by an arrow on the *y*-axis. The figure is based on the initial responses made by animals as they left the start area of the maze. (From Potash & Kelly, 1980, by permission of the publisher and authors; © 1980 by the American Psychological Association.)

pup approach responding. Therefore, further observations were made to determine whether or not the responses were dependent on binaural cues.

Our results show that infant approach responding in rats is dependent upon the balance of auditory input to the two ears, a factor which is known to be important for sound localization in adults (Potash & Kelly, 1980). Approach responses by infant rats to low-intensity social calls can be disrupted by blocking the external meatus of one ear with a wax ear plug. This monaural obstruction of the ear canal has the effect of shifting responses towards the side of the unobstructed ear and thus reducing the percentage of approach responses to near chance levels (see Fig. 10). Binaural ear blocks, on the other hand, which affect the auditory input equally in the two ears, do not result in substantial disruptions of directional responding. With both ear blocks in place the infants are still able to hear the stimulus and determine its position in space. This result confirms our previous observation that rat pups are capable of sound localization shortly after the onset of auditory sensitivity and strongly indicates that binaural cues are important during this developmental period.

Similar results have been obtained in other mammalian species (Kelly,

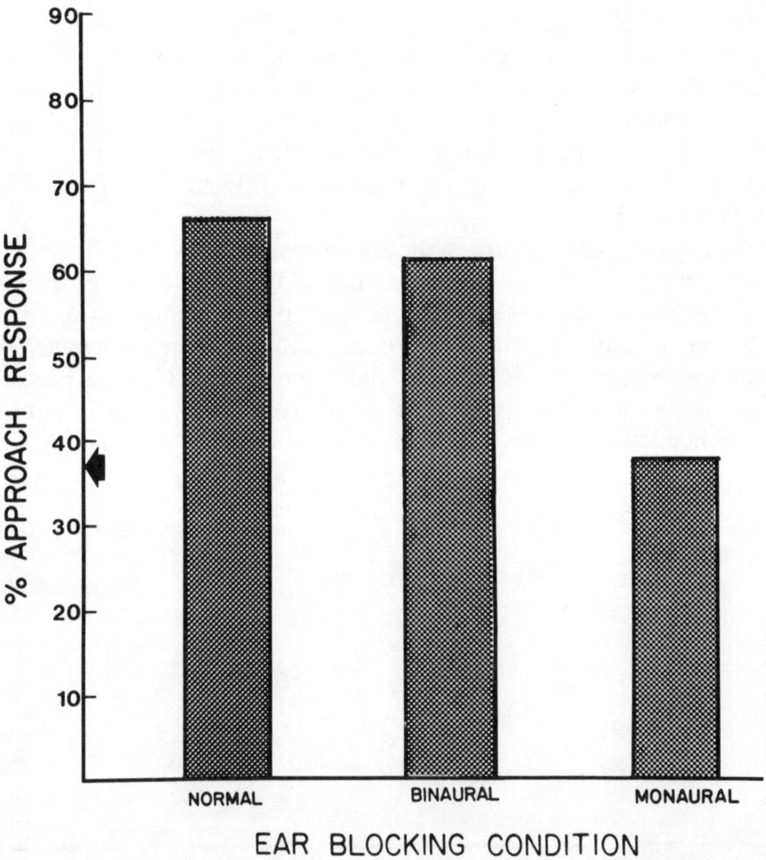

Figure 10. The effects on auditory approach responses of placing wax ear blocks in the external meatus. The mean percentages of initial approach responses are shown for rats without ear plugs (NORMAL), for rats with both ears plugged (BINAURAL), and for rats with one ear plugged (MONAURAL). The level of performance expected by chance (37.5%) is indicated by an arrow on the *y*-axis. (From Potash & Kelly, 1980, by permission of the publisher and authors; © 1980 by the American Psychological Association.)

1982). Kelly and Potash (1986) have examined auditory approach responses in gerbils, *Meriones unguiculatus,* between 16 and 23 days of age. The testing procedures were essentially the same as described for the albino rat, except different stimuli were used to induce behavioral responses. The studies with gerbils employed a tape loop of a gerbil social call which was recorded from a litter of 11-day-old infants huddled in their home cage, a broadband noise stimulus, and a blank tape which was included for control purposes. These tape-recordings were played back at either low- or high-intensity levels. The social call contained a wide range of frequencies between 2–32 kHz with a peak around 8 kHz. The sound pressure level at that frequency was approximately 80 dB SPL for the high-intensity playback and 55 db SPL for the low-intensity playback. The temporal characteristics for the call can be seen in Figure 11. The noise stimulus had a broader representation of high frequencies with a peak at 4 kHz. The maximum sound pressure was approximately 85 dB SPL for the high intensity playback and 35 dB SPL for the low-intensity playback.

Gerbil pups tended to approach the low-intensity playback of the gerbil social call more readily than the high-intensity playback or either of the noise conditions. There was also some tendency to approach the noise stimulus. As can be seen in Figure 12, general approach responses to the low-intensity social call were recorded on 64% of the trials, compared to 37.5% expected by chance. On the more demanding measure of direct approach, a score of 27% was obtained, compared to 12.5% expected by chance. Thus, a clear direc-

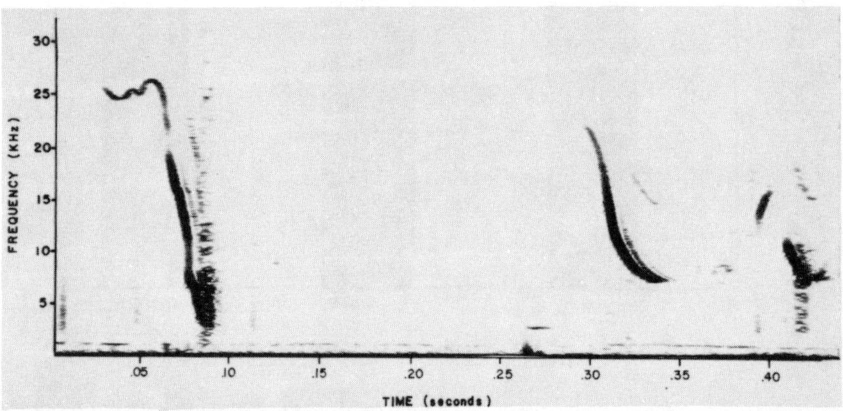

Figure 11. A sonagram of part of the gerbil social call used in studies of directional approach responding. Frequency is indicated in kilohertz, and time is shown in seconds. The relative intensity of the different components of the call is reflected in the darkness of the print. Two descending frequency modulated chirps can be seen as part of this call. (From Kelly & Potash, 1986, by permission of the publisher and authors; © 1986 by the American Psychological Association.)

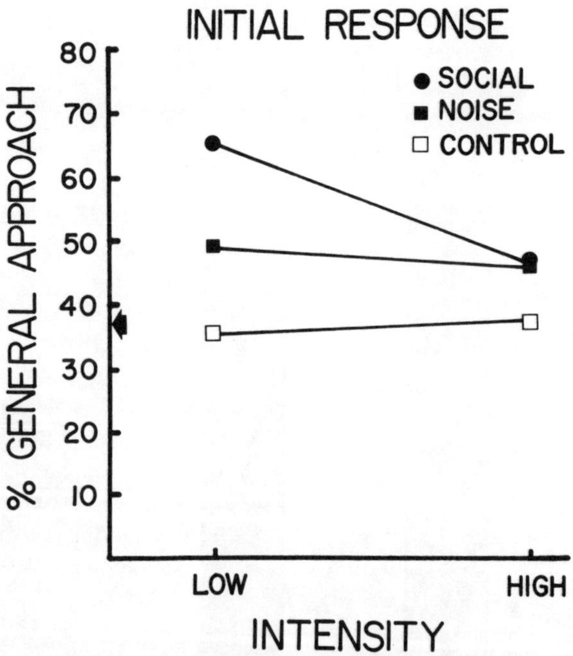

Figure 12. Average performance levels of gerbils for executing a general approach response are shown for low- and high-intensity social calls compared to white noise and blank-tape control conditions. The performance level expected by chance is 37.5% as indicated by the arrow on the *y*-axis. (From Kelly & Potash, 1986, by permission of the publisher and authors; © 1986 by the American Psychological Association.)

tional tendency was demonstrated, although the accuracy of the response was not great.

In a further study it was demonstrated that 16–23-day-old gerbil pups depend upon binaural input for maintaining approach responses. Animals with obstruction of one external ear canal failed to show any signs of approaching a low-intensity social call, whereas animals without ear obstruction clearly went toward the source of stimulation. Animals with both ears blocked showed some reduction in performance but were still better than chance (see Fig. 13). These results confirm that gerbil pups are capable of responding on the basis of the location of a sound source and indicate that binaural cues are important.

The directional ability shown in gerbils between 16 and 23 days of age follows closely upon the development of cochlear sensitivity and central responses to sounds. The earliest cochlear microphonic and eighth-nerve action potentials occur at around 12 and 14 days of age, respectively, in response to stimuli in excess of 80 dB SPL. Responses to more moderate

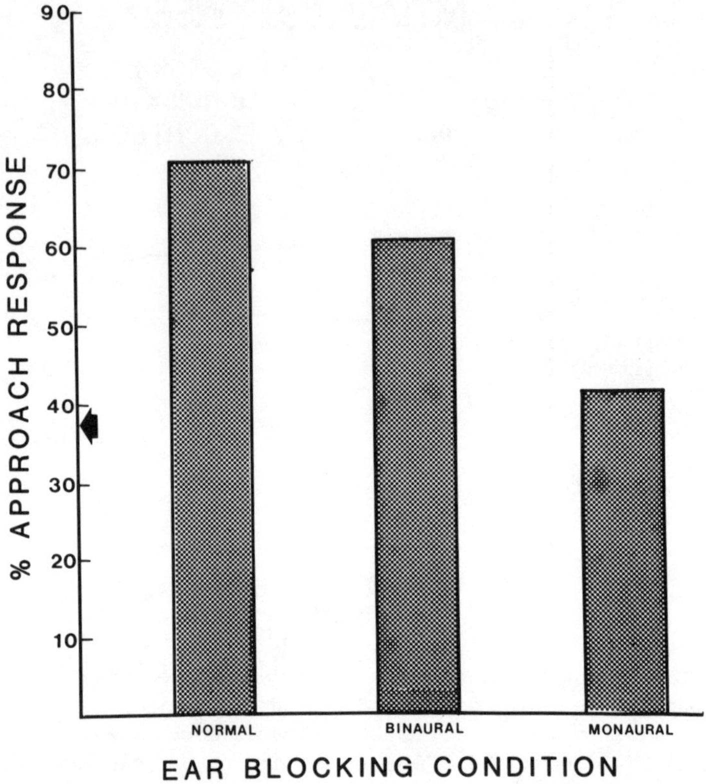

Figure 13. Average performance levels of gerbils for executing a general approach response under conditions without ear blocks (NORMAL), with both ears blocked (BINAURAL), and with one ear blocked (MONAURAL). The performance level expected by chance is 37.5% as indicated by the arrow on the *y*-axis. (From Kelly & Potash, 1986, by permission of the publisher and authors; © 1986 by the American Psychological Association.)

sound pressures do not appear until around day 16 (Finck et al., 1972). Functional activity (2-DG) in the central auditory system undergoes a caudal-to-rostral sequence of development between days 12 and 16 and is seen in the inferior colliculus and medial geniculate for the first time around day 16 in response to sound pressures of 105 dB SPL (Ryan et al., 1982). Thus, given the sound pressures used in behavioral studies of auditory approach responses, directional sensitivity to sound was manifested very soon after the onset of general responsiveness.

Guinea pigs, *Cavia porcellus,* also show early directional responses to sounds. In this highly precocial species, tests of approach responding are possible almost immediately after birth. Using the same circular apparatus described above for rats and gerbils, Clements and Kelly (1978a) have shown that guinea pigs tested over the period from 1–4 days postpartum will approach the source of an auditory stimulus, in this case, a tape-recording of vocalizations obtained from a guinea pig litter played back over a loudspeaker at approximately 50 dB SPL. As in the case of other rodents tested so far, it was found that monaural ear blocking reduced the level of approach responding to near chance levels, whereas binaural ear blocking did not (see Kelly, 1982, for further discussion of guinea pig studies).

Physiological studies indicate that the guinea pig is sensitive to sounds well before birth. Limited cochlear microphonic responses can be recorded for the first time around 15 days before birth and eighth nerve action potentials appear 2 days later. By around the time of birth the amplitude and latency of these potentials have reached near adult values (Romand, 1971). Cortical evoked potentials can also be recorded at about the same time and reach adultlike values soon after birth (Chaloupka, Záhlava, Mysliveĉek, & Hassmannova, 1968). Because of the prolonged prenatal development of the auditory system in this species, it is impossible to determine the relation between the onset of auditory function and directional responses to sound beyond concluding that directional responses occur as soon as they are possible in normal development.

Approach responses have also been examined in kittens using a two-choice procedure with reinforcement for correct responses (Clements & Kelly, 1978b). With a tape-recorded kitten purr (75 dB SPL) as a stimulus, it was possible to show significant levels of approach responding at around 18–24 days of age. This estimate is very similar to the reports by Villablanca and Olmstead (1979; Olmstead & Villablanca, 1980) on the development of reliable auditory approach responses in kittens at around 16 days of age. In contrast to what has been reported for rats and gerbils, the onset of spatial approach responses in kittens seems to be delayed relative to the onset of general sensitivity. Cochlear microphonic responses in cats are already present a few days before birth, and eighth-nerve action potentials can be recorded at the time of birth, although the thresholds for eliciting responses are high and the range of effective frequencies is limited (Pujol & Hilding, 1973; Romand, 1971; Romand, 1983; Rubel, 1978). The subsequent development of cochlear responses is rather slow. The microphonic potential reaches adultlike characteristics around the second week after birth, and the action potential attains maturity toward the end of the first month (Romand, 1971). Central responses including evoked potentials and single unit activity can be recorded from various levels of the auditory pathway beginning a few days after birth. Dynamic maturational changes continue over a period of approximately a month before adultlike responses are obtained (see Brugge, 1983; Moore, 1983; Rubel, 1978). Nondirectional behavioral responses such as pinna movements or facial responses have been demonstrated within the first four or five days after birth (Olmstead & Villablanca, 1980; Ehret & Romand, 1981). The earliest responses were elicited by sound pressures in excess of 100 dB SPL over a limited frequency range between 0.2 and 4.0 kHz. Sensitivity increased dramatically between 6 and 10 days of age, and a continued development of sensitivity with an extension of the upper range of effective frequencies was observed until between 22 and 30 days of age (Ehret & Romand, 1981). Thus, in the cat directional approach responses to sounds may be delayed relative to the development of general auditory sensitivity.

Head Orientation

Directional responses have also been examined using head orientation rather than spatial approach responses to sounds. The head orientation response has the advantage of being more readily elicited by a wide range of stimuli including short duration tones and noise bursts and can be produced in adults as well as infants. The generality of the response makes it a useful tool for analytical assessments of the development of sensory capacity associated with sound localization.

Judge and Kelly (1981) have employed a simple procedure for evaluating auditory orientation in rat pups from 11 to 20 days of age. The animals were placed in a small wire cage located inside a sound-attenuated chamber and were exposed to sudden, brief, auditory stimuli presented occasionally against an essentially quiet background. Behavioral responses were observed through an overhead television camera with a monitor located outside the sound-proof room. Sounds were presented on an animal's left or right side at approximately +90° or −90° azimuth, and directional responses were measured in terms of the percentage of trials with a response toward the sound source. A baseline of spontaneous responding was established for each animal using a series of "mock trials" in which "directional responses" were evaluated, but actual stimulus presentation was omitted. In this way, possible contamination of results by false positive responses was eliminated.

It is important in these studies that stimuli be presented infrequently in order to avoid the possible influence of habituation of responses. By using intervals of not less than 5 minutes between trials and restricting the number of trials to five per day, a high level of responding could be maintained. The same animals were tested on two successive days to obtain an estimate of head orientation based on 10 trials. Separate animals were tested at five different ages begining on days 8, 11, 14, 17, and 20. The stimulus was a 65-dB SPL noise burst of brief (520 ms) duration. At this sound pressure level there was no evidence of head orientation at either 8 or 11 days of age. The first indication of a reliable directional response was seen on day 14. Increased orientation toward the sound source was apparent on days 17 and 20 (see Fig. 14A). The asymptotic level of orientation by 20-day-old animals was around 90% compared to very low levels of spontaneous responding.

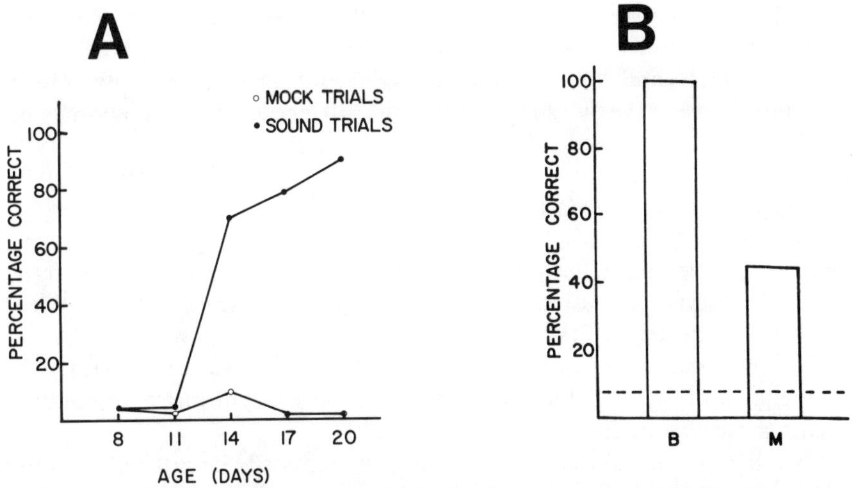

Figure 14. Average performance levels of rat pups in tests of head orientation. A. The percentage of trials in which orientation toward the sound source was observed is shown for different postnatal ages. Performance levels on trials in which a SOUND was presented (filled circles) are compared with levels of "false positive" responding on MOCK TRIALS in which no sound was presented (open circles). B. The effect on performance of obstructing the external auditory meatus is shown for two conditions: BINAURAL, both ears were obstructed so that sound pressure was attenuated equally in the two ears; MONAURAL, one ear was obstructed so that an imbalance of auditory input to the two ears was produced. The dashed line represents the level of "correct" responding during mock trials.

Judge and Kelly (1981) have also shown that orientation at 17 days of age is based upon binaural cues. Animals with surgical obstruction (ligation of the external meatus) of one ear did not show any differential response based on the position of the stimulus. Rather, these animals frequently oriented toward the side of the unobstructed ear regardless of where the sound was located. When a stimulus was presented on the side of the obstructed ear, the animals oriented toward the opposite side on 85% of the trials. Thus, the performance scores for these animals fell to 46.6% as can be seen in Figure 14B. Animals with both ears obstructed were still capable of hearing the stimulus and showed a consistent orientation toward the side of the sound source.

More recently, we have examined the development of head orientation in rats to low and high frequency tones using the behavioral measures described above (Fraser, 1984). In this study separate groups of animals were tested with either 2-kHz or 16-kHz tone bursts, with repeated testing on a daily basis from postnatal day 12 through 16. The sound pressure level of the tone bursts was adjusted to compensate for the sensitivity curve of the *adult* rat as defined in psychophysical tests by Kelly and Masterton (1978) and verified in auditory orientation tests with adults. The sound pressures selected were 55 dB SPL for the 2-kHz stimulus and 35 dB SPL for the 16-kHz tone. Presentation of these stimuli to adult rats elicited head orientation at very nearly identical levels (82% and 78% for low and high frequencies, respectively). Given the equivalence of the two stimuli for adults, differences in orientation by infants might be attributed to developmental trends in auditory sensitivity to low and high frequency tones or to differences in the use of different frequencies for directional orientation.

The results of this study are shown in Figure 15. Generally the data reveal an onset of orientation between days 11 and 14, which is consistent with the previous observations using broadband stimuli. A difference was noticed, however, in the age of first appearance of directional responses to high and low frequencies. On days 12 and 13 reliable orientation was found with high-frequency stimulation but not with low. Thus, the onset of spatial responding occurs somewhat earlier for 16 kHz than 2 kHz.

This difference in onset of orientation cannot easily be attributed to the relative sensitivity of infants to high and low frequencies. While there is no question that the infant's sensitivity to pure tones is quite different from the

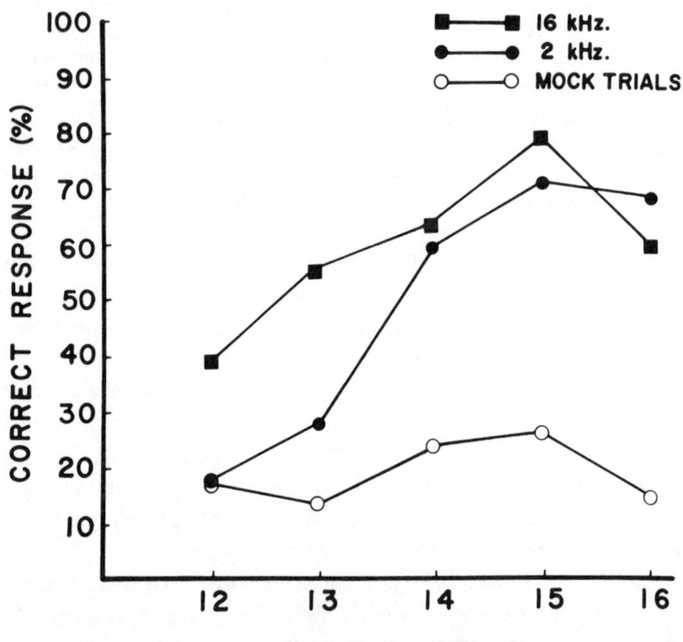

Figure 15. The percentage of head orientation responses shown for rat pups at different ages using 2-kHz (filled circles) or 16-kHz (filled squares) tone pips. The averaged level of false positive responses on trials without any auditory stimulus is also indicated (open circles).

adult's, it is now well established that the direction of development is from low to high frequencies. Infants are first sensitive to tones in the low-frequency range including 2 kHz and only later develop sensitivity to high frequencies including 16 kHz. An infant rat, therefore, is likely to hear a 2-kHz tone before he hears a 16-kHz tone, even if the sound pressure levels are equated. If the high frequency is attenuated by 20 dB relative to the low as in the present study, this expectation becomes a virtual certainty. The finding that *directional responses* occur earlier for 16 kHz than 2 kHz is, therefore, inconsistent with the development of high- and low-frequency sensitivity.

A more likely explanation of this result requires consideration of the mechanisms involved in sound localization. Between days 11 and 17 there are several factors which might influence the central processing of binaural cues and which could differentially affect high- and low-frequency localization. First, as pointed out by Saunders and Garfinkle (1982) and Moore and Irvine (1979b), binaural cues in infants are affected by changing head size. As an infant grows, the binaural intensity cues are altered, particularly at midrange frequencies, because of the greater shadowing effect of the head, and binaural time cues undergo changes because of the increasing interaural distance. In the context of our experiment, however, binaural intensity cues are probably not implicated, because our high-frequency stimulus is above the range most affected by growth, and the low-frequency stimulus is not greatly influenced by the sound shadowing effect even in adults. Binaural time cues might be altered, although it is difficult to envision changes large enough to account for the rapid development of head orientation between days 11 and 17.

A second, more likely possibility is that developmental changes taking place in the cochlea, eighth nerve, and/or structures of the lower brainstem affect the representation of binaural cues centrally. For example, during the period immediately after the onset of auditory sensitivity there are dramatic changes in the latencies and temporal characteristics of physiological responses to sounds which could have a profound impact on the analysis of binaural cues centrally. Changes associated with myelination of the eighth nerve and trapezoid body could have an influence on the integration of binaural cues by altering conduction times to central structures such as the superior olive. These changes in the timing of neural activity might be expected to selectively disrupt central processing of binaural time of arrival cues. Head orientation to a 16-kHz tone, based largely on binaural intensity cues, might be relatively unaffected by changes in timing and latency of neural activity, whereas orientation to a 2-kHz tone, based predominantly on binaural time cues, might be delayed by such changes.

Also, it should be pointed out that because of the basal to apical sequence of development in the cochlea, the earliest activity which registers in the central nervous system will likely activate structures which in adults are associated with high-frequency localization. Even though the auditory system responds first to low-frequency stimuli, the pathways involved are those associated with activation of the basal turns of the cochlea in adults. These pathways innervate structures such as the lateral superior olive, which are specialized for the analysis of high frequency cues. The recruitment of neural structures involved in the analysis of low-frequency cues, e.g., the medial superior olive, would presumably take place at a later date, when more apical turns of the cochlea are activated due to a shift in the mechanical properties of the cochlea at different ages (Rubel, 1984). Therefore, in the early stages of auditory development there is a *mismatch* between the peripheral cues for localization and the central nervous system mechanisms adapted for binaural analysis. This mismatch may result in a developmental delay in the ability of infants to localize low-frequency stimuli.

The development of head orientation to sounds has also been investigated in humans by Muir and Field (1979) and Muir, Abraham, Forbes, and Harris (1979). The first indication of reliable head turning toward the source of a broadband auditory stimulus, a rattle sound, was seen in babies as soon as testing was possible at 2 or 3 days after birth. Furthermore, more recent studies by Muir and colleagues have shown the presence of auditory orientation in preterm infants at 32–36 weeks gestational age, with performance levels equivalent to normal newborns (Muir, 1982). The ability to localize sounds, therefore, exists in infants around the time of birth.

Clifton, Morrongiello, Kulig, and Dowd (1981) have extended the studies of Muir and Field to include frequency-restricted stimuli. By filtering the sound produced by a rattle, it was possible to compare the effectiveness of a low-pass (< 1600 Hz), midrange (1000–3000 Hz), and high-pass (> 1800 Hz) stimulus in eliciting directional head movements. In newborn infants the high-pass condition was found to be as likely as an unfiltered stimulus to produce a correct orientation response, but the low-pass stimulus was relatively ineffective. Tests at 5 months of age revealed a marked improvement in low-frequency orientation, but only slight improvements in middle- and high-frequency localization. These results suggest the possibility that infants use binaural intensity cues earlier than binaural time cues for sound localization.

CONCLUSIONS

1. Directional aspects of hearing develop early in ontogeny in the albino rat. At about the time that infants first become sensitive to moderately intense sounds, between the 11th and 14th postnatal day, some capacity for sound localization can be demonstrated in tests of head orientation and directional approach responding.

Generally, the behavioral observations are consistent with physiological data which indicate an early onset of function of central nervous system structures involved in sound localization, including neural responses to binaural input. Physiological studies which can be related directly to sound localization, however, are so far quite limited in number. Virtually nothing is known about the development of different cues for sound localization or about binaural responses at levels of the auditory pathway other than the inferior colliculus. Physiological studies of free-field stimuli have not been reported for the rat, although such studies have been useful in suggesting developmental trends in other species, e.g., the bat.

2. Behavioral studies of both auditory approach responding and directional head orientation in rats indicate the importance of binaural input in early infancy. Infants with monaural ear blocks consistently misdirect their responses toward the side of the unobstructed ear. This result is consistent with the perceptual shift which results from monaural hearing loss in adults and indicates that infant sound localization is based upon binaural mechanisms similar to those found in adults. The behavioral results do not reveal, however, whether or not the infant's ability to localize sounds is as refined or accurate as binaural localization in adults. Indeed, in infants the accuracy of approach responses is rather low, and performance in head orientation tests increases as a function of age. Because of the nature of the behavioral responses, however, it is uncertain whether these data reflect a limitation of sensory capacity in early infancy.

3. The course of development of auditory orientation in the rat is dependent upon the frequency of the sound source. Directional head turning can be elicited earlier by a high-frequency (16-kHz) than a low-frequency (2-kHz) tone. This effect cannot be attributed merely to the functional onset of sensitivity to different tones but seems to be related to the development of central mechanisms for sound localization. Corresponding physiological studies of the relative development of directional responses to high and low frequency stimuli are completely lacking. However, it seems likely that central process ing of binaural time and intensity cues, which are largely responsible for localization of low and high frequency tones, respectively, would develop at different rates. Specifically, it is suggested that the lack of synchrony and extended latencies of early auditory responses might more readily affect the processing of binaural time than intensity cues. Furthermore, the early development of low-frequency responses in the basal rather than apical end of the cochlea would result in a mismatch of the appropriate cue, namely the binaural time cue, and the central structures responsible for its analysis in sound localization. This mismatch would result in a delay in the development of directional responding to low frequency sounds.

4. Early development of sound localization is found in a number of mammals other than the albino rat. In the rapidly developing altricial mammal, *Meriones unguiculatus,* there is a tendency toward directional auditory approach responses soon after the onset of hearing. The pattern of behavior is quite similar to that seen in rats. The precocial rodent, *Cavia porcellus,* exe-

cutes approach responses toward auditory stimulation almost immediately after birth, and human infants also show directional responses to sound at birth. In the cat, directional responses are seen early in development, around days 16 or 17, but there is some indication that these responses are delayed relative to the onset of general sensitivity to sounds. Further studies of the development of sound localization would benefit from the use of relatively slowly developing mammals which might reveal sequential trends in the functional ontogeny of the auditory system.

REFERENCES

Aitkin, L.M., & Reynolds, A. (1975). Development of binaural responses in the kitten inferior colliculus. *Neuroscience Letters, 1,* 315–319.

Beer, C.G. (1970). Individual recognition of voice in the social behavior of birds. In D.S. Lehrman & R.A. Hinde (Eds.), *Advances in the study of behavior.* New York: Academic Press.

Bosher, S.K., & Warren, R.L. (1971). A study of the electrochemical and osmotic relationships of the cochlear fluids in the neonatal rat at the time of development of the endocochlear potential. *Journal of Physiology (London), 212,* 739–761.

Brown, P.E., Grinnell, A.D., & Harrison, J.B. (1978). The development of hearing in the pallid bat (*Antrozous pallidus*). *Journal of Comparative Physiology, 126,* 169–182.

Brugge, J.F. (1983). Development of the lower brainstem auditory nuclei. In R. Romand (Ed.), *Development of auditory and vestibular systems.* New York: Academic Press.

Brugge, J.F., Javel, E., & Kitzes, L.M. (1978). Signs of functional maturation of peripheral auditory system in discharge patterns of neurons in anteroventral cochlear nucleus of kitten. *Journal of Neurophysiology, 41,* 1557–1579.

Carlier, E., Lenoir, M., & Pujol, R. (1979). Development of cochlear frequency selectivity tested by compound action potential tuning curves. *Hearing Research, 1,* 197–201.

Chaloupka, Z., Záhlava, J., Myslivec̆ek, J., & Hassmannova, J. (1968). Development of functional abilities of the auditory system. In L. Jilek & S. Trojan (Eds.), *Ontogenesis of the brain* (pp. 387–393). Prague, Czechoslovakia: Universita Karlova.

Clements, M., & Kelly, J.B. (1978a). Auditory spatial responses of young guinea pigs (*Cavia porcellus*) during and after ear blocking. *Journal of Comparative and Physiological Psychology, 92,* 34–44.

Clements, M., & Kelly, J.B. (1978b). Directional responses by kittens to an auditory stimulus. *Developmental Neurobiology, 11,* 505–511.

Clifton, R., Morrongiello, B., Kulig, J., & Dowd, J. (1981). Developmental changes in auditory localization in infancy. In R.N. Aslin, J.R. Alberts, & M.R. Petersen (Eds.), *Development of perception: Psychobiological perspectives, Vol. 1* (pp. 141–160). New York: Academic Press.

Clopton, B.M., & Silverman, M.S. (1977). Plasticity of binaural interaction. II. Critical period and changes in midline response. *Journal of Neurophysiology, 40,* 1275–1280.

Clopton, B.M., & Winfield, J.A. (1973). Tonotopic organization in the inferior colliculus of the rat. *Brain Research, 56,* 355–358.

Collias, N.E., & Collias, E.C. (1956). Some mechanisms of family integration in ducks. *Auk, 73,* 378–400.

Crowley, D.E., & Hepp-Raymond, M.C. (1966). Development of cochlear function of the ear of the infant rat. *Journal of Comparative and Physiological Psychology, 62,* 427–432.

Ehret, G., & Romand, R. (1981). Postnatal development of absolute auditory thresholds in kittens. *Journal of Comparative and Physiological Psychology, 95,* 304–311.

Evans, R.M. (1970). Imprinting and control of mobility in young ring-billed gulls (*Larus delawarensis*). *Animal Behaviour Monographs, 3,* 193–248.

Fernández, C., & Hinojosa, R. (1974). Postnatal development of endocochlear potential and stria vascularis in the cat. *Acta Otolaryngologica, 78,* 173–186.

Finck, A., Schneck, C.D., & Hartman, A.F. (1972). Development of cochlear function in the neonate mongolian gerbil (*Meriones unguiculatus*). *Journal of Comparative and Physiological Psychology, 78,* 375–380.

Fraser, I.H. (1984). *Development of reflexive head orientation to high and low frequency tones in the rat.* Unpublished honours thesis, Carleton University, Ottawa, CANADA.

Gottlieb, G. (1965). Imprinting in relation to parental and species identification by avian neonates. *Journal of Comparative and Physiological Psychology, 59,* 345–356.

Jewett, D.L., & Romano, M.N. (1972). Neonatal development of auditory system potentials averaged from the scalp of rat and cat. *Brain Research, 36,* 101–115.

Judge, P.W., & Kelly, J.B. (1981). Development of the auditory orientation response in rats. *Journal of the Acoustical Society of America, 69,* 645.

Kelly, J.B. (1981). Behavioral and anatomical studies of central auditory development. In Josef Syka & Lindsay Aitkin (Eds.), *Neuronal mechanisms in hearing.* New York: Plenum Press.

Kelly, J.B. (1982). Developmental aspects of sound localization. In R.W. Gatehouse (Ed.), *Localization of sound: Theory and application.* Groton, CT: Amphora Press.

Kelly, J.B., & Masterton, R.B. (1977). Auditory sensitivity of the albino rat. *Journal of Comparative and Physiological Psychology, 91,* 930–936.

Kelly, J.B., & Potash, M. (1986). Directional responses to sounds in young gerbils (*Meriones unguiculatus*). *Journal of Comparative Psychology, 100,* 37–45.

Kelly, J.B., & Skeen, L.C. (1979). Development of central auditory function in the rat: A [^{14}C]-deoxyglucose study. *Neuroscience Abstracts, 5,* 23.

König, N., & Marty, R. (1974). On functions and structure of deep layers of immature auditory cortex. *Journal of Physiology (Paris), 68,* 145–155.

Moore, D.R. (1983). Development of inferior colliculus and binaural audition. In R. Romand (Ed.), *Development of auditory and vestibular systems* (pp. 121–166). New York: Academic Press.

Moore, D.R., & Irvine, D.R.F. (1979a). The development of some peripheral and central auditory responses in the neonatal cat. *Brain Research, 163,* 49–59.

Moore, D.R., & Irvine, D.R.F. (1979b). A developmental study of the sound pressure transformation by the head of the cat. *Acta Otolaryngologica, 87,* 434–440.

Moore, D.R., & Irvine, D.R.F. (1981). Development of responses to acoustic interaural intensity differences in the cat inferior colliculus. *Experimental Brain Research, 41,* 301–309.

Mourek, J., Himwich, W.A., Myslivec̆ek, J., & Callison, D.A. (1967). The role of undernutrition in the development of evoked cortical responses in the rat. *Brain Research, 6,* 241–251.

Muir, D. (1982). The development of human auditory localization in infancy. In R.W. Gatehouse (Ed.), *Localization of sound: Theory and applications* (pp. 220–243). Groton, CT: Amphora Press.

Muir, D., Abraham, W., Forbes, B., & Harris, L. (1979). The ontogenesis of an auditory localization response from birth to four months of age. *Canadian Journal of Psychology, 33,* 320–333.

Muir, D., & Field, J. (1979). Newborn infants orient to sounds. *Child Development, 50,* 431–436.

Myslivec̆ek, J. (1983). Development of the auditory evoked responses in the auditory cortex in mammals. In R. Romand (Ed.), *Development of auditory and vestibular systems* (pp. 167–209). New York: Academic Press.

Olmstead, C.E., & Villablanca, J.R. (1980). Development of behavioral audition in the kitten. *Physiology and Behavior, 24,* 705–712.

Plum, F., Gjedde, A., & Samson, F.E. (1976). Neuroanatomical functional mapping by the radioactive 2-deoxy-D-glucose method. *Neurosciences Research Program Bulletin, 14,* 456–518.

Potash, M., & Kelly, J.B. (1980). Development of directional responses to sounds in the rat (*Rattus norvegicus*). *Journal of Comparative and Physiological Psychology, 94,* 864–877.

Pujol, R. (1972). Development of tone-burst responses along the cat's auditory pathway. *Acta Otolaryngologica, 74,* 383–391.

Pujol, R., & Hilding, D. (1973). Anatomy and physiology of the onset of auditory function. *Acta Otolaryngologica, 76,* 1–10.

Pujol, R., & Marty, R. (1970). Postnatal maturation in the cochlea of the cat. *Journal of Comparative Neurology, 139,* 115–126.

Romand, R. (1971). Maturation des potentiels cochléaires dans la période périnatale chez le chat et chez le cobaye. *Journal of Physiology (Paris), 63,* 763–782.

Romand, R. (1983). Development of the cochlea. In R. Romand (Ed.), *Development of the auditory and vestibular systems* (pp. 47–88). New York: Academic Press.

Romand, R., Granier, M-R., & Marty, R. (1973). Développement postnatale de l'activité provoquée dans l'olive supérieure latérale chez le chat par la stimulation sonore. *Journal of Physiology (Paris), 66,* 303–315.

Romand, R., & Marty, R. (1975). Postnatal maturation of the cochlear nuclei in the cat: A neurophysiological study. *Brain Research, 83,* 225–233.

Rubel, E.W. (1978). Ontogeny of structure and function in the vertebrate auditory system. In M. Jacobson (Ed.), *Handbook of sensory physiology, Vol. 9* (pp. 135–237). New York: Springer Verlag.

Rubel, E.W. (1984). Ontogeny of auditory system function. *Annual Review of Physiology, 46,* 213–229.

Ryan, A.F., Woolf, N.K., & Sharp, F.R. (1982). Functional ontogeny in the central auditory pathway of the mongolian gerbil. *Experimental Brain Research, 47,* 428–436.

Saunders, J.C., & Garfinkle, T.J. (1982). Peripheral anatomy and physiology I. In W.F. Willott (Ed.), *The auditory psychobiology of the mouse.* Springfield, IL: Thomas.

Schmidt, R.S., & Fernández, C. (1963). Development of mammalian endocochlear potential. *Journal of Experimental Zoology, 153,* 227–235.

Schneirla, T.C. (1965). Aspects of stimulation and organization in approach/withdrawal processes underlying vertebrate behavioral development. In D.S. Lehrman & R.A. Hinde, *Advances in the study of behavior, (Vol. 1).* New York: Academic Press.

Uziel, A., Romand, R., & Marot, M. (1981). Development of cochlear potentials in rats. *Audiology, 20,* 89–100.

Villablanca, J.R., & Olmstead, C.E. (1979). Neurological development of kittens. *Developmental Psychobiology, 12,* 101–127.

Wada, T. (1923). Anatomical and physiological studies on the growth of the inner ear of the albino rat. *American Anatomical Memoirs, 10,* 1–74.

Author Index

Subject Index